RADIATION PROTECTION
in Medical Radiography

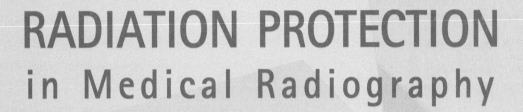

RADIATION PROTECTION
in Medical Radiography

Third Edition

Mary Alice Statkiewicz-Sherer
A.S., R.T.(R), F.A.S.R.T

Paul J. Visconti, Ph.D.

E. Russell Ritenour, Ph.D.

with 163 illustrations

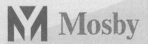 Mosby

St. Louis Baltimore Boston Carlsbad Chicago Minneapolis New York Philadelphia Portland
London Milan Sydney Tokyo Toronto

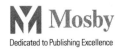

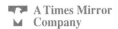

Publisher: Don E. Ladig
Senior Editor: Jeanne Rowland
Developmental Editor: Carole Glauser
Editorial Assistant: Tamara Myers
Project Manager: Linda McKinley
Production Editors: Jennifer Furey, René Spencer
Designer: Renée Duenow
Manufacturing Supervisor: Karen Boehme
Cover Design: Color Associates Creative Imaging Group

THIRD EDITION
Copyright© 1998 by Mosby, Inc.
Previous editions copyrighted 1993, 1983.

Printed in the United States of America
Composition by Graphic World Inc.
Lithography by Graphic World Inc.
Printing/Binding by Von Hoffmann Press

Mosby, Inc.
11830 Westline Industrial Drive
St. Louis, Missouri 63146

International Standard Book Number 0-8151-2896-7

98 99 00 01 02/ 9 8 7 6 5 4 3 2 1

In memory of my parents,
Felix J. *and* Elizabeth M. Krohn.

To my sons,
Joseph F. Statkiewicz, Christopher R. Statkiewicz,
and Terry R. Sherer, Jr., *with love,*

and
To all with whom I may share my knowledge.

About the Authors

Mary Alice Statkiewicz-Sherer, A.S., R.T. (R), F.A.S.R.T., the primary author of this text, is a private radiography education, radiation safety, and medical publishing consultant. She also performs diagnostic imaging procedures for Summit Medical Center in Hermitage, Tennessee. Ms. Statkiewicz-Sherer was previously employed at Memorial Hospital of Burlington County in Mount Holly, New Jersey, where she served for over 16 years as program director for the facility's radiography program and then as educational administrative assistant for the Department of Radiology for over a year.

After earning an A.R.R.T. certification in 1965, Ms. Statkiewicz-Sherer filled several technical and teaching positions in the New Jersey area and graduated with an associate degree in science from the College of Allied Health Professions, Hahnemann Medical College and Hospital of Philadelphia (now Hahnemann University) in 1980. She has been an active and leading member of several professional organizations, having served on committees and task forces of the American Society of Radiologic Technologists, as president of the Twenty-eighth Mid-Eastern Conference of Radiologic Technologists, and as president and chairman of the Board of Directors of the New Jersey Society of Radiologic Technologists. Services to the A.S.R.T. include functioning as chairman of the *Radiologic Technology* editorial review board for the membership year 1989-91 and participating as a member of the Committee on Memorial Lectures for the membership year 1989-91 and for 1991-93. In June 1990, Ms. Statkiewicz-Sherer was elevated to Fellow of the American Society of Radiologic Technologists for her services and contributions to the profession.

In addition to being the primary author of the first edition, *Radiation Protection for Student Radiographers*, the second edition, *Radiation Protection in Medical Radiography*, and also this edition, Ms. Statkiewicz-Sherer co-authored the textbook *Radiation Protection for Dental Radiographers*, which was published by Multi-Media Publishing, Denver, in 1984. Articles written by Ms. Statkiewicz-Sherer have been published in *Radiologic Technology, The Journal of the American Society of Radiologic Technologists,* and *ADVANCE for Radiologic Science Professionals,* a national biweekly newspaper published by Merion Publications, King of Prussia, Pennsylvania. She has also served as a consultant to ADVANCE.

Paul J. Visconti, Ph.D. has been director of medical physics and radiation safety officer at Memorial Hospital of Burlington County in Mount Holly, New Jersey, since 1982. Dr. Visconti received a Ph.D. in physics from the City University of New York in 1971. He was a full-time instructor in the Physics Department at the City College of New York for several years thereafter. Dr. Visconti began his career in medical physics at Montefiore Hospital and Medical Center in New York City, where he remained for 5 years as an associate physicist. During that time, he lectured extensively in radiologic physics to both diagnostic radiology residents and student radiographers. Dr. Visconti is a member of the Society of the Sigma Xi, the American Association of Physicists in Medicine, the American College of Medical Physics, and the American College of Radiology and is certified in therapeutic radiological physics by the American Board of Radiology.

Russell Ritenour, Ph.D., is associate professor and director of the physics section, Department of Radiology, University of Minnesota School of Medicine. He is also director of graduate studies for the program in biophysical sciences at the University of Minnesota. Dr. Ritenour received his Ph.D. in physics from the University of Virginia, completed a postdoctoral fellowship in medical physics sponsored by the National Institutes of Health, and was a faculty member at the University of Colorado School of Medicine for 10 years, serving as director of the graduate medical physics training program until moving to Minnesota. He has served as radiation safety officer for several hospitals and research foundations, been a consultant to the Army for resident training programs, and written a number of audiovisual training programs for radiologic technologists, radiology residents, and medical physicists. He has been active on committees of the American College of Radiology, the American Board of Radiology, and the American Association of Physicists in Medicine and is a past president of the Rocky Mountain Chapter of the Health Physics Society and the North Central Chapter of the American Association of Physicists in Medicine.

Foreword

I am pleased to write a foreword to the third edition of this excellent book on radiation protection. My relationship to Ms. Statkiewicz-Sherer and Dr. Ritenour goes back to 1983, when as a publisher (Multi-Media Publishing, Inc.), I was able to work with them on the first edition of this book, then titled *Radiation Protection for Student Radiographers.*

I had co-authored several audiovisual programs with Dr. Ritenour, including a seven-unit radiation physics series, and found him to be one of those unique individuals with both a high level of intellectual knowledge and the ability to explain and describe concepts and principles in a practical and easy-to-understand manner. Ms. Statkiewicz-Sherer, an experienced educator and program director, provided input and assumed coordination responsibilities as the primary author of this edition. Dr. Ritenour and Ms. Statkiewicz-Sherer were later joined by Dr. Visconti, who became the third member of this author team for the expanded second and third editions.

I am pleased that the authors have retained the basic concepts related to radiation protection required by student radiographers. They have also expanded and updated the information on radiation safety, regulations, and radiation biology as related to radiation safety to make this an excellent resource for both students and practicing radiographers.

I believe future radiographers will need to be more knowledgeable about radiation hazards and saftey practices, including the possible documentation of patient doses per exam. They will need to know how to minimize dosage levels to the patients and to themselves and fellow occupational workers. This text can help prepare students and radiographers for this eventuality. I am pleased to see expanded information on topics such as various types of shielding, repeat radiographs, unnecessary radiologic procedures, pediatric considerations, and techniques for limiting exposure during fluoroscopy, including mobile C-Arm fluoroscopy.

The authors have also added chapter outlines and chapter objectives, which help both instructors and students in the use of this book as a textbook for radiation protection courses.

I congratulate the authors on this excellent updated and expanded new edition.

Kenneth L. Bontrager, M.A., R.T. (R)

Preface to the Third Edition

When the second edition of *Radiation Protection in Medical Radiography* was published in 1993, the scope of the text was changed not only to meet the educational needs of the student radiographer in a structured radiography program but also to assist practicing radiographers, radiology residents, medical physicists, and physicians by functioning as a resource and reference guide to the safe use of x-rays in diagnostic imaging. The third edition continues the expansion of the scope of the text by building on the foundations of the first and second editions. The third edition covers the fundamentals of radiation protection and radiation biology in greater detail and includes material of interest to more experienced radiation workers as well. This edition contains practical material that describes the way radiographers deal with the day-to-day implementation of radiation safety, regulations, and theory. The latest information concerning regulations and guidelines from the major standards setting and advisory agencies are discussed. The authors have endeavored to present this material in a succinct but reasonably complete fashion that is intended to meet the needs of the various members of the health care sector.

In Chapter 7 a section discussing "high-level," (i.e., high dose-rate) fluoroscopy has been added. Information concerning radiation safety in pediatric radiologic procedures has been updated and expanded. Revised data governing patient dose in mammography have also been included in this section. In Chapter 8, material on radiation protection design for diagnostic suites has been incorporated to provide more advanced reading material. A comprehensive chapter on radiation biology is also presented to provide the reader with a solid foundation in this discipline. This unit emphasizes the relevance of radiation biology to radiation protection. A complete listing of textbook content can be found in the table of contents.

In general, the presentation of the third edition presumes that the reader has some background in physics, human anatomy, and medical and imaging terminology. Basic knowledge of simplified mathematics, units of measurement (metric and English), basic atomic structure, the physical concepts of energy, electric charge, subdivision of matter, electromagnetic radiation, x-ray production (both quality and quantity), and the process of ionization are useful but not mandatory. The reader may build on this knowledge by assimilating information presented in this volume.

The format of the book has been changed somewhat. Each chapter in this edition begins with an outline, followed by a list of key terms and then a list of learning objectives. An introductory paragraph describes the essence of the material to be covered in each chapter. Chapter content is followed by multiple-choice review questions with which the reader can assess the knowledge acquired. Footnotes containing additional information and references to other important material or sources are provided throughout each chapter. Each chapter also contains an updated and expanded bibliography. **Bold print** has been used to focus the reader's attention on the key terms of each chapter.

Throughout the text, radiation units are stated in metric units of measurement (System International) with traditional radiation units following in parentheses. Existing tables have been updated, and many new tables have been added throughout the book. Numerous new illustrations and color photographs are included. Color has also been added to enhance the visual appearance of new and existing tables and illustrations. (Historical photographs, however, remain in black and white.) The new text contains six appendices. Appendix A describes the chance of a 50 keV photon to interact with atoms of tissue as it travels through 5 cm of soft tissue. Appendix B presents the relationship between photons, electromagnetic waves, wavelength, and energy. Appendix C discusses Compton interaction. Appendix D presents the periodic table of the elements in color. Appendix E gives the metric system equivalents for length, and Appendix F reprints the Consumer-Patient Radiation Health and Safety Act of 1981. The glossary has been updated and expanded to include many new terms.

To facilitate a working knowledge of the principles of radiation protection, study materials presented in the third edition remain sophisticated enough to be true to the complexity of the subject yet simple and concise enough to permit comprehension by all readers. For student radiographers and radiology residents, this text is *not* intended as a complete self-learning tool; rather, it should be used in conjunction with formal instruction from a qualified instructor. The practicing radiographer, medical physicist, and physician may use this book as a self-teaching instrument to broaden and reinforce existing knowledge of the subject matter and also as a means to acquaint themselves with changing concepts and new material. The book can serve as a resource for continuing education because it provides an extensive range of information.

By mastering the material covered in this radiation protection resource and applying this knowledge in the performance of radiologic procedures, the reader will help to ensure the safety of the patient and all diagnostic imaging personnel.

Mary Alice Statkiewicz-Sherer

Acknowledgments

Very special acknowledgment is given to my three sons, Joseph, Christopher, and Terry. Their unselfish love provides the ongoing strength that I need to accomplish my goals. They always provide encouragement and are always supportive of my endeavors. I want to thank them for being there for me when I needed their love and support. My family also includes four small furry friends (our little dogs), who are always near me while I work. Pixie Lee, Coco, Tips, and Sonya are fondly remembered for their constant affection and loyalty.

I also extend special thanks to my many caring friends who have been supportive of my writing endeavors. I sincerely thank Evelyn Golden, R.T. (R), for technical discussions and personal encouragement and friendship. I am grateful to Arlene Chadwick for ongoing support and friendship throughout the completion of this project. Heartfelt appreciation is extended to William B. McLendon, M.D., Radiologist at Summit Medical Center, Hermitage, Tennessee, for many, many technical discussions and constant encouragement. Dr. McLendon's sense of humor, blended with his vast knowledge, has made discussion of even the most complex subject matter enjoyable. Another physician at Summit Medical Center whom I want to thank for many discussions and personal encouragement is emergency department physician Brian R. McMurray, M.D. Dr. McMurray has shared personal experiences and observations from recent visits to the Ukraine, where he was engaged in life-saving humanitarian operations. He provided current information about the status of that population in the aftermath of the Chernobyl nuclear power station accident. Dr. McMurray also provided several radiation–protection–oriented articles for reference purposes in this edition.

I also thank the radiologists, radiographers, and ancillary personnel at Summit Medical Center for their immense support. I am proud to acknowledge each of them not only as professional associates but also as personal friends. Their support is greatly appreciated. I am also grateful to the emergency department physicians and staff at Summit Medical Center for support and encouragement.

Sincere appreciation for writing the foreword to this edition is given to author/publisher, Kenneth L. Bontrager, M.A., R.T. (R). Mr. Bontrager is well-known in the field of medical imaging education for many fine publications. It was through Mr. Bontrager's publishing company that the first edition of this text was published.

The technical integrity of this edition has been ensured through the collaborative efforts of two very knowledgeable medical physicists, Paul J. Visconti, Ph.D., and E. Russell Ritenour, Ph.D. Both have contributed their time and expertise to make this book well-rounded and accurate. I am deeply indebted to Dr. Visconti for numerous technical recommendations, contributions of materials such as the section in Chapter 8 on radiation protection design for diagnostic suites, many hours of intense discussion of various technical material, review of all chapter drafts, valuable advice concerning selective materials in this edition, and constant personal encouragement. Dr. Visconti is also recognized for his significant contribution to the second edition. The technical and scientific value of both the previous and the current edition has been greatly enhanced by Dr. Visconti's noteworthy contributions to the manuscript. I am also deeply indebted to E. Russell Ritenour, Ph.D., for his valuable contributions of technical material, numerous new illustrations and photographs, hours of intense discussion concerning various technical data, input into future advancements for the section on radiation protection design for diagnostic suites, continuous review of chapter drafts, numerous technical recommendations, development of definitions for various technical terms, and advice concerning selective materials in this edition. Dr. Ritenour has been a source of support and encouragement not only from the inception of this project but also throughout the development of the first and second editions. His contributions to all three editions have made this text a valuable resource for radiation protection and radiation biology.

Very special thanks is given to the professional staff of Mosby, with special acknowledgment to senior editor, Jeanne Rowland; developmental editor, Carole Glauser; production editor, Jennifer Furey; editorial assistant, Tamara Myers; and freelancer, Linda Woodard for assistance in the preparation and publication of this text. Their publishing expertise has guided this manuscript from its initial stages to the development of the final product.

Reviewers

Sandra L. Alsop, R.T. (R)
Clearfield Hospital
Clearfield, Pennsylvania

Gerald A. Baker, M.Ed., R.T. (R)
Washtenaw Community College
Ann Arbor, Michigan

Alberto Bello, Jr., M.Ed., R.T. (R)
Oregon Institute of Technology
Klamath Falls, Oregon

Susyn Dees, M.S., R.T. (R)
Champlain College
Burlington, Vermont

Donna Goetz, M.S., R.T. (R), L.R.T.
Bronx Community College
Bronx, New York

Christopher J. Gould, M.S., R.T. (R)
San Jacinto College Central
Pasadena, Texas

Edna Jones-Holmes, M.P.A., R.T. (R)
Lake Michigan College
Benton Harbor, Michigan

John P. Lampignano, M.Ed., R.T. (R) (CT)
Gateway Community College
Phoenix, Arizona

Josephine M. Latini, M.S., R.T. (R)
Lock Haven Hospital
Lock Haven, Pennsylvania

Cynthia L. Liotta, M.S., R.T. (R)
Gannon University
Erie, Pennsylvania

Cyndi McCauley, M.Ed., R.T. (R)
Columbia East Houston Medical Center
Houston, Texas

Kathy McGarry, Ph.D., R.T. (R) (QM)
Burdette Tomlin Memorial Hospital
Cape May Court House, New Jersey

Rob McLaughlin, M.A., R.T. (R)
Louisiana State University at Eunice
Eunice, Louisiana

Christine M. Mehlbaum, B.S., R.T. (R)
Pennsylvania State University Schuykill Campus
Schuykill Haven, Pennsylvania

Stan Olejniczak, B.H.S., R.T. (R)
University of Arkansas for Medical Sciences
Area Health Education Center
Northwest Radiologic Technology
Fayetteville, Arkansas

Robert J. Parelli, M.A., R.T. (R)
Cypress College
Cypress, California

Linda Pearson, M.Ed., R.T. (R)
Midwestern State University
Wichita Falls, Texas

Angela Pickwick, M.S., R.T. (R) (M)
Montgomery College
Takoma Park, Maryland

M. Gary Sayed, Ph.D., R.T. (N)
Nuclear Medicine Institute
the University of Findlay
Findlay, Ohio

Stephen Schulz, M.Ed., R.T. (R)
Oregon Institute of Technology
Klamath Falls, Oregon

Linda Shields, M.Ed., R.T. (R) (M)
El Paso Community College
El Paso, Texas

George M. Uschold, Ed.D., R.T. (T)
University of Rochester
Rochester, New York

Zoland (Skip) Zile, M.S., R.T. (R)
Northampton Community College
Bethlehem, Pennsylvania

The time and effort expended by the reviewers is most appreciated. The input made it possible for the authors to view the manuscript from another point of view. Through their constructive feedback, we have been able to strengthen various areas of the text. We also appreciate their many positive comments and words of encouragement. They have contributed to the overall success of this writing project. Thanks is also given to the individuals who participated in the third edition photo shoot held in the radiology department of Anna Jaques Hospital in Newburyport, Massachusetts. Special acknowledgment is given to Judith Tunstall, R.T. (R) (CT), the radiographer/model. Her participation in this capacity helped to make our visual material current and fashionable. We also sincerely appreciate Ms. Tunstall's efforts in obtaining permission for the photo shoot from the hospital. The participation of this health care facility contributed greatly to improving the photographic integrity of the third edition. Special thanks is also due to Tom Lochhaas, photo shoot coordinator, and Pat Watson, the photographer. Gratitude for arranging for shadow shield photos to be shot at the Mayo Clinic in Rochester, Minnesota is also expressed to Eugene D. Frank, M.A., R.T. (R), F.A.S.R.T. His help and ongoing support is very much appreciated.

Radiography students and radiology residents are the future of the medical imaging profession. To those who will use this text, it is my hope that the materials contained in this edition will greatly contribute to enhancing your knowledge of radiation protection and radiation biology.

Appreciation is extended to those who have given permission to reproduce illustrations, diagrams, quotations, and pictures from their work. Their material enhances this manuscript. In particular, special thanks for use of materials is given to Stewart C. Bushong, Sc.D; Philip W. Ballinger, M.S., R.T. (R); and Professor Elizabeth LaTorre Travis.

Acknowledgments and thanks for permission to reproduce photographic materials are also given to the National Council on Radiation Protection and Measurements (Bethesda, Maryland); the U.S. Department of Energy, Office of LWR Safety and Technology and the Office of Nuclear Energy (Washington, D.C.); and the U.S. Department of Energy, Nevada Operations Office (Las Vegas, Nevada). Many manufacturers of products and commercial suppliers provided technical information about their products and gave permission for the reproduction of photographs and other illustrations. Thanks for the use of these materials is given to the following companies: Baird Corporation (Bedford, Massachusetts); Dosimetry Corporation of America (Cincinnati, Ohio); Eberline Instruments (Santa Fe, New Mexico); Landauer, Inc. (Glenwood, Illinois); Machlett Labs, Inc. (Stamford, Connecticut); Nuclear Associates (Carle Place, New York); Solon Technologies, Inc. (Solon, Ohio); Victoreen, Inc. (Solon, Ohio); and X-Rite, Inc. (Grandville, Michigan).

Finally, a very special remembrance is noted to my parents, the late Felix and Elizabeth (Markovitch) Krohn, for all they did for me. Their many words of wisdom and lifelong personal encouragement remain with me. The education they made possible helped me gain the knowledge necessary to prepare this book. My accomplishments serve as a tribute to them.

Mary Alice Statkiewicz-Sherer

Contents

5

Overview of Cell Biology, *72*

6

Radiation Biology, *92*

7

Protection of the Patient During Diagnostic Radiologic Procedures, *146*

8

Protecting Occupationally Exposed Personnel During Diagnostic Radiologic Procedures, *188*

9

Radiation Monitoring, *214*

RADIATION PROTECTION
in Medical Radiography

1

Introduction to Radiation Protection

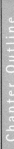

Chapter Outline

biologic damage
cellular damage
diagnostic efficacy
dose equivalent (DE)
enhanced natural sources
Environmental Protection Agency (EPA)
high-quality radiographs
ionizing radiation
manmade, or artificial, radiation
natural background radiation
nuclear power
organic damage
radiation
radiation protection
radon
rem
sievert (Sv)
terrestrial radiation

*After completing this chapter, the reader will be able
to perform the following:*

- Define radiation protection and discuss reasons for employing it.

- Explain the justification and responsibility for radiologic procedures.

- Define ionizing radiation.

- Describe the potential for ionizing radiation to cause biologic damage.

- Define sievert and rem and explain their functions.

- Identify the various sources of natural background ionizing radiation and the different sources of manmade, or artificial, ionizing radiation.

- Describe the magnitude of medical radiation exposure.

- Explain the responsibility for radiation protection in the field of radiology.

Since the early 1900s, scientists have been aware of both the *beneficial* and *destructive* potential of ionizing radiation. By using the knowledge of radiation hazards that has been gained over the years and employing effective methods to limit or eliminate those hazards, human beings can exercise greater control over the use of "radiant energy." **Radiation protection** consists of tools and techniques employed by radiation workers to protect patients and personnel from exposure to ionizing radiation. Various methods of radiation protection may be applied to ensure safety for persons employed in radiation industries, including medicine, and for the population at large. This book focuses on radiation protection for patients, diagnostic imaging personnel, and the general public.

Justification and Responsibility for Radiologic Procedures

Radiation exposure should always be kept at the lowest possible level for the general public. In certain cases of illness or injury, however, a patient may be exposed to ionizing radiation for the purpose of obtaining essential diagnostic medical information. Ionizing radiation possesses both a beneficial and a destructive potential; when employed in the healing arts for the welfare of the patient, the potential benefits of exposure to ionizing radiation should far outweigh the potential risks (the possibility of inducing radiogenic cancer or genetic defects after irradiation) (Fig. 1-1). The **diagnostic efficacy** (the degree to which the diagnostic study accurately reveals the presence or absence of disease in the patient) of the examination is maximized when essential radiographs are produced under recommended radiation protection guidelines.

After determining the justification for an x-ray examination or procedure, the referring physician must accept basic responsibility for protecting the patient from radiation exposure. The physician may exercise this responsibility by employing competent technical personnel. As qualified professionals, radiographers must accept a portion of the responsibility for patient welfare by providing quality patient care and imaging services (Fig. 1-2). The radiologist and radiographer share in keeping patient medical radiation exposure at the lowest level possible. By keeping exposure as low

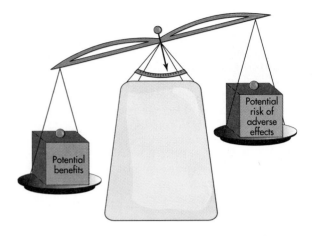

Potential benefits versus potential risk of adverse effects

Fig. 1-1 The potential benefits of exposing the patient to ionizing radiation must far outweigh the potential risk of adverse effects.

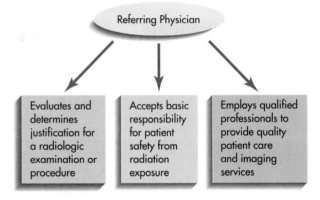

Referring Physician

| Evaluates and determines justification for a radiologic examination or procedure | Accepts basic responsibility for patient safety from radiation exposure | Employs qualified professionals to provide quality patient care and imaging services |

Fig. 1-2 Physician's responsibility in providing quality care.

as reasonably achievable (ALARA), imaging professionals help ensure that both occupational and nonoccupational dose equivalents (upper boundary doses of ionizing radiation that result in a negligible risk of bodily injury or genetic damage) remain well below maximal allowable levels. (See Chapter 4 for more information on the concept of ALARA.) This can best be accomplished by using the lowest exposure factors that will produce useful radiographs, and by producing **high-quality radiographs** with the first exposure; repeated examinations made necessary by technical error or carelessness (Fig. 1-3) must be

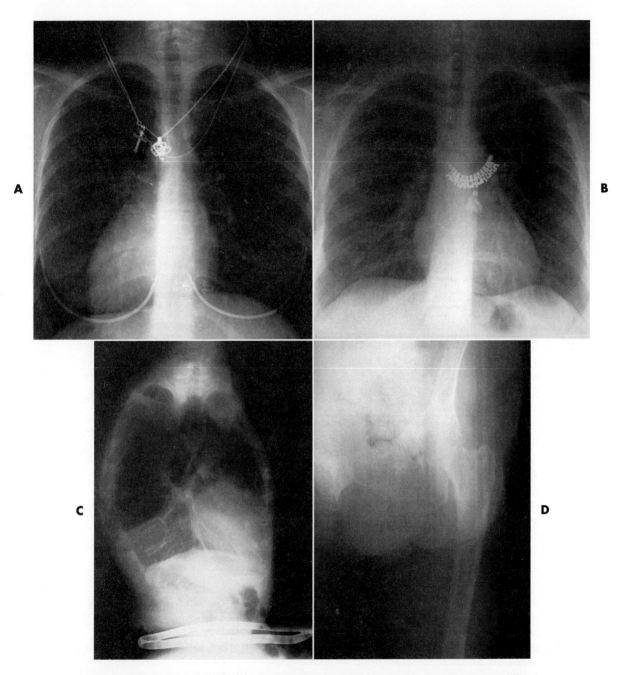

Fig. 1-3 **A,** A posteroanterior (PA) chest radiograph requiring a repeat examination because of multiple external foreign bodies (several necklaces and an underwire bra) that should have been removed before the radiographic examination. **B,** A PA chest radiograph requiring a repeat examination because of an external foreign body (necklace) that should have been removed before the radiographic examination. **C,** A double exposure (PA and lateral projections of the chest superimposed) requiring a repeat examination. **D,** Radiograph of a left hip demonstrating an "off-level" grid error. This occurs when the patient's weight is not evenly distributed on the grid, causing the grid to tilt so that it is not properly aligned to the x-ray tube.

avoided because they significantly increase radiation exposure for both the patient and the radiation worker.

Ionizing Radiation

Definition

Radiation is energy in transit from one location to another. Some types of radiation such as microwaves can deposit energy in a material and produce heat. Higher-energy radiation such as x-rays or gamma rays can remove electrons from materials (ionization), thereby producing direct chemical changes. **Radiation** is a transfer of energy that results from a change occurring naturally within an atom (e.g., radioactive decay, whereby the nucleus of an unstable atom disintegrates by the spontaneous emission of charged particles or photons) or a process caused by the interaction of a particle with an atom. The latter occurs most commonly when a beam of high-energy electrons bombards the atoms composing the target of an x-ray tube (Fig. 1-4). If radiation produces positively and negatively charged particles (ions) as it passes through matter, it is called **ionizing radiation.**

Not all forms of radiation, however, are capable of causing ionization. In fact, an entire spectrum of radiation that encompasses such familiar entities as the colors of the rainbow, microwaves, radio waves, and ultraviolet rays does not produce ionizing radiation. X-radiation may be considered a special type of radiation because of its ability to create electrically charged particles by liberating orbital electrons from the atoms with which it interacts. These electrically charged particles possess the potential to cause **biologic damage** (damage to living tissue) in humans by recombining disadvantageously; the liberated, fast-moving electrons and x-ray photons that emerge from such interactions can cause further damage by producing additional ionization.

Radiation quantity unit for dose equivalent

Sievert (Sv) is the International System of Units radiation quantity unit for **dose equivalent (DE),** and the **rem** is the traditional radiation quantity unit for DE. These units help define the biologic effects of various types of radiation in human beings. The DE is a concept that enables the calculation of the effective absorbed dose for all types of ionizing radiation. Both occupational and nonoccupational DEs may be stated in Sv (rem). Radiation quantities and units are discussed in substantial detail in Chapter 3.

Biologic damage potential

Ionizing radiation produces damage while penetrating body tissues primarily by ejecting electrons from the atoms comprising tissues. Destructive radiation interaction at the atomic level results in molecular change, and this in turn can cause **cellular damage** leading to abnormal cell function or loss of cell function. If excessive cellular damage occurs, the living organism exhibits genetic or somatic changes such as mutations, cataracts, and leukemia. Changes in blood count are a classic example of **organic damage** resulting

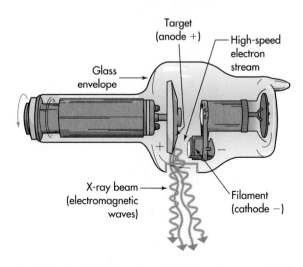

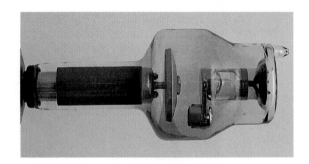

Fig. 1-4 Radiant energy is emitted from the x-ray tube in the form of waves (or particles).

from significant exposure to ionizing radiation. A DE of x-radiation as low as 0.25 Sv (25 rem) delivered to the whole body may within a few days cause a decrease in the number of lymphocytes (white blood cells that defend the body against foreign antigens by producing antibodies to combat disease) in the blood. Table 1-1 provides some basic information on the known biologic effects of different radiation DEs. Because this potential to cause biologic damage exists, the use of ionizing radiation should be limited whenever possible.

Sources of radiation

Human beings are continuously exposed to sources of ionizing radiation. Some people are exposed to a wide variety, whereas others are exposed to a limited number. Sources of ionizing radiation may be natural or manmade (artificial). Table 1-2 provides quick reference for average annual radiation DEs of Americans resulting from both natural background and manmade sources of radiation.

Table 1-1
Radiation Dose Equivalent and Subsequent Biologic Effects

Radiation dose equivalent	Subsequent biologic effect
0.25 Sv (25 rem)	Blood changes (e.g., measurable hematologic depression, decreases in the number of lymphocytes present in the circulating blood)
1.5 Sv (150 rem)	Nausea, diarrhea
2.0 to 6.0 Sv (200 to 600 rem)*	Erythema (diffuse redness over an area of skin after irradiation)
2.5 Sv (250 rem)	If dose is to gonads, temporary sterility
3.0 Sv (300 rem)	50% chance of death; lethal dose for 50% of population over 30 days (LD 50/30)
6.0 Sv (600 rem)	Death

Modified from *Radiologic health,* unit 4, slide 17, Denver, Multi-Media Publishing (slide program).
*2.0 Sv is a threshold for erythema as a result of an acute exposure, whereas a dose of 6.0 Sv is required to elicit the same effect if the exposure is chronic.[1]

Table 1-2
Average Annual Radiation Dose Equivalent of Americans

Overall 5 360 mrem (100%)* All percentages listed below are percentages of 360 mrem (~1 mrem/day).

Category	Type of radiation	Dose (mrem)	Percentage of dose equivalent (%)
Natural	Radon	198	55
	Cosmic, terrestrial, internal	97	27
		295	82
Manmade	Medical x-rays	40	11
	Nuclear medicine	14	4
	Consumer products	11	3
		65	18
Other	Occupational	1.1	0.3
	Fallout	<1.1	<0.3
	Nuclear fuel cycle	0.4	0.1
	Miscellaneous	0.4	0.1
		3.0	0.8

Adapted from National Council on Radiation Protection and Measurements (NCRP): *Report #93, ionizing radiation exposure of the population of the United States,* Bethesda, Md, 1987, NCRP.
*360 mrem = 0.36 rem = 3.6 mSv

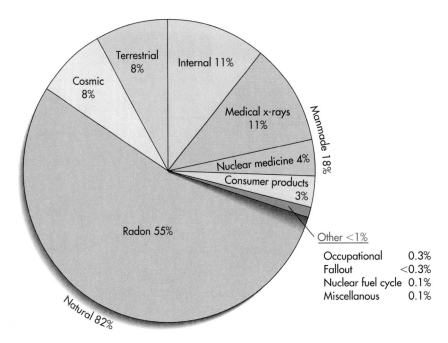

Fig. 1-5 Various radiation sources contribute to the total average effective DE for inhabitants of the United States. This diagram demonstrates the percentage contribution of each natural and manmade radiation source. (From National Council on Radiation Protection and Measurements [NCRP]: *Report No. 93, ionizing radiation exposure of the population of the United States,* Bethesda, Md, 1987, NCRP.)

Natural radiation

Natural sources of ionizing radiation have always been a part of the human environment. Ionizing radiation from environmental sources is called **natural background radiation** and has three components:

1. Terrestrial radiation from radioactive materials in the earth
2. Cosmic radiation from the sun (solar) and beyond the solar system (galactic)
3. Biologic, from radionuclides deposited in the human body through natural processes.

If any of these natural sources become increased because of accidental or deliberate human actions, they are termed **enhanced natural sources.**

Terrestrial radiation. Long-lived radioactive elements such as uranium, radium, and thorium that emit densely ionizing radiations are present in variable quantities in the earth. These sources of ionizing radiation are classified as **terrestrial radiation.** The quantity of terrestrial radiation present in an area depends on the composition of the soil or rocks in that geographic area. Approximately 55% of the gross common exposure of human beings to natural background radiation comes from **radon** (Fig. 1-5). It is by far the largest contributor to background radiation. The average U.S. resident receives approximately 1.98 mSv (198 mrem) per year from indoor and outdoor levels of radon. Radon, the first decay product of radium, is a colorless, odorless, and heavy radioactive gas that along with its decay products is always present to some degree in the air. Because it is a gas, radon can penetrate soil. It enters buildings through cracks or holes in their frameworks. In homes, it may gain access through crawlspaces under the living areas, through floor drains and sump pumps, and through porous cement block foundations (Fig. 1-6). In many cases, a pressure gradient exists between a house and the soil on which it rests so that in effect the house draws on the ground like a vacuum cleaner.

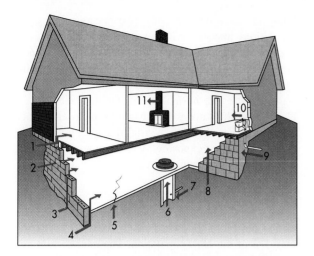

Fig. 1-6 Radon gas can penetrate through soil and enter a home through holes or cracks in its framework, crawlspaces under the living areas, floor drains, sump pumps, and porous cement block foundations. *1,* Spaces behind brick veneer on top of block foundation; *2,* pores and cracks in concrete block foundation; *3,* open top of block foundation walls; *4,* floor to wall joints; *5,* cracks in concrete floor; *6,* exposed soil as in basement sump; *7,* weeping drain tile draining into open sump; *8,* mortar joints; *9,* loose-fitting pipe wall penetration; *10,* well water from some wells; *11,* some building materials such as stone. (Courtesy U.S. Environmental Protection Agency, Washington, D.C.)

Radon concentrations in a particular structure vary across days and seasons. In the cooler months, when homes and buildings are tightly closed, radon levels are usually higher. This is the best time to perform tests for radon.*

High indoor concentrations of radon have the potential to cause serious health hazards for human beings. After being inhaled, this airborne, radioactive gas produces daughter radioactive isotopes that remain for lengthy periods in the epithelial tissue of the lungs. As these secondary isotopes decay, they give off radiation, which may injure lung tissues, thereby increasing the risk for lung cancer. Smokers exposed to high radon levels face a higher risk of lung cancer than

do nonsmokers. One reason for this may be that smokers have already been exposed to higher concentrations of radioactivity from the lead 210 (^{210}Pb) and polonium 210 (^{210}Po) isotopes contained in tobacco and tobacco smoke.

The **Environmental Protection Agency (EPA)** considers radon to be the second leading cause of lung cancer in the United States, responsible for approximately 20,000 cancer deaths per year. (For more information on the EPA see Chapter 4.) The EPA recommends that action be taken to reduce elevated levels of radon to below 4 picocuries† per liter (pCi/L) of air (a concentration that specifies the number of radioactive processes per second that occur on average in 1 L of air). This level of radon presence is considered to be statistically safe by the agency. The EPA estimates that 10% of the homes in the United States exceed the recommended limit of 4 pCi/L. Hence, accurate radon testing and appropriate structural repair, if required, are essential to reduce the risk of lung cancer from radon.

Cosmic radiation. Cosmic rays are of extraterrestrial origin and result from nuclear interactions that have taken place in the sun and other stars. The intensity of cosmic rays varies with altitude relative to the earth's surface. The greatest intensity occurs at high altitudes, and the lowest intensity occurs at sea level. The earth's atmosphere and magnetic field help shield it from cosmic rays. The shielding is diminished at higher elevations, where less atmosphere separates the earth from cosmic rays. The average U.S. inhabitant receives a DE of approximately 0.3 mSv (30 mrem) per year from extraterrestrial radiation. Cosmic radiations consist predominantly of high-energy protons; as a result of interactions with molecules in the earth's atmosphere, these protons may be accompanied by alpha particles, atomic nuclei, mesons, gamma rays, and high-energy electrons. These other forms of radiation are collectively referred to as a *secondary cosmic radiation.* The gamma rays among them are energetic enough to penetrate several meters of lead.

Biologic radiation. The tissues of the human body contain many naturally existing radioactive nuclides that have been ingested in minute quantities from various foods or inhaled as particles in the air. Potassium 40 (^{40}K), carbon 14 (^{14}C), hydrogen 3 (^{3}H; tritium), and

---

*Detection kits are relatively easy to use and may be purchased at retail stores or obtained free of charge from the National Safety Council in Washington D.C. by calling 1-800-SOS-RADON.
†1 picocurie $= 10^{-12}$ curie.

strontium 90 (^{90}Sr) are examples of radionuclides that exist in small quantities within the body. Radionuclides in the soil and air also add to the human internal radiation DE burden. The average member of the general population receives more than 0.67 mSv (67 mrem) per year from combined exposure to radiations from the earth's surface and from radiation within the human body. In total, the radon (1.98 mSv [198 mrem]), cosmic ray radiations (0.3 mSv [30 mrem]), and internally deposited radionuclides (0.67 mSv [67 mrem]) that comprise the natural background radiation in the United States result in an estimated average annual individual DE of approximately 2.95 mSv (295 mrem). The quantity of natural radiation that human beings are exposed to cannot be controlled.

Manmade (artificial) radiation

Ionizing radiation created by humans for various uses is classified as **manmade, or artificial, radiation.** Sources of artificial ionizing radiation include the following:

1. Consumer products containing radioactive material
2. Air travel
3. Nuclear fuel for generation of power
4. Atmospheric fallout from nuclear weapons
5. Accidents in nuclear power plants
6. Medical radiation

Manmade radiation contributes about 0.65 mSv (65 mrem) to the average annual radiation exposure of the U.S. population. Of this DE, 0.4 mSv (40 mrem) results from medical diagnostic x-ray procedures, 0.14 mSv (14 mrem) results from nuclear imaging, and 0.11 mSv (11 mrem) results from consumer products.

Consumer products containing radioactive material. Consumer products containing radioactive material include airport surveillance systems; early televisions; smoke detector alarms; static eliminators; timepieces with luminous dials and numbers containing promethuim 147, radium 226, strontium 90, and tritium; and video display terminals that use cathode-ray tubes. These products contribute a small fraction of the total average effective DE to each member of the general population.

When color television monitors were first made available to consumers, radiation exposure levels from these devices was substantial. As a result of techno-

logic advances over the past two decades and strict regulations imposed within the United States by the Food and Drug Administration (FDA) regarding such devices, the radiation exposure to the general public may now be considered negligible.

Air travel. The normal use of the airplane at high elevations brings many human beings in closer contact with high-energy extraterrestrial radiation and consequently increases exposure. A flight in a typical commercial airliner results in a DE rate of .005 to .01 mSv/hr (0.5 to 1 mrem/hr).

Nuclear fuel for generation of power. Nuclear power plants that produce nuclear fuel for the generation of power do not contribute significantly to the annual DE of the U.S. population. The nuclear fuel cycle contributes approximately 0.1% to the total average effective DE rate for persons living in the United States.

Atmospheric fallout from nuclear weapons. An accurate estimate of the total annual DE from fallout cannot be made because actual radiation measurements do not exist. The dose commitment (the dose that may ultimately be delivered from a given intake of radionuclide)[2] may be estimated by using a series of approximations and simplistic models that are subject to considerable speculation. The actual radiation dose to the global population from atmospheric fallout from nuclear weapons testing is not received all at once. It is instead delivered over a period of years at changing dose rates. The changes in the dose rates depend on factors such as characteristics of the fallout field and the elapsed time since the test occurred. No atmospheric nuclear testing has occurred since 1980.

When spread over the inhabitants of the United States, fallout from nuclear weapons tests (Fig. 1-7) and other environmental sources contributes less than 0.011 mSv (1.1 mrem) annually to the DE of each person. This annual DE is considered to have a negligible impact on the U.S. population.

Accidents in nuclear power plants. Although **nuclear power** benefits human beings by creating a needed supply of electricity, unfortunate accidents involving nuclear reactors can occur. This can lead to additional, unplanned radiation exposure for human beings and the environment. For example, on March 28, 1979, the Three Mile Island-2 (TMI-2) pressurized water reactor, located near Harrisburg, Pennsylvania,

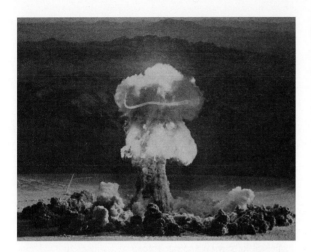

Fig. 1-7 The United States performed above-ground nuclear weapons tests before 1963. During the Priscilla Test, this atomic cloud resulted from an explosion of a 37-kiloton testing device exploded from a balloon at the Nevada test site on June 24, 1957. The atomic cloud top, which contains man-made ionizing radiation, ascended approximately 43,000 feet. (Courtesy U.S. Department of Energy, Nevada Operations Office, Las Vegas, NV.)

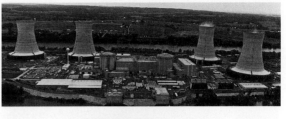

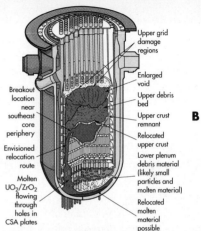

Fig. 1-8 A, Nuclear power stations such as the one located on Three Mile Island (TMI) near Harrisburg, Pennsylvania, house nuclear reactors. The large, round containment buildings holding the reactors retain radioactive liquids and gases even in a high-pressure environment. **B,** TMI-2 end-state core conditions, illustrating the damage to the radioactive nuclear reactor core after the loss of coolant accident on March 28, 1979. Some of the original core mass formed an upper layer of debris. A hard crust supports this material. Zones of previously molten material and standing fuel rod segments account for some of the core mass lying beneath the upper debris bed. The lower reactor vessel head contains some of the melted core material. Closed-circuit television, mechanical probing, and core-boring operations contributed to assessing the TMI-2 end-state core conditions. (Courtesy U.S. Department of Energy, Washington, DC.)

suffered a loss of coolant that resulted in severe over-heating (at a temperature greater than 5000° F) of the radioactive reactor core. Consequently a significant melting of the core occurred. The U.S. Department of Energy estimated that about 40% of the material in the TMI-2 nuclear reactor core reached a molten state. Approximately 15% of the melted uranium dioxide fuel of the core actually flowed through the undamaged portions of the core and settled on the bottom of the reactor vessel. This melted material in the nuclear reactor core and bottom of the reactor vessel formed crusts on its outside surfaces and in time cooled to form resolidified debris (Fig. 1-8). Although significant melting of the core and flowing of the molten radioactive material into intact portions of the reactor vessel occurred, fortunately no "melt-through" of the reactor vessel resulted. To remedy the hazardous condition, TMI has initiated a program to clean up the radioactive waste.

Although the potential existed for release of significant amounts of radioactive material, according to the General Public Utilities Nuclear Corporation (GPU), the company that owns and operates TMI, the quantity of radiation that actually escaped during the accident was not sufficient to cause health problems for persons occupationally exposed or for the 2 million people living within 50 miles of the plant. According to conventional methods of risk assessment, between zero and one additional case of fatal cancer will occur in this population as a result of radiation exposure from this accident.[3] Therefore excess cancer deaths are not expected to occur in this exposed population as a consequence of it having received a dose equivalent of .02 mSv (2 mrem).

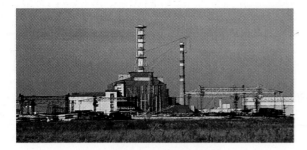

Fig. 1-9 Nuclear power plant in Chernobyl, former Soviet Union. Site of the 1996 radiation accident. (Courtesy Ken Graham Photography.)

Table 1-3	
Permissible Skin Entrance Exposures for Various Radiographic Examinations	
Examination	Skin exposure (milliroentgens [mR] per projection)*
Chest (posteroanterior [PA])	12 to 26
Skull (lateral)	105 to 240
Abdomen (anteroposterior [AP])	375 to 698
Retrograde pyelogram	475 to 829
Cervical spine (AP)	35 to 165
Thoracic spine (AP)	295 to 485
Limb	8 to 327
Dental (bite wing and periapical)	227 to 425

Modified from Ballinger PW: *Merrill's atlas of radiographic positions and radiologic procedures,* ed 8, vol 1, St Louis, 1995, Mosby.
*These ranges are liberal and reflect the equipment and techniques used in state-of-the-art technology.

An explosion at a nuclear power plant in Chernobyl (near Kiev in Ukraine in the former Soviet Union) (Fig. 1-9) in April 1986 resulted in the release of a number of radioactive nuclides, including 46 megacuries of iodine 131 (^{131}I), 136 megacuries of xenon radioisotopes, and 2.3 megacuries of cesium 137 (^{137}Cs). This is far more than one million times the amount of radioactive material released at TMI, which was approximately 15 curies of iodine 131 (^{131}I). More than 200 people working at the Chernobyl plant received a whole-body DE exceeding 1 Sv (100 rem). More than two dozen workers died as a result of explosion-related injuries and the effects of receiving DEs greater than 4 Sv (400 rem). The average DE to the approximately quarter of a million individuals living within 200 miles of the reactor was 0.2 Sv (20 rem), with thyroid doses (from drinking milk containing radioactive iodine) in some individuals possibly exceeding several Sv. Adverse health effects from radiation exposure are expected to occur for many years as a consequence of the total collective DE received by the affected population.

Because human beings are unable to control natural background radiation, exposure from artificial sources must be limited to protect the general population from further biologic damage.

Medical radiation. Medical radiation exposure results from the use of diagnostic x-ray machines and radiopharmaceuticals in medicine. Diagnostic medical x-ray and nuclear medicine procedures are the two largest sources of artificial radiation, collectively accounting for 15% of the total average effective DE of the population of the United States (see Fig. 1-5). These two types of medical radiation account for about 0.54 mSv (54 mrem) of the average annual individual DE of ionizing radiation. The average annual effective total DE from manmade and natural radiation, including radon, is 3.6 mSv (360 mrem). Although the amount of natural background radiation remains fairly constant from year to year, the frequency of exposure to manmade radiation in medical applications is rapidly increasing among all age groups in the United States for a number of reasons. Because of medicolegal considerations, physicians in general are relying more on radiologic diagnoses to assist them in patient care. Greater accuracy in radiologic diagnosis resulting from educational and technologic improvements makes this increased usage understandable. However, to reduce the possibility of the occurrence of genetic damage in future generations, this increase in frequency of radiation exposure in medicine must be counterbalanced by limiting the amount of patient exposure in individual procedures. This can best be accomplished through application of appropriate radiation protection measures and techniques on the part of the radiographer.

Because of the large variety of radiologic equipment, differences in radiologic procedures, and indi-

Table 1-4

Typical Skin Exposure and Mean Tissue Glandular Dose for Screen/Film Mammography Examinations

Examination	Skin exposure per projection (mR)	Approximate mean glandular dose per projection (mrad)*
Screen/film	200 to 1000	75

Modified from Ballinger PW: *Merrill's atlas of radiographic positions and radiographic procedures,* ed 8, vol 1, St Louis, 1995, Mosby.
*The millirad (mrad) is equal to 1/1000 of a rad. The rad is the traditional unit of absorbed dose. See Chapter 3 for further information.

Table 1-5

Typical Bone Marrow Doses for Various Radiographic Examinations

X-ray examination	Mean marrow dose (mrad)
Skull	10
Cervical	20
Chest	2
Stomach and upper gastrointestinal	100
Gallbladder	80
Lumbar spine	60
Intravenous urography	25
Abdomen	30
Pelvis	20
Extremity	2

From Ballinger PW: *Merrill's atlas of radiographic positions and radiologic procedures,* ed 8, vol 1, St Louis, 1995, Mosby.

Table 1-6

Typical Gonad Doses from Various Radiographic Examinations

X-ray examination	Gonad dose (mrad)* Male	Female
Skull	<1	<1
Cervical spine	<1	<1
Full-mouth dental	<1	<1
Chest	<1	<1
Stomach and upper gastrointestinal	2	40
Gallbladder	1	20
Lumbar spine	175	400
Intravenous urography	150	300
Abdomen	100	200
Pelvis	300	150
Upper limb	<1	<1
Lower limb	<1	<1

From Ballinger PW: *Merrill's atlas of radiographic positions and radiologic procedures,* ed 8, vol 1, St Louis, 1995, Mosby.
*For some radiologic examinations the female gonad dose is greater than the dose received by the male because the female reproductive organs are located within the pelvic cavity, unlike the male reproductive organs, which are located outside and below the pelvic cavity. The distribution of biologic tissue overlying the ovaries also affects the dose received for a given radiologic examination.

Table 1-7

Typical Fetal Dose Factors as a Function of Skin Entrance Exposure

X-ray examination	Fetal dose factor (mrad/R)
Skull	<0.01
Cervical	<0.01
Full-mouth dental	<0.01
Chest	2
Stomach and upper gastrointestinal	25
Gallbladder	3
Lumbar spine	250
Intravenous urography	265
Abdomen	265
Pelvis	295
Limb	<0.01

From Ballinger PW: *Merrill's atlas of radiographic positions and radiologic procedures,* ed 8, vol 1, St Louis, 1995, Mosby.

vidual radiologist or radiographer technical skills, patient dose for each examination varies according to the institution. Patient dose may be indicated in terms of entrance skin exposure (ESE), skin dose, bone marrow dose, and gonadal dose. In pregnant females, fetal dose also may be estimated. A more complete discussion of patient dose may be found in Chapter 7. Tables 1-3 through 1-7 indicate permissible patient ESEs and skin, bone marrow, gonadal, and fetal doses for several different radiologic examinations.

Summary

In this chapter rationales for protection of human beings from unnecessary exposure to ionizing radiation have been identified. The responsibility of professional radiation workers for providing radiation protection also has been explained. Radiation exposure must always be kept as low as reasonably achievable (ALARA) to keep both occupational and nonoccupational dose equivalents well below maximal allowable levels. Referring physicians must justify the need for every radiation procedure. The potential benefits of exposing the patient to ionizing radiation must far outweigh the potential risk of the possibility of radiogenic cancer or genetic defects after irradiation. When a patient undergoes a diagnostic radiologic procedure, the radiographer should select the lowest exposure factors that will produce useful radiographs and produce a high-quality diagnostic image with the first exposure.

Ionizing radiation is radiation that passes through matter, producing positively and negatively charged particles. These electrically charged particles can cause biologic damage in humans. The sievert (rem) is the radiation quantity unit for DE, a concept that enables the calculation of the effective absorbed dose for all types of ionizing radiation. This unit considers the biologic effects of various types of radiation in man. It may be used to express both occupational and nonoccupational DEs. The ejection of electrons from the atoms of biologic tissue by ionizing radiation causes damage. This damage can occur on three levels: molecular, cellular, and organic. Damage at the organic level results from large amounts of ionizing radiation exposure. Because of this biologic damage potential, the use of ionizing radiation must be limited whenever possible.

Sources of ionizing radiation may be natural or manmade (artificial). Natural sources are part of the human environment; hence they are called *natural background radiation*. They include terrestrial radiation from radioactive materials in the earth, cosmic radiation from the sun (solar) and beyond the solar system (galactic), and biologic radiation from radionuclides deposited in the human body through natural processes. Whenever accidental or deliberate human actions increase these natural sources, they become enhanced natural sources. Manmade or artificial radiation sources include consumer products containing radioactive material, air travel, nuclear fuel for generation of power, atmospheric fallout from nuclear weapons, accidents in nuclear power plants, and medical radiation from diagnostic x-ray machines and radiopharmaceuticals in nuclear medicine. Because human beings are unable to control radiation from natural sources, they must control radiation from manmade sources to protect the global population from further biologic damage.

Review Questions

1. Which of the following is an acceptable reason for a person to undergo a radiologic procedure?
   A. Individual feels routine radiologic procedures should be performed each year.
   B. People should have some exposure to ionizing radiation each year because it kills cancer cells that normally exist in the human body.
   C. Physician ordering the radiologic procedure feels that the potential benefits of the procedure in terms of knowledge gained far outweigh the potential risks of exposure to ionizing radiation.
   D. No acceptable reasons exist for an individual to be exposed to ionizing radiation.

2. Of the following, who has the responsibility for ordering a radiologic examination?
   1. Radiographer
   2. Physician
   3. Patient
   A. 1 only
   B. 2 only
   C. 3 only
   D. 1, 2, and 3

3. Radiation exposure to the patient and the radiographer is increased by which of the following?
   A. Producing a high-quality diagnostic radiograph with the first radiographic exposure
   B. Using appropriate radiation protection safety principles
   C. The repetition of radiographic exposures because of technical error or carelessness
   D. The radiologist ordering a limited radiographic examination

4. Which of the following is a special form of radiation that is capable of creating electrically charged particles by removing orbital electrons from the atoms with which it interacts?
   A. Ionizing radiation
   B. Nonionizing radiation
   C. Subatomic radiation
   D. Ultrasonic radiation

5. Through which of the following routes can radon enter houses?
   1. Crawlspaces under living areas
   2. Floor drains
   3. Porous cement block foundations
   A. 1 and 2 only
   B. 1 and 3 only
   C. 2 and 3 only
   D. 1, 2, and 3

6. A DE of x-radiation as low as 0.25 Sv (25 rem) delivered to the whole body may cause which of the following within a few days?
   A. An increase in the number of lymphocytes in the circulating blood
   B. A decrease in the number of lymphocytes in the circulating blood
   C. The lymphocyte count to drop immediately to zero
   D. A large increase in the number of platelets

7. Which of the following are natural sources of ionizing radiation?
   A. Medical x-radiation and cosmic radiation
   B. Radioactive elements in the earth and in the human body
   C. Radioactive elements in the human body and a diagnostic x-ray machine
   D. Radioactive fallout and environs of atomic energy plants

8. What do airport surveillance systems, smoke detector alarms, luminous-dial timepieces, and nuclear power plants have in common?
   A. All are sources of natural background radiation.
   B. They each contribute 0.05 mSv (5 mrem) per year to the DE received by the global population.
   C. They are not sources of ionizing radiation.
   D. All are sources of manmade radiation.

9. From which of the following sources do humans receive the *largest* dose of ionizing radiation?
   A. Radioactive fallout from atomic weapons
   B. Medical radiation procedures
   C. Cosmic rays
   D. Environs of nuclear reactors

10. Why is radiologic diagnosis more accurate today than in previous years?
    1. Improvements in education of medical personnel
    2. Improvements in education of technical personnel
    3. Greater sophistication in the design of diagnostic imaging equipment
    A. 1 only
    B. 2 only
    C. 3 only
    D. 1, 2, and 3

11. Of the estimated 0.65 mSv (65 mrem) that man-made radiation contributes to the average annual radiation exposure of the U.S. population, what portion of this DE results from consumer products?
    A. 0.01 mSv (1 mrem)
    B. 0.11 mSv (11 mrem)
    C. 0.21 mSv (21 mrem)
    D. 0.31 mSv (31 mrem)

12. Which of the following is the average effective total DE from manmade and natural radiation?
    A. 0.3 mSv (30 mrem) per year
    B. 0.6 mSv (60 mrem) per year
    C. 1.8 mSv (180 mrem) per year
    D. 3.6 mSv (360 mrem) per year

13. Terrestrial radiations include which of the following sources?
    A. Radioactive elements such as uranium, radium, and thorium, which are present in variable quantities in the earth
    B. Radioactive fallout from nuclear weapons tests in which detonation occurred above ground
    C. The sun and other stars
    D. Video display terminals and television receivers

14. Occupational and nonoccupational DEs will remain well below maximal allowable levels when which of the following occur?
    A. Radiographers and radiologists keep exposure as low as reasonably achievable (ALARA).
    B. Referring physicians discontinue ordering x-ray examinations.
    C. Orders for radiologic examinations are determined only by medical insurance companies.
    D. Patients assume responsibility for ordering all radiologic procedures.

15. Which of the following protects the world's population from exposure to essentially all high-energy, bombarding cosmic rays?
    A. Clouds
    B. Fog
    C. Earth's atmosphere
    D. Smog

16. Radon accounts for approximately what percent of the gross common exposure to human beings from natural background radiation?
    A. 15
    B. 25
    C. 55
    D. 75

17. According to the Environmental Protection Agency (EPA), radon levels in homes should not exceed what level?
    A. 200 pCi/L
    B. 135 pCi/L
    C. 47 pCi/L
    D. 4 pCi/L

18. Which of the following is considered by the EPA to be the second leading cause of lung cancer in the United States?
    A. An annual chest x-ray examination
    B. Cosmic rays
    C. Radon
    D. A fluoroscopic examination of the esophagus

19. The degree to which the diagnostic study reveals the presence or absence of disease in the patient defines which of the following?
    A. Radiation protection
    B. Radiographic pathology
    C. Effective diagnosis
    D. Diagnostic efficacy

20. Manmade radiation contributes what amount of mSv and mrem to the annual exposure of the U.S. population?
    A. 0.3, 30
    B. 0.65, 65
    C. 1.2, 120
    D. 3.6, 360

21. Cosmic radiation occurs in which two forms?
    A. Solar and manmade
    B. Artificial and galactic
    C. Natural background and artificial
    D. Solar and galactic

22. Which of the following statements concerning the 1979 nuclear reactor accident at TMI-2 is *not* true?
    A. Excess cancer deaths have been predicted to occur in the 2 million people living within 50 miles of the plant.
    B. Excess cancer deaths have not been predicted to occur in the 2 million people living within 50 miles of the plant.
    C. The DE received by 2 million people in the vicinity of the reactor is .02mSv (2mrem).
    D. No "melt-through" of the reactor vessel occurred.

23. When exposed to high radon levels in the home, which of the following groups of people have the *highest* risk of lung cancer?
    A. Newborn infants
    B. Young children
    C. Nonsmokers
    D. Smokers

24. Acute melting of the uranium dioxide fuel of a nuclear reactor core requires how great a temperature?
    A. Less than 500° F
    B. At least 1000° F
    C. 2000° F
    D. Greater than 5000° F

25. In the 1990s, how serious does the FDA consider the risk radiation exposure received by the U.S. population from color television monitors?
    A. Above average
    B. Below average
    C. Negligible
    D. Substantial

26. Which of the following groups of people are predicted to suffer adverse health effects as a consequence of radiation exposure?
    A. Employees at TMI-2 at the time of the 1979 nuclear power plant accident
    B. People living within 50 miles of the TMI-2 nuclear reactor at the time of the 1979 accident
    C. People living near Kiev in the former Soviet Union at the time of the 1986 Chernobyl nuclear power plant accident
    D. News reporters visiting the former Soviet Union after the 1986 Chernobyl nuclear power plant accident

27. When natural sources of ionizing radiation become increased because of accidental or deliberate human actions, what are they called?
    A. Artificial sources
    B. Enhanced natural sources
    C. Extraterrestrial sources
    D. Manmade sources

28. Which of the following occurrences places human beings in closer contact with extraterrestrial radiation?
    A. Having a chest x-ray examination
    B. Going deep-sea diving
    C. Taking a flight on a commercial airplane
    D. Visiting a nuclear power plant

29. Medical radiation exposure and radiopharmaceuticals in medicine account for about what amount of the average annual individual DE of ionizing radiation?
  - A. 0.25 mSv (25 mrem)
  - B. 0.54 mSv (54 mrem)
  - C. 0.78 mSv (78 mrem)
  - D. 0.92 mSv (92 mrem)

30. The frequency of exposure to manmade radiation in medicine is rapidly increasing among all age groups in the United States because of which of the following?
  1. Medicolegal considerations
  2. Physicians relying more on radiologic diagnoses to assist them in patient care
  3. Medical insurance company requirements for increases in the number of radiologic procedures they order
  - A. 1 and 2 only
  - B. 1 and 3 only
  - C. 2 and 3 only
  - D. 1, 2, and 3

References

1. Wagner LK et al: *Radiation bioeffects and management test and syllabus,* Reston, Va., 1991, American College of Radiology.
2. National Council on Radiation Protection and Measurements (NCRP): *Report #93, ionizing radiation exposure of the population of the United States,* Bethesda, Md, 1987, NCRP.
3. Bushong SC: *Radiologic science for technologists: physics, biology and protection,* ed 6, St Louis, 1997, Mosby.

Bibliography

American College of Radiology Bulletin 52(1):4, 1996.

Arena V: *Ionizing radiation and life,* St Louis, 1971, Mosby.

Ballinger PW: *Merrill's atlas of radiographic positions and radiologic procedures,* ed 8, vol 1, St Louis, 1995, Mosby.

Balter M: Children become the first victims of fallout, *Science* 272:357, 1996.

Bonte FJ: Chernobyl retrospective, *Semin Nucl Med* 18(1):16, 1988.

Bushong S: *Radiologic science for technologists: physics, biology and protection,* ed 5, St Louis, 1993, Mosby.

Carlton RR, Adler AM: *Principles of radiographic imaging: an art and a science,* Albany, NY, 1992, Delmar.

Fried S: Fear itself, *Philadelphia Magazine* 77(9):126, 1986.

Hall EJ: *Radiobiology for the radiologist,* ed 4, Philadelphia, 1994, Lippincott.

Hendee WR, Ritenour ER: *Medical imaging physics,* ed 3, St Louis, 1992, Mosby.

Herlitz Publications: Ionizing radiation exposure levels show less than estimated, *Oncology Times* 10(2):4, 1988.

Hildreth R: *From x-ray martyrs to low level radiation,* Kalamazoo, In, 1981, Industrial Graphics Services.

Hiss SS: *Understanding radiography,* ed 3, Springfield, Il, 1993, Charles C. Thomas.

International Commission of Radiation Units and Measurements (ICRU): *Report *33, radiation quantities and units,* Washington, D.C., 1980, ICRU.

Kilthau GF: Cancer risk in relation to radioactivity in tobacco, *Radiol Technol* 67(3): 217, 1996.

Merion Publications: Radon returns to prominence on agency's list of dangers, *Adv Radiol Technol* 3(12):17, 1990.

Miller PE: Biological effects of diagnostic irradiation, *Radiol Technol* 48:11, 1976.

National Council on Radiation Protection (NCRP): *Commentary #13, an introduction to efficacy in diagnostic radiology and nuclear medicine (justification of medical radiation exposure),* Bethesda, Md, 1996, NCRP.

National Council on Radiation Protection and Measurements (NCRP): *Report #39, basic radiation protection criteria,* Washington, D.C., 1971, NCRP.

National Council on Radiation Protection and Measurements (NCRP): *Report #43, review of the current state of radiation protection philosophy,* Washington, D.C., 1975, NCRP.

National Council on Radiation Protection and Measurements (NCRP): *Report #91, recommendations on limits for exposure to ionizing radiation,* Bethesda, Md, 1987, NCRP.

National Council on Radiation Protection and Measurements (NCRP): *Ionizing radiation exposure of the population of the United States,* Report No. 93, Bethesda, Md, 1987, NCRP.

National Council on Radiation Protection and Measurements (NCRP): *Report #116, limitation of exposure to ionizing radiation,* Bethesda, Md, 1993, NCRP.

New Jersey Department of Health, Division of Occupational and Environmental Health: *Facts and recommendations on exposure to radon,* 1987.

Radford EP, Hunt VR: Cigarettes and polonium-210, *Science* 144:366, 1964.

Radford EP, Hunt VR: Polonium-210: a volatile radioelement in cigarettes, *Science* 143:247, 1964.

Ritenour ER: *Radiation protection and biology: a self-instructional multimedia learning series, instructor manual,* Denver, 1985, Multi-Media Publishing.

Scheele RV, Wakley J: *Elements of radiation protection,* Springfield, Ill, 1975, Charles C. Thomas.

Seeram E: *Radiation protection,* Philadelphia, 1997, Lippincott.

Selman J: *Elements of radiobiology,* Springfield, Ill, 1983, Charles C. Thomas.

Selman J: *The fundamentals of x-ray and radium physics,* ed 7, Springfield, Ill, 1985, Charles C. Thomas.

Shapiro J: *Radiation protection: a guide for scientists and physicians,* ed 3, Cambridge, Mass, 1990, Harvard University Press.

Standard Education Society: *New standard encyclopedia,* vols Q-R, Chicago, 1960, Standard Education Society.

Stone R: The explosions that shook the world, *Science* 272:352, 1996.

Travis EL: *Primer of medical radiobiology,* ed 2, Chicago, 1989, Mosby.

US Department of Defense: *The effects of nuclear weapons,* revised edition, Glasstone S, editor, reprinted Feb. 1964, US Atomic Energy Commission.

US Department of Health and Human Services, Public Health Service, Food and Drug Administration, Bureau of Radiological Health: *The correlated lecture laboratory series in diagnostic radiological physics,* HHS Publications FDA81-8150, Rockville, Md, 1981, HHS.

Vann JM: *Radiation effects of Three Mile Island,* lecture, New Jersey Society of Radiologic Technologists, Nov. 28, 1979, State of NJ Nuclear Engineer, Bureau of Radiation Protection.

Williams N, Balter M: Chernobyl research becomes international growth industry, *Science* 272:355, 1996.

2

Basic Interactions of X-Radiation with Matter

Chapter Outline

absorbed dose
absorption
annihilation radiation
attenuation
characteristic photon
coherent scattering
Compton scattering
contrast media
effective atomic number
electron volt (eV)
exit or image-formation
   photons
fluorescent radiation
fluorescent yield
kilovolt (kV)

mass density
pair production
peak kilovoltage (kVp)
photoelectric absorption
photoelectron
positron emission tomography (PET)
primary photons
primary radiation
radiographic density
radiographic fog
radiographic image receptor
Rayleigh scattering
scattered photon
small-angle scatter

*After completing this chapter, the reader will be able
to perform the following:*

- Define the terms *primary radiation, exit or image formation radiation,* and *attenuation.*

- Discuss the way x-rays are produced and explain the
range of energies present in the x-ray beam.

- List the events that occur when x-radiation passes
through matter.

- Discuss the probability of photon interaction with
matter.

- Describe and illustrate by diagram the x-ray photon
interactions with matter that are important in diagnostic radiology.

- State the impact of contrast media with regard to
photoelectric absorption and identify its effect on
absorbed dose in the body structure that contains it.

- Describe the effect of kilovoltage (kVp) on radiographic image quality and patient absorbed dose.

19

In this chapter, basic physics concepts that relate to radiation protection are reviewed. The mechanisms by which radiation is absorbed and scattered by atoms help explain many important concepts in radiography and radiation protection. The processes of interaction between radiation and matter are emphasized.

X-rays are carriers of energy. If x-rays enter a material such as human tissue, they may interact with the atoms of the biologic material or pass through the biologic material without interacting. If they interact, energy is transferred from the x-rays to the atoms of the biologic material. This transference of energy is called **absorption** (Fig. 2-1), and the amount of energy absorbed per unit mass is referred to as the **absorbed**

dose. The more energy received by the atoms of the patient's body, the greater the risk of biologic damage in the patient. For the patient's safety the amount of energy transferred should be kept as small as possible. However, without the phenomenon of absorption and differences in the absorption properties of different body structures, diagnostically useful radiographs in which different structures may be perceived and distinguished would not be possible to produce. The radiographer also benefits when patient dose is minimal because less radiation is scattered from the patient.

X-Ray Beam Production and Energy

A diagnostic x-ray beam is produced by bombarding a positively charged target with a stream of high-speed electrons in a highly evacuated glass tube. This target, also known as the anode, is usually made of tungsten, a metal, or rhenium tungsten, a metal alloy. These materials have high melting points and high atomic numbers. As the electrons interact with the atoms of the target, x-ray photons (particles associated with electromagnetic radiation that have neither mass nor electric charge) emerge from the target with a broad spectrum or range of energy and leave the x-ray tube through a glass window. The glass window permits passage of all but the lowest components of the x-ray spectrum. It therefore acts as a filter for diagnostically useless, very–low-energy x-rays. The emerging x-ray photon beam is collectively referred to as **primary radiation** (Fig. 2-2).

Although all photons in a diagnostic x-ray beam do not have the same energy, the most energetic photons in the beam can have no more energy than the electrons that bombard the target. The energy of the electrons inside the x-ray tube is expressed in terms of the electrical voltage applied across the tube. For diagnostic radiology, this is expressed in thousands of volts, or **kilovolts (kV).** Moreover, because the voltage across the tube fluctuates, it is usually expressed in **peak kilovoltage, or kVp.** If an electron is drawn across an electrical potential difference of 1 volt, it has acquired an energy of 1 **electron volt, or eV.** Thus a technique factor of 100 kVp means that the electrons bombarding the target have an energy of 100,000 electron volts, or 100 keV. X-rays of various energies are

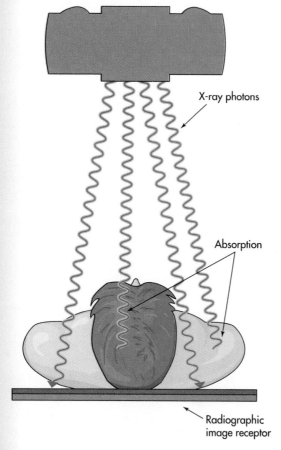

Fig. 2-1 X-ray photons can interact with atoms of the patient's body and transfer energy to the tissue. This transference of energy is called *absorption.*

X-ray photons

Absorption

Radiographic
image receptor

produced, but the most energetic x-ray photon can have no more energy than 100 keV. For a typical diagnostic x-ray unit the energy of the average photon in the x-ray beam is about one third the energy of the most energetic photon. Therefore a 100-kVp beam contains photons having energies of 100 keV or less, with an average energy of about 33 keV.

Attenuation

Fig. 2-3 illustrates the passage of four x-ray photons through an object. Before the four photons produced by the x-ray source enter the object, they are referred to as **primary photons**. Only two photons emerge from the object and strike the **radiographic image receptor** below it. They are referred to as **exit or image-formation photons** (formerly termed *remnant photons*) because they remain in the x-ray beam after it has passed through the object. The two that do *not* strike the image receptor are attenuated. The term **attenuation** is rather broad; with respect to x-rays, it is used to refer

to any process decreasing the intensity of the primary photon beam that was directed toward a destination. The destination of the photons in Fig. 2-3 is the image receptor. Therefore photon #3, which has deviated from its path (i.e., it has been "scattered") to the extent that it will not strike the image receptor, is said to have

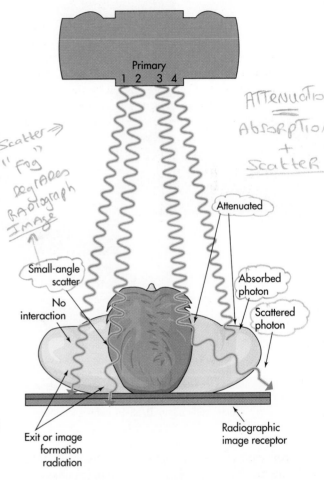

Fig. 2-3 Primary, exit, and attenuated photons. Primary photons (photons *#1*, *#2*, *#3*, and *#4*) are photons that emerge from the x-ray source. Exit or image formation photons (photons *#1* and *#2*) are photons that pass through the object being radiographed (the patient) and reach the radiographic image receptor. Attenuated photons (photons *#3* and *#4*) are photons that have interacted with atoms of the object (the patient) and been scattered or absorbed such that they do not reach the radiographic image receptor.

Fig. 2-2 Primary radiation emerges from the x-ray tube target and consists of x-ray photons of various energies. It is produced when the positively charged target is bombarded with a stream of high-speed electrons and these electrons interact with the atoms of the target.

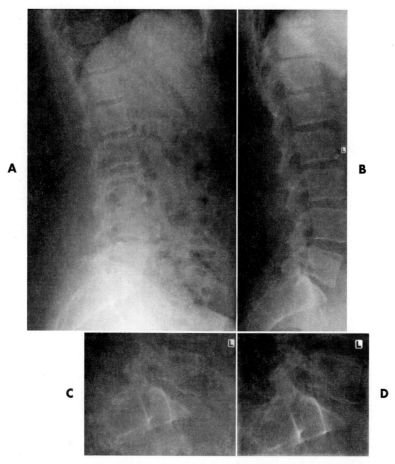

Fig. 2-4 A, Lateral view of the lumbar vertebrae showing improper collimation, which results in the production of radiographic fog and a consequent lack of radiographic clarity. **B,** Lateral view of the lumbar vertebrae showing proper collimation, which eliminates radiographic fog and consequently increases radiographic clarity. **C,** Lateral view of the L5-S1 lumbosacral junction demonstrating inadequate collimation. **D,** L5-S1 lumbosacral junction demonstrating adequate collimation.

Continued

been attenuated. Photon #4 seems to disappear. It has transferred all its energy to the atoms of the object and has therefore been eliminated. Because a photon has no mass, no charge, and no attribute other than energy, it ceases to exist when it gives up its energy.

The term *attenuation,* then, refers to both absorption and scatter that prevent photons from reaching a predefined destination. Fig. 2-3 shows that the path of photon #2 was bent but not so much that the photon missed its target. Insofar as photon #2 reached the im-

age receptor, it is part of the exit or image-formation radiation, but the bending of its path represents what is called **small-angle scatter.** These scattered photons have essentially the same energy as the incident unscattered photons. Small-angle scatter degrades the appearance of a radiograph. Sharp outlines of dense objects are smeared by the effects of such scatter. Moreover, because millions of such small-angle scatter events occur, a radiosensitive film darkens overall, interfering with the radiologist's ability to distinguish

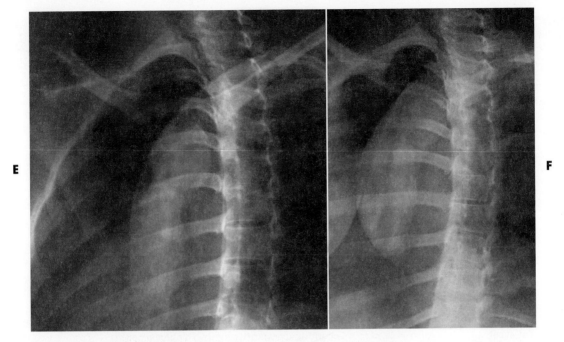

E

F

Fig. 2-4, cont'd. E, Right anterior oblique view of the sternum demonstrating poor collimation.
F, Right anterior oblique view of the sternum demonstrating good collimation.

different structures in the image. This extended darkening is called **radiographic fog**. Reducing the amount of tissue irradiated reduces the amount of fog produced by small-angle scatter. Therefore adequately collimating the x-ray beam is one way to reduce fog (Fig 2-4). Other methods used to reduce the image-degrading effects of scatter are discussed later.

Probability of Photon Interaction with Matter

Because the interaction of photons with biologic matter is random, radiologists cannot predict with certainty what will happen to a single photon when it enters biologic matter. When they deal with a large number of photons, however, they can predict what will happen on the average, and this is more than adequate to determine the characteristics of the radiograph that results from such interactions (Table 2-1). For example, in a beam of x-ray photons a 50 keV photon has a 66% likelihood of interacting with the atoms of the tissue when it travels through 5 cm of soft tissue (see Appendix A); 34% of the time the photon will simply pass through the tissue. Another way to say this is that if 100 photons travel through 5 cm of soft tissue, 66 interactions may be expected to occur. Of the 66 interactions, 11% should be of a type called photoelectric; thus about 7 out of 100 (11% of 66) interactions would be of the photoelectric type. In the photoelectric interaction a photon is completely absorbed by the atoms of the tissue (i.e., removed from the beam). If this were the only interaction possible, irradiating 5 cm of soft tissue with 50 keV photons would create a light area on a radiographic film, which would be the result of 7% fewer photons reaching that portion of the film. In reality the process is much more complicated because several additional effects occur, and a typical x-ray beam is composed of photons with a continuous spectrum of energies. In the remainder of this chapter the different interactions of photons with individual atoms and the effect of a particular type of interaction on the radiograph are examined.

Table 2-1				
Interaction of X-Radiation with Matter—Overview*				
X-ray photon energy range	Site of interaction	X-ray photon	Most probable type of interaction	Byproducts of the interaction
1 to 50 kVp†	An atom	Energy: unchanged; direction after interaction: slight change (less than 20 degrees)	Coherent scattering	None
1 to 50 kVp‡	Inner-shell electron (usually K shell)	Energy: absorbed; direction after interaction: not applicable	Photoelectric absorption	Photoelectron (characteristic photon)
60 to 90 kVp§	Outer-shell electron	Energy: reduced; direction after interaction: changed (x-ray photon energy partially absorbed)	Compton scattering	Compton scattered electron
200 kVp to 2 meV‖	Outer-shell electron	Energy: reduced; direction after interaction: changed	Compton scattering	Scattered x-ray photon of lower energy and energetic ionizing electron
Begins at about 1.022 MeV; becomes important at 10 MeV; becomes predominant at 50 MeV and above	Nucleus of atom	Energy: disappears after interaction with nucleus; transformed into two new particles that annihilate each other; direction after interaction: energy reappears in form of two 0.511-MeV photons, each moving in opposite directions	Pair production	Positive electron (positron); ordinary electron (negatron); two 0.511-MeV photons

*For more information, refer to the latest editions of the following textbooks: Bushong SC: *Radiologic science for technologists: physics, biology, and protection*, St Louis, 1996, Mosby and Hendee WR, Ritenour ER: *Medical imaging physics*, St Louis, 1992, Mosby.
†Most probable where photoelectric absorption is most important, but much less probable than photoelectric absorption at these energies.
‡Most important interaction in soft tissue.
§Compton and photoelectric absorption in soft tissue are of equal importance.
‖Compton interaction alone is present in soft tissue.

Processes of Interaction

Four basic types of interaction between x-radiation and matter are possible: coherent scattering, Compton scattering, photoelectric absorption, and pair production.

Coherent scattering (classical or unmodified scattering)

If a photon with energy significantly less than 100 keV interacts with an atom, the electrons of the atom as a whole may be caused to vibrate momentarily.

This is analogous to the behavior of electrons in the antenna of a receiver intercepting a radio signal. Because they are charged particles, each of the atom's vibrating electrons radiates energy in the form of electromagnetic waves. These waves coherently (i.e., cooperatively) combine with each other to form a scattered wave. This represents the **scattered photon.** Its wavelength is the same as that of the incident photon. Thus no net energy has been absorbed by the atom (see Appendix B). However, a change in the direction of the emitted photon is very likely. In general this

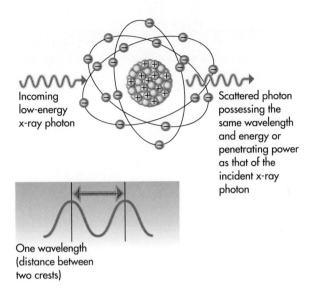

One wavelength
(distance between
two crests)

Fig. 2-5 Coherent scattering. The incoming low-energy x-ray photon interacts with an atom, causing the electrons of the atom to vibrate momentarily. The electrons then radiate energy in the form of electromagnetic waves. These waves nondestructively combine with each other to form a scattered wave. This represents the scattered photon. Its wavelength and energy, or penetrating power, is the same as the incident photon. Generally the emitted photon may change in direction less than 20 degrees with respect to the direction of the original photon. (Wavelength is the distance from one crest to the next.)

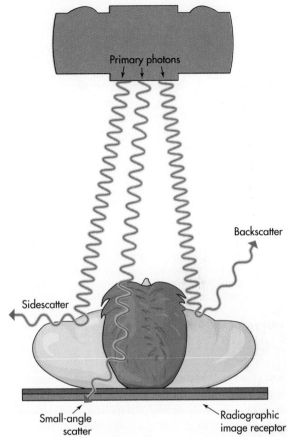

Fig. 2-6 Compton scattering results in all-directional scatter. The scatter created may be directed onward as small-angle scatter, backward as backscatter, and to the side as sidescatter. The direction of travel of the scatter is a major factor in planning protection for members of the medical radiography team during a radiologic examination.

change in direction is less than 20 degrees with respect to the initial direction of the original photon. This is the net effect of **coherent scattering,** also known as **Rayleigh scattering** in honor of the scientist who first explained it before the concept of the photon by using wave analysis. Although coherent scattering is most likely to occur below 30 kVp, some unmodified scattering occurs throughout the diagnostic range and may result in small amounts of radiographic fog (Fig. 2-5).

Compton scattering (incoherent or modified scattering)

Compton scattering, also known as incoherent or modified scattering, is responsible for most of the scattered radiation produced during radiologic procedures. This scatter is isotropic, meaning it may be directed forward as small-angle scatter, backward as

backscatter, and to the side as sidescatter. The direction the scatter travels is a major factor in planning protection for members of the medical radiography team during a radiologic examination (Fig. 2-6).

In the Compton process an incoming x-ray photon interacts with a loosely bound outer-shell electron of an atom of the irradiated object (Fig. 2-7). On encountering the electron, the incoming x-ray photon surrenders a portion of its kinetic energy to dislodge the electron from its outer-shell orbit (see Appendix C for an extended discussion of this type of interaction). The freed electron, called a Compton scattered elec-

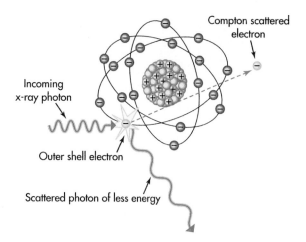

Fig. 2-7 Compton scattering. On encountering a loosely bound outer-shell electron, the incoming x-ray photon surrenders a portion of its kinetic energy to dislodge the electron from its orbit. The energy-degraded x-ray photon then continues on its way but in a new direction. The high-speed electron ejected from its orbit is called a *Compton scattered electron,* or *"recoil" electron.*

tron, possesses excess kinetic energy and is capable of ionizing atoms. It loses its kinetic energy by a series of collisions with nearby atoms and finally recombines with an atom that needs another electron. This usually occurs within a few micrometers of the site of the original Compton interaction.

The x-ray photon that surrendered some of its energy (see Appendix C) to free the electron from its orbit continues on its way but in a new direction. It has the potential to interact with other atoms either by the process of photoelectric absorption or by Compton scattering. It also may emerge from the patient, in which case it may contribute to degradation of the radiographic image (see **small-angle scatter,** p 22) or present a health hazard to the radiographer or radiologist (Box 2-1).

In diagnostic radiology the probability of occurrence of Compton scattering relative to that of the photoelectric interaction increases as the energy of the x-ray photon increases. Compton scattering and photoelectric absorption in tissue are equally probable at about 35 keV. Therefore in a 100-kVp x-ray beam a significant number of Compton events occur.

Photoelectric absorption

Within the energy range of diagnostic radiology (30 to 150 kVp), photoelectric absorption is the most important mode of interaction between x-ray photons and the atoms of the patient's body for producing useful patient images.

Photoelectric absorption is an interaction between an x-ray photon and an inner-shell electron (usually in the K shell) tightly bound to an atom of the absorbing medium (Figure 2-8). To dislodge an inner-shell electron from its atomic orbit, the incoming x-ray photon must be able to transfer a quantity of energy as large as or larger than the amount of energy that binds the electron in its orbit. On interacting with an inner-shell electron, the x-ray photon surrenders all its energy to the orbital electron and ceases to exist. The electron is ejected from its inner shell, creating a vacancy. The ejected orbital electron, called a **photoelectron,** possesses kinetic energy equal to the energy of the incident photon less the binding energy of the electron shell. This photoelectron may interact with other atoms, causing excitation or ionization, until all its kinetic energy has been spent. The photoelectron is usually absorbed within a few micrometers of the medium through which it travels. In the human body, this energy transfer results in increased patient dose and contributes to biologic damage of tissues.

As a result of the photoelectric effect, in general a vacancy exists in the inner shell of the parent atom. To fill this opening, an electron from an outer shell drops down to the vacated inner-shell opening by releasing energy (equivalent to the energy level difference between the two shells) in the form of a photon. This photon is termed a **characteristic photon.** It possesses relatively low energy in human tissue and is locally absorbed in the irradiated object. Ensuing vacancies in successive shells are filled and photons emitted in a like fashion until the atom regains electrical equilibrium (Box 2-2). A characteristic photon created as a result of a K-shell vacancy may not escape the confines of the atom but may instead produce its own photoelectric effect by releasing its energy to an electron of lower binding energy, thereby ejecting that electron from the atom. Unbound electrons generated in this manner are known as Auger electrons. This internal photoelectric effect reduces the intensity of characteristic radiation (also called **fluorescent radiation**) emitted from atoms as a result of photoelectric interactions. The term **fluorescent yield** refers to the number of characteristic x-rays emitted per K-shell vacancy. The fluorescent yield per photoelectric interaction in general is lower in materials composed of higher atomic number atoms (see Fig. 2-8, *C*).

The probability of occurrence of photoelectric absorption depends on the energy of the incident x-ray photons and the atomic number of the atoms composing the irradiated object; it increases markedly as the energy of the incident photons decreases and the atomic number of the irradiated atoms increases, ap-

$$P.E \propto \frac{Z^4}{E^3}$$

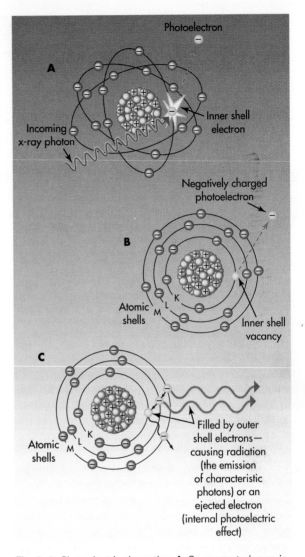

Fig. 2-8 Photoelectric absorption. **A,** On encountering an inner shell or K-shell electron, the incoming x-ray photon surrenders all its energy to the electron and the photon ceases to exist. **B,** The atom responds by ejecting the electron, called a *photoelectron,* from its inner shell, creating a vacancy in the shell. **C,** To fill the opening, an electron from an outer shell drops down to the vacated inner shell by releasing energy in the form of a characteristic photon. Then, to fill the new vacancy in the outer shell, another electron from the shell next farthest out drops down and another characteristic photon is emitted, and so on until the atom regains electrical equilibrium. A K-shell vacancy characteristic photon also may interact with an outer-shell electron, ejecting it from the atom. (See Table 2-2.)

Table 2-2								
Electron Shell Occupancies for Some Common Atoms								

Atom	Symbol	Atomic number	Shell					
			K	L	M	N	O	P
Hydrogen	H	1	1					
Helium	He	2	2					
Lithium	Li	3	2	1				
Carbon	C	6	2	4				
Oxygen	O	8	2	6				
Sodium	Na	11	2	8	1			
Aluminum	Al	13	2	8	3			
Calcium	Ca	20	2	8	8	2		
Copper	Cu	29	2	8	18	1		
Molybdenum	Mo	42	2	8	18	13	1	
Tungsten	W	74	2	8	18	32	12	2
Lead	Pb	82	2	8	18	32	18	4
Radon	Rn	86	2	8	18	32	18	8

proximately Z^4/E^3 per atom, Z^3/E^3 per electron. Thus in the radiographic kilovoltage range, compact bone (effective atomic number 13.8) with a high content by weight (14.7%) of calcium (atomic number 20) undergoes much more photoelectric absorption (approximately 12 times per atom) than an equal mass of soft tissue (effective atomic number approximately 7.4) and air (effective atomic number 7.6).

The density (**mass density** measured in grams per cubic centimeter) of different body structures also influences attenuation. A difference in density leads to a corresponding increase in photon absorption. In any given sample of material, both density and atomic number play a role in determining attenuation. For example, if radiography is performed on equal thicknesses of bone and soft tissue, the bone, which is approximately twice as dense as soft tissue, will absorb about 9 times as many photons in the diagnostic energy range as will the soft tissue. A factor of 4.5 is caused by the higher atomic number of the bone, and a factor of 2 is caused by the higher density of bone. The total effect is 2 times 4.5, for an overall factor of 9.

Thickness of body parts also plays a role. The thickness factor is approximately linear. If two structures have the same density and atomic number but one is twice as thick as another, the thicker structure absorbs twice as many photons. Consequently, if a 2-cm-thick bone sample was radiographed next to a 4-cm-thick tissue sample, the density and thickness factors would cancel each other out. The bone is half as thick in this example, but it is approximately twice as dense. The remaining factor, the higher atomic number of bone, causes the bone to absorb approximately 4.5 times as many photons as the soft tissue.

Such differences in absorption properties between different body structures make diagnostically useful radiographs possible. In other words the ability to perceive and distinguish between different body structures in a radiograph depends on the presence of differences in the amount of x-radiation these structures permit to pass through them to reach the radiographic image receptor.

The less a given structure attenuates radiation, the darker (i.e., the greater the **radiographic density**) its image on the finished radiograph will be, and vice versa. Thus bone, with a higher **effective atomic number** and greater mass density than either soft tissue or air cavities, absorbs more radiation and appears white on a diagnostic radiograph, whereas soft tissue presents a gray image and air-containing structures (e.g., lungs, stomach) appear black (Fig. 2-9).

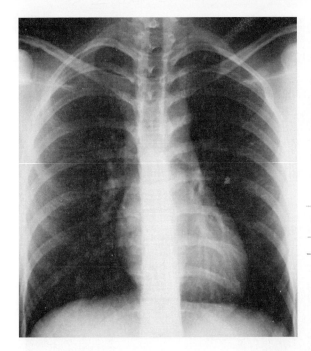

Fig. 2-9 The less a given structure attenuates radiation, the darker (i.e., the greater its radiographic density) its image will be on the finished radiograph, and vice versa. Thus compact bone, with a higher effective atomic number and greater mass density than either soft tissue or air cavities, absorbs more radiation and appears white on a diagnostic radiograph, whereas soft tissue presents a gray image and air-containing structures such as the lungs appear black.

In Figure 2-10, two posteroanterior (PA) hand radiographs illustrate age-related changes in bone density resulting from changes in calcium content. Radiograph *A* exhibits substantial calcium deposits in the bones of a young person. Radiograph *B* exhibits the demineralized bones of an elderly person. The lack of x-ray absorption results from the decrease in bone calcium. Hence the elderly person's bones are almost transparent in radiographic appearance. Pathologic conditions such as degenerative arthritis also contribute to differences in absorption. Radiographic exposure factors must be adjusted to compensate for such changes.

Within the energy range of diagnostic radiology, the greater the difference in the amount of photoelectric absorption, the greater the contrast will be in the radiographic image between adjacent structures. However, as absorption increases, so does the potential for biologic damage. For those regions in which the photoelectric absorption occurs most frequently (e.g., in dense atomic number areas such as cortical bone), the absorbed dose to the patient may be greater by a factor of 6 to 9 than in adjacent low-atomic-number and less dense regions. Thus to ensure both radiographic image quality and patient safety, the radiologist or radiographer should choose the highest energy x-ray beam that permits adequate radiographic film contrast.

If tissues or structures that are similar in atomic number must be distinguished, the photoelectric interaction by itself will not be sufficient to produce adequate contrast. To resolve the problem, the use of **contrast media** has been adopted. Very simply, contrast media consist of high atomic solutions (e.g., barium or iodine based) that are either ingested or injected into the tissues or structures to be visualized. The high atomic number of the contrast media (barium = 56, iodine = 53) significantly enhances the occurrence of photoelectric interaction relative to similar adjacent structures that do not have the contrast media. These contrast-enhanced structures appear brighter than adjacent structures that did not receive the contrast media. Caution must be exercised in the use of contrast media because some patients may not be able to tolerate their presence. The use of contrast media also leads to an increase in absorbed dose in the body structure that has the contrast media.

Pair production

Pair production does not occur unless the energy of the incident photon is at least 1.022 million electron volts (MeV). Although this energy range is far above that used in diagnostic radiology, a brief description of pair production is included in this chapter for the purpose of furnishing the reader with a broader understanding of the basic interactions of x-radiation with matter.

In pair production (Fig. 2-11) the incoming photon strongly interacts with the nucleus of an atom of the irradiated object and disappears. In the process the energy of the photon is transformed into two new particles, a negatron (an ordinary electron) and a positron (a positively charged electron). The negatron and the

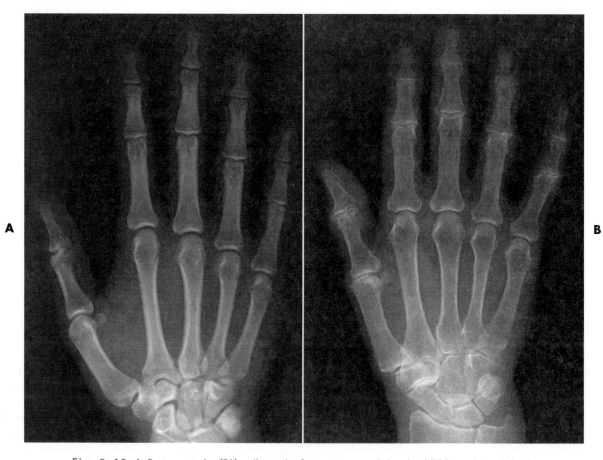

A

B

Fig. 2-10 **A,** Posteroanterior (PA) radiograph of a young person's hand exhibiting substantial calcium deposits in the bones. **B,** PA radiograph of an elderly person's hand exhibiting demineralized bone as a consequence of a decrease in bone calcium. This and other degenerative changes account for the almost transparent appearance of the bones.

Fig. 2-11 Pair production. The incoming photon (equivalent in energy to at least 1.022 MeV) strongly interacts with the nucleus of the atom of the irradiated object and disappears. In the process the energy of the photon is transformed into two new particles, a negatron (electron) and a positron. The negatron eventually recombines with any atom that needs another electron. The positron interacts destructively with a nearby electron. During the interaction the positron and the electron annihilate each other with their rest masses being converted into energy, which appears in the form of two 0.511-MeV photons, each moving in the opposite direction.

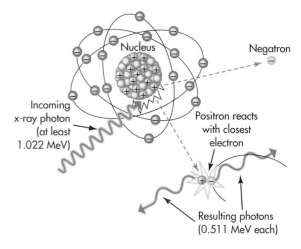

positron have the same mass and magnitude of charge; the only difference is in the "sign" of their electrical charges. The incoming photon must have enough energy to produce the combined mass of these two particles. The *minimum* energy required to produce an electron-positron pair is 1.022 MeV.

$$\text{Mass (electron or positron)} = 9.1 \times 10^{-31} \text{ kg}$$

$$c = 3 \times 10^8 \text{ m/s}$$

$$E \text{ (total)} = E \text{ (electron)} + E \text{ (positron)} =$$

$$mc^2 \text{ (electron)} + mc^2 \text{ (positron)} = 16.38 \times 10^{-14} \text{ J}$$

$$1 \text{ Mev} = 1.602 \times 10^{-13} \text{ J}$$

$$\text{Therefore } E = 16.38 \times 10^{-14} \div$$

$$1.602 \times 10^{-13} = 1.022 \text{ MeV}.$$

For this reason, pair production does not occur at lower energies. The electron loses its kinetic energy by exciting and ionizing atoms in its path. The electron eventually loses enough energy that it may be captured by an atom in need of another electron.

As far as is known, no large quantities of positrons freely exist in the universe. The positron is classified as a form of antimatter. It interacts destructively with a nearby electron. During the interaction the positron and the electron annihilate each other, and in their place, energy appears that is carried off by two 0.511-MeV photons moving in opposite directions. Here, *mass has been transformed into energy.*

Although pair production does not have any direct use in diagnostic radiology, **annihilation radiation** is used in **positron emission tomography (PET)**. In PET scanning the source of the positrons are atomic nuclei that are unstable because they contain too many protons relative to their number of neutrons. To relieve this instability, the surplus proton is replaced in the nucleus by a neutron while a positron and another particle called a neutrino are ejected from the nucleus. This process is called positron decay. Within a very short distance (several micrometers or less) the emitted positron interacts with a local electron, and the two mutually annihilate, converting mass into energy in the process. This energy is carried off by a pair of photons emerging in opposite directions from the electron-positron interaction site. These annihilation photons are intercepted by a ring of detectors surrounding the patient and are used to build a cross-sectional image of the radioactivity within the patient. Some examples of unstable nuclei used in PET scanning are fluorine 18 (18F), carbon 11 (11C), and nitrogen 13 (13N).

Summary

In this chapter, basic physics concepts that relate to radiation protection have been reviewed. Biologic damage in the patient may result from the absorption of x-ray energy. Moreover, different body structures differ in their absorption properties. These variations in x-ray absorption in biologic tissue make radiographic visualization of human anatomy possible. When an x-ray beam passes through matter, the intensity of the primary photons decreases as a result of the processes of absorption and scatter. This is termed *attenuation*. The energy absorbed by the patient per unit mass is the absorbed dose, whereas the scatter contributes to radiographic fog or becomes a biologic hazard to the radiographer. Several factors influence the probability of interaction of photons in matter. An overview of these factors is shown in Table 2-3.

Table 2-3

Factors that Influence the Probability of Interaction of Photons with Energy E in Materials with Density p

Interaction	Photon energy	Atomic number	Electron density p_e (e$^-$/g)	Physical density p (g/cm^3)
Photoelectric	$1/E^3$	Z^3	Independent	p
Compton	$1/E$	Independent	p_e	p
Pair production	E	Z	Independent	p

The number of photons absorbed or scattered from a beam of x-rays depends on the energy of the photons and the composition of the material in the path of the x-ray beam. The photoelectric effect is the basis of radiographic imagery, whereas the Compton effect is its bane. When kVp is decreased, the number of photoelectric interactions increases and the number of Compton interactions decreases. Therefore maintaining low kVp would seem to be logical. However, when kVp is decreased, more energy is absorbed by the patient (the entire energy of the photon is absorbed when the photoelectric interaction occurs, whereas only part of the photon's energy is absorbed when a Compton interaction occurs); consequently, patient dose is increased. Clearly, a compromise between image quality and patient safety is necessary. For a given examination an optimal technique (kVp and mAs combination) exists that minimizes the dose to the patient and produces a radiograph of acceptable quality. The kVp selections are usually based on the type of procedure and body part being radiographed. Other factors such as film or screen type, patient thickness, degree of muscle tissue, and so forth affect the technique selected and cannot always be determined by referring to standard charts. The radiographer must balance these variables to arrive at the technique that will provide an acceptable image in keeping with the standards of radiation protection.

Review Questions

1. What comprises exit or image formation radiation?
   A. Primary photons and Compton scattered electrons
   B. Noninteracting and small-angle scattered photons
   C. Attenuated photons
   D. Absorbed photons

2. When a technique factor of 90 kVp is selected, which of the following occurs?
   A. The highest energy photon in the beam has an energy of 30 keV.
   B. The electrons are accelerated from the cathode to the anode with an energy of 30 keV.
   C. The energy of the average photon in the beam is 90 keV.
   D. The energy of the average photon in the beam is 30 keV.

3. Which of the following contributes *significantly* to the exposure of the diagnostic radiographer?
   A. Positrons
   B. Electrons
   C. Compton scattered photons
   D. Compton scattered electrons

4. Which of the following defines *attenuation?*
   A. Absorption and scatter
   B. Absorption only
   C. Scatter only
   D. Compton electrons

5. Which of the following is *not* a type of interaction between x-radiation and biologic matter?
   A. Compton scattering
   B. Bremsstrahlung
   C. Pair production
   D. Photoelectric absorption
   E. None of the above

6. In which of the following x-ray interactions with matter is the energy of the incident photon *completely* absorbed?
   A. Compton scattering
   B. Photoelectric absorption
   C. Bremsstrahlung
   D. Rayleigh scattering

7. In which of the following x-ray interactions with matter is the energy of incident photon *partially* absorbed?
   A. Compton scattering
   B. Photoelectric effect
   C. Coherent scattering
   D. Pair production

8. What is the result of coherent scattering?
   A. A simple change in direction of the incident x-ray photon
   B. A transfer of all the energy of the incident x-ray photon to the atoms of the irradiated object
   C. The production of a negatron and a positron
   D. A transfer of only some of the energy of the incident x-ray photon to the atoms of the irradiated object

9. A Compton scattered electron does which of the following?
   A. Annihilates another electron
   B. Is absorbed within a few microns of the Compton interaction
   C. Causes photoelectric interactions
   D. Is an exit photon

10. In photoelectric absorption, the kinetic energy of the incoming x-ray photon must be _____ to be able to dislodge an inner-shell electron from its orbit.
    A. Less than the energy that binds the atom together
    B. Ten times as great as the energy that binds the atom together
    C. The same as or slightly greater than the energy that binds the electron in its orbit
    D. Equal to or greater than 1.02 MeV, regardless of the energy that binds the electron in its orbit.

11. Which of the following interactions between photons and matter involves a matter-antimatter annihilation reaction?
    A. Compton scattering
    B. Coherent scattering
    C. Pair production
    D. Photoelectric absorption

12. The probability of the occurrence of photoelectric absorption _____ as the atomic number of the irradiated material _____.
    A. Increases, decreases
    B. Decreases, increases
    C. Increases, increases
    D. Stays the same, increases

13. Which of the following terms refers to the radiation that occurs when an electron moves from an outer orbit to fill a vacancy in an inner orbit?
    A. Characteristic radiation
    B. Bremsstrahlung
    C. Photoelectric radiation
    D. Primary radiation

14. Most of the scattered radiation produced during radiographic procedures is the direct result of which of the following?
    A. Photoelectric effect
    B. Nuclear decay
    C. Image-formation electrons
    D. Compton interactions

15. Which of the following is *not* another term for coherent scattering?
    A. Characteristic
    B. Classical
    C. Rayleigh
    D. Unmodified

16. What is the effective atomic number of bone?
    A. 13.8
    B. 7.6
    C. 7.4
    D. 5.9

17. Before interaction with matter, an incoming x-ray photon may be referred to as which of the following?
    A. Attenuated photon
    B. Primary photon
    C. Exit photon
    D. Scattered photon

18. Which of the following are byproducts of photoelectric absorption?
    A. Photoelectron and Compton scattered electron
    B. Low-energy scattered x-ray photon and characteristic photon
    C. Low-energy scattered x-ray photon and Compton scattered electron
    D. Photoelectron and characteristic x-ray photon

19. Which two interactions between x-radiation and matter may result in the production of small-angle scatter?
   A. Photoelectric absorption and Compton scattering
   B. Coherent scattering and Compton scattering
   C. Photoelectric absorption and pair production
   D. Coherent scattering and pair production

20. Which of the following particles is considered to be a form of antimatter?
   A. Electron
   B. Positron
   C. X-ray photon
   D. Scattered x-ray photon

21. Which of the following interactions results in the conversion of mass into energy?
   A. Classical scattering
   B. Photoelectric absorption
   C. Modified scattering
   D. Annihilation reaction

22. With which of the following is *Compton scattering* synonymous?
   A. Coherent scattering
   B. Incoherent scattering
   C. Photoelectric absorption
   D. Pair production

23. To which of the following does the radiation permeability of a structure refer?
   A. Ionizing properties
   B. Penetrability by radiation
   C. Radiosensitivity
   D. Radioinsensitivity

24. During the process of coherent scattering, with what does the incident x-ray photon interact?
   A. A single inner-shell electron, ejecting it from its orbit
   B. A single outer-shell electron, ejecting it from its orbit
   C. An atom's electrons, causing them to vibrate and emit radiation
   D. A scattered photon of lesser energy, annihilating it

25. What characteristic primarily differentiates the probability of occurrence of the various interactions of x-radiation with human tissues?
   A. Energy of the incoming photon
   B. Direction of the incident photon
   C. X-ray beam intensity
   D. Difference in the binding energy of the atom's electron shells

26. What is the term for the number of characteristic x-rays emitted per K-shell vacancy during photoelectric absorption?
   A. Characteristic absorption
   B. Classical gain
   C. Fluorescent yield
   D. Modified pair production

27. Which of the following influence attenuation?
   1. Effective atomic number of the absorber
   2. Mass density
   3. Thickness of the absorber
   A. 1 and 2 only
   B. 1 and 3 only
   C. 2 and 3 only
   D. 1, 2, and 3

28. Which of the following result in all-directional scatter?
   A. Classical interaction
   B. Coherent interaction
   C. Photoelectric interaction
   D. Compton interaction

29. Mass density may best be described by which of the following?
   A. It identifies the probability of occurrence for Compton interactions in the diagnostic radiology ranges.
   B. It is the same as radiographic density.
   C. It relates the way the effective atomic number of biologic tissues influences absorption.
   D. It is measured in grams per cubic centimeter.

Bibliography

Ball JL, Moore AD: *Essential physics for radiographers,* London, 1980, Blackwell Scientific.

Bushong S: *Radiologic science for technologists: physics, biology, and protection,* ed 6, St Louis, 1997, Mosby.

Carlton RR, Adler AM: *Principles of radiographic imaging: an art and a science,* Albany, NY, 1992, Delmar Publishers.

Christensen EE, Curry III TS, Dowdey JE: *An introduction to the physics of diagnostic radiology,* ed 2, Philadelphia, 1978, Lea & Febiger.

Cullinan AM, Cullinan JE: *Producing quality radiographs,* ed 2, Philadelphia, 1994, Lippincott.

Curry III TS, Dowdey JE, Murry Jr RC: *Christensen's introduction to the physics of diagnostic radiology,* ed 3, Philadelphia, 1984, Lea & Febiger.

Donohue DP: *An analysis of radiographic quality: lab manual and workbook,* ed 2, Rockville, Md, 1984, Aspen.

Frankel R: *Radiation protection for radiologic technologists,* New York, 1976, McGraw-Hill.

Graham BJ, Thomas WN: *An introduction to physics for radiologic technologists,* Philadelphia, 1975, WB Saunders.

Hall, EJ: *Radiobiology for the radiologist,* ed 4, Philadelphia, 1994, Lippincott.

Hendee WR, Ritenour ER: *Medical imaging physics,* ed 3, St Louis, 1992, Mosby.

Hewitt PG: *Conceptual physics: a new introduction to your environment,* ed 4, Boston, 1981, Little, Brown.

Malott JC, Fodor III J: *The art and science of medical radiography,* ed 7, St Louis, 1993, Mosby.

Noz ME, Maguire Jr GQ: *Radiation protection in the radiologic and health sciences,* ed 2, Philadelphia, 1985, Lea & Febiger.

Pizzarello DJ, Witcofski RL: *Basic radiation biology,* ed 2, Philadelphia, 1975, Lea & Febiger.

Ritenour ER: *Radiation protection and biology: a self-instructional multimedia learning series—instructor manual,* Denver, 1985, Multi-Media Publishing.

Scheele RV, Wakley J: *Elements of radiation protection,* Springfield, Ill, 1975, Charles C. Thomas.

Selman J: *The fundamentals of x-ray and radium physics,* ed 7, Springfield, Ill, 1985, Charles C. Thomas.

Stanton L: *Basic medical radiation physics,* New York, 1969, Appleton-Century-Crofts, Educational Division, Meredith Corporation.

Thompson MA et al: *Principles of imaging science and protection,* Philadelphia, 1994, WB Saunders.

US Department of Health and Human Services, Public Health Service, Food and Drug Administration, Bureau of Radiological Health: *The correlated lecture laboratory series in diagnostic radiological physics,* HHS Publication FDA818150, Rockville, Md, 1981, HHS.

3

Radiation Quantities and Units

Chapter Outline

absorbed dose (D)
alpha particles
atomic number
beta particles
collective effective dose
    equivalent (S_E)
coulomb (C)
coulomb per kilogram (C/kg)
dose equivalent (H)
effective atomic number
effective dose equivalent
    (H_E)
erg
exposure *(X)*
free-air ionization chamber
General Conference of
    Weights and Measures
gray (Gy)
International Commission on
    Radiation Units and
    Measurement (ICRU)

International System of
    Units (SI)
joule (J)
linear energy transfer (LET)
neutrons
protons
quality factor (QF)
rad
rem
roentgen (R)
sievert (Sv)
skin erythema dose
somatic damage
stochastic effects
tissue weighting factor (W_T)
traditional units

*After completing this chapter, the reader will be able
to perform the following:*

- Describe the historical evolution of radiation quantities and units.

- Define the radiation terms *exposure, absorbed dose,* and *dose equivalent* and identify the appropriate symbol for each quantity.

- List and explain the International System (SI) and traditional units for radiation exposure, absorbed dose, and dose equivalent.

- State the purpose of the radiation quantities effective dose equivalent and collective effective dose equivalent.

- Explain the importance of linear energy transfer (LET) as it applies to biologic damage resulting from irradiation of human tissue.

- Define the term *quality factor (QF)* and identify this factor for each of the ionizing radiations.

- State the formula for determining dose equivalent.

- Determine the dose equivalent in terms of SI and traditional units when given the quality factor and absorbed dose for different ionizing radiations.

As the potentially harmful effects of ionizing radiation became known, the medical community sought to reduce radiation exposure throughout the world by developing standards for measuring and limiting this exposure. To be able to measure patient and personnel exposure in a consistent and uniform manner, diagnostic imaging personnel should be familiar with the standardized radiation quantities and units discussed in this chapter. Chapter 4 describes the standardized dose limits on radiation exposure expressed in these units, which are designed to minimize the associated risk and the potentially harmful effects of such exposure.

Historical Evolution of Radiation Quantities and Units

Wilhelm C. Roentgen announced the discovery of x-rays in December 1895. In the months that followed, experimentation with this new "wonder ray" resulted in acute biologic damage to some patients and radiation workers. Cases of **somatic damage** (biologic damage to the body of the exposed individual) caused by exposure to ionizing radiation were reported in Europe as early as 1896. In the United States, Clarence Dally, glassblower, tube maker, and assistant to Thomas A. Edison, became the first American radiation fatality. Dally died of radiation-induced cancer in 1904 at age 39. Among physicians, cancer deaths attributable to x-ray exposure were reported as early as 1910. Many radiologists and dentists developed cancerous skin lesions on their hands as a result of occupational exposure (Fig. 3-1). Blood disorders such as aplastic anemia and leukemia were more common among early radiologists than among nonradiologists.

Alarmed by the increasing number of radiation injuries reported, the medical community decided to investigate methods for reducing radiation exposure. In 1921 the British X-Ray and Radium Protection Committee was formed to perform this task. The committee planned to formulate guidelines for the manufacture and use of radium and x-ray equipment and devices to eliminate the chance of occupational injury. Unfortunately, because they could not agree on a workable unit of radiation exposure, the members of the committee were unable to fulfill this responsibility.

The unit in use at that time (1900 to 1930) was called the **skin erythema dose,** defined as the received quantity of radiation that causes diffused redness over an area of skin after irradiation. This amount of absorbed radiation corresponds roughly to a modern dose of several gray (several hundred rads). Because the amount of radiation required to produce the erythema reaction varied from one person to another, it was a crude and inaccurate way to measure radiation exposure. Scientists felt compelled to continue searching for a more reliable unit. The new unit selected was to be based on some exactly measurable effect produced by radiation such as ionization of atoms or energy absorbed in the irradiated object.

The **International Commission on Radiation Units and Measurements (ICRU)** was formed in 1925. In 1928 this commission was charged by the Second International Congress of Radiology to define a unit of exposure. In 1937 the commission finished its assignment, and although not accurately defined, the roentgen (R) became internationally accepted as the unit of measurement for exposure to x-radiation and gamma radiation (short-wavelength, high-energy electromagnetic waves emitted by the nuclei of radioactive substances). The roentgen was redefined in 1962 to increase accuracy and acceptability.

In 1948 the **General Conference of Weights and Measures,** which was responsible for the development and international unification of the metric system, assigned its International Committee for Weights and Measures the responsibility of developing guidelines for the units of measurement. To fulfill this responsibility, the committee developed the **International System of Units (SI).** This system makes possible the interchange of units among all branches of science throughout the world. In 1980 the ICRU adopted the SI units for use with ionizing radiation and urged full implementation of these units as soon as possible. Many developed countries, particularly in Europe, have already made this transition. In the United States the SI units, the gray (Gy) and centigray (cGy), are used routinely in therapeutic radiology to specify absorbed dose. Even though the National Council on Radiation Protection and Measurements (NCRP) (see

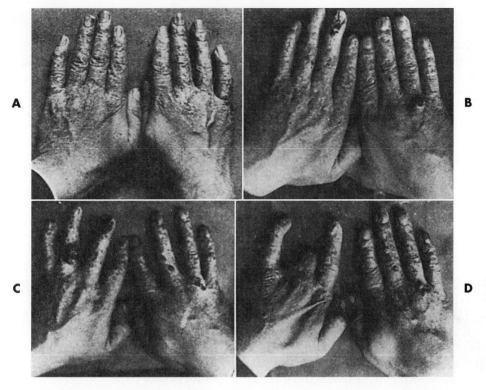

Fig. 3-1 The hands of x-ray pioneer Mihran Kassabian (1870-1910) of Philadelphia demonstrate lesions induced by ionizing radiation. **A,** After sustaining some exposure, the hands, photographed in 1903, exhibited "tanned skin." **B,** By 1908 the cracked, fissured, and reddened skin had developed chronic roughening. **C,** Later, malignancy of the skin had developed. **D,** By 1909 a series of surgeries and amputations became necessary. Kassabian eventually died of metastases. (From Eisenberg RL: *Radiation: an illustrated history*, St Louis, 1992, Mosby.)

Chapter 4) adopted the internationally accepted SI units for use in 1985, quantities and **traditional units** associated with radiation protection and dosimetry, namely the **roentgen (R)** and the **rem,** are still widely employed. For example, personnel monitoring reports (see Chapter 9) continue to specify dose equivalent (addressed later in this chapter) in millirem. Fluoroscopic entrance exposure rates are measured in roentgens per minute (R/min), and essentially all radiation survey instruments provide readings in traditional units. In addition, many regulatory criteria are described in terms of traditional units. Because both SI and traditional units are still being used, the current generation of radiation workers must understand both unit systems for the safety of patients and personnel.

Therefore SI and traditional units are presented where applicable throughout this text. The traditional units are identified in parentheses after the SI units. Table 3-1 presents an overview of the important dates in the historical evolution of radiation quantities and units.

The SI unit of absorbed dose (discussed later in this chapter) was named after the English radiobiologist Louis Harold Gray (1901-1965), who was instrumental in developing what is arguably the most important theory in all of radiation dosimetry. The Bragg-Gray theory relates the ionization produced in a small cavity within an irradiated medium or object to the energy absorbed in that medium as a result of its radiation exposure. Thus with the use of appropriate correction factors the theory essentially links the determination

Table 3-1	
Overview of Important Dates in the Historical Evolution of Radiation Quantities and Units	

Year	Event
1895	X-rays are discovered, and the discovery is announced.
1896	Initial cases of somatic damage caused by exposure to ionizing radiation are reported in Europe.
1904	Clarence Dally becomes the first American radiation fatality.
1910	First cancer deaths among physicians that are attributed to x-ray exposure are reported.
1921	British X-Ray and Radium Protection Committee is formed to investigate methods for reducing radiation exposure.
1925	International Commission on Radiation Units and Measurements (ICRU) is formed.
1928	ICRU is charged by the Second International Congress of Radiology to define a unit of exposure.
1937	Roentgen (R) becomes internationally accepted as the unit of measurement for exposure to x-radiation and gamma radiation.
1948	International System (SI) of units is developed.
1962	Roentgen (R) is redefined to increase accuracy and acceptability.
1980	ICRU adopts the SI Units for use with ionizing radiation.
1985	National Council of Radiation Protection (NCRP) adopts the SI units for use.

of the absorbed radiation dose in a medium to a relatively simple measurement of ionization charge. Gray also was responsible for many pioneering papers in radiation biology. Rolf Maximilian Sievert (1896-1966), the Swedish physicist for whom the SI unit of dose equivalent was named, is best known for his method (the Sievert Integral) to determine the exposure rates at various points near linear radium sources (tubes).

Radiation Quantities

Exposure (X)

When a volume of air is irradiated with x-rays or gamma rays, the interaction that occurs between the x-rays and neutral air atoms results in some electrons being liberated from those atoms. Consequently, the ionized air can function as a conductor and carry electricity because of the negatively charged free electrons and positively charged associated ions that have been created. As the intensity of x-ray exposure of the air volume increases, the number of electron-ion pairs increases. Thus the amount of radiation responsible for the ionization of a well-defined volume of air may be determined by measuring the number of electron-ion pairs. This radiation ionization in the air is termed **exposure (X)**.

The reader must understand the concept of the radiation quantity exposure to differentiate it from other quantities used in medical imaging. *Exposure* may be defined as the total electrical charge per unit mass that x-ray and gamma ray photons with energies up to 3 mega electron volts (MeV) generate in air only. In a simplified sense, exposure may be viewed as the amount of ionizing radiation that may strike an object such as the human body when in the vicinity of a radiation source.

For precise measurement of radiation exposure in medical radiography, the total amount of ionization an x-ray beam produces in a known mass of air must be obtained. This type of direct measurement is accomplished in an accredited calibration laboratory by using a standard or **free-air ionization chamber** (Fig. 3-2). The chamber contains a known quantity of air with precisely measured temperature, pressure, and humidity. If in that specific volume of dry (i.e., nonhumid) air the total charge of all the ions of one sign (either all pluses or all minuses) produced are collected and measured, the total amount of radiation

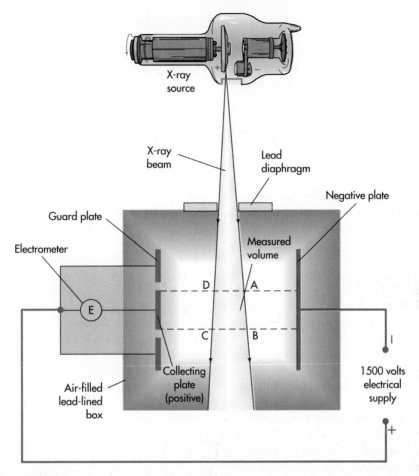

Fig. 3-2 This device determines radiation exposure by measuring the amount of ionization an x-ray beam produces within its air collection volume. The instrument consists of a box containing a known quantity of air, two oppositely charged metal plates, and an electrometer, an instrument that measures the total amount of charge collected on the positively charged metal plate. The chamber measures the total amount of electrical charge of all the electrons produced during the ionization of a specific volume of air at standard atmospheric pressure and temperature. The electrical charge is measured in units called coulombs (C) (charge of an electron = -1.6×10^{-19} C). A collected electrical charge of 2.58×10^{-4} C/kg of irradiated air constitutes an exposure of 1 roentgen (R).

exposure may be accurately determined. The chamber response is modified to correspond to standard temperature and pressure of dry air of 760 mm Hg or 1 atm at sea level and 22° C.

Such an instrument, however, is not a practical device at locations other than a standardization laboratory. As a result, much smaller and less complicated instruments have been developed for use away from the laboratory. Although very conve-

nient, these instruments must be periodically recalibrated in a standardization laboratory against a free-air chamber.

Absorbed dose (D)

As ionizing radiation passes through an object, some of the energy of that radiation is transferred to the object. Some of the radiation that is transferred to the object is absorbed (i.e., it stays within the object). The quantity

absorbed dose is defined as the amount of energy per unit mass absorbed by the irradiated object. This absorbed energy is responsible for any biologic damage resulting from the tissues being exposed to radiation.

Anatomic structures in the body possess different absorption properties; some structures can absorb more radiant energy than others. The amount of energy absorbed by a structure depends on the **atomic number** of the tissue composing the structure, the mass density of the tissue, and the energy of the incident photon; absorption increases as atomic number and mass density increase and photon energy decreases. In other words, low-energy photons are generally more easily absorbed in a material such as biologic tissue than are high-energy photons.

The **effective atomic number** of a given tissue is a composite of the atomic numbers of the many different chemical elements composing the tissue. Bone has a higher effective atomic number (13.8) than does soft tissue (7.4) because bone contains calcium (atomic number = 20) and phosphorus (atomic number = 15), whereas soft tissue comprises mostly fat (atomic number = 5.9) and structures with atomic numbers close to that of water (atomic number = 7.4). Bone absorbs more ionizing radiation than soft tissue in the diagnostic energy range of 30 to 150 kilovolts peak (kVp) because the photoelectric process for bone is the dominant mode of energy absorption within this range. The probability of photoelectric interaction is strongly dependent on the atomic number of the irradiated material. The higher the atomic number of a material, the greater will be the amount of energy absorbed by that material.

In the therapeutic radiology range of 100 keV and above, however, the difference in absorption between bone and soft tissue gradually decreases (Fig. 3-3). This is because the amount of photoelectric absorption decreases and the amount of Compton scattering relative to the photoelectric interaction increases as the energy of the x-ray beam increases; the amount of Compton scattering in a material does not depend on the atomic number of the material. Hence, as energy increases, the difference in amount of absorption between any two tissues of different atomic number decreases. Because the process of absorption is responsible for biologic damage and absorption properties vary with the quality of the radiation and the type of tissue irradiated, tissue dosage in therapeutic radiology is generally specified in terms of absorbed dose rather than in terms of exposure.

Dose equivalent (H)

Dose equivalent provides a method with which to calculate the effective absorbed dose for all types of ionizing radiation, including **protons** (basic nuclear particles that carry a positive electrical charge equal in magnitude to that of electrons and have a mass over 1800 times that of an electron) and **neutrons** (basic, electrically neutral particles with a mass just slightly greater than that of the proton) as well as x-rays. Equal absorbed doses of different types of radiation produce different amounts of biologic damage in body tissue. For example, a 1-gray (100-rad) absorbed dose of fast neutrons causes more biologic damage than a 1-gray (100-rad) absorbed dose of x-rays. The dose equivalent takes this biologic impact into consideration by using a specific modifying or **quality factor (QF)** to adjust the absorbed dose value. This is accomplished by multiplying the absorbed

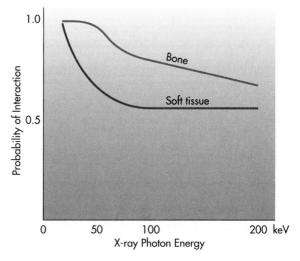

Fig. 3-3 Probability of interaction of x-rays when a 5-cm-thick layer of soft tissue or bone is encountered. The probability is greater at lower energies and is greater for bone than soft tissue, particularly at low energies.

dose by the quality factor and any other applicable modifying factor. The product obtained is the dose equivalent. The following formula is commonly used to make the calculation:

$$DE \text{ (dose equivalent)} = AD \text{ (absorbed dose)} \times QF \text{ (quality factor)}$$

X-rays, **beta particles** (high-speed electrons), and gamma rays produce virtually the same biologic effects in body tissue for equal absorbed doses. In terms of quality factor, these radiations have been given a value of 1 and are the base or standard against which to compare the effectiveness of other types of ionizing radiation in producing biologic damage. The quality factors of different kinds of ionizing radiations are listed in Table 3-2. The concept of **linear energy transfer (LET)** helps explain the need for a quality factor. LET is the amount of energy transferred on average by incident radiation to an object per unit length of travel through the object and is expressed in units of keV/μm (see Appendix E).

Radiation with a high LET transfers a large amount of energy into a small area and can therefore do more biologic damage than radiation with a low LET. Thus

a high-LET radiation has a quality factor that is greater than the quality factor for a low-LET radiation. LET and its relationship to biologic damage will be discussed again in Chapter 6.

Other dosimetric quantities

In addition to dose equivalent, other dosimetric quantities have been derived and implemented for use in radiation protection to describe internal and external dose measurements. These include the quantity effective dose equivalent (H_E), which is used to relate the absorbed dose to different organs of the body when radiation exposure is localized, and the quantity collective effective dose equivalent (S_E), which is used to describe radiation exposure of a population from different sources.

The **effective dose equivalent (H_E)** may be either of the following:
1. H_{wb}, the dose equivalent when the whole body is irradiated in a uniform fashion without variation
2. H_T, the weighted sum of the dose equivalents to each of the tissues (T) of the body

Stochastic effects are nonthreshold, randomly occurring biologic effects of ionizing radiation such as cancer and genetic abnormalities. If the effective dose equivalent involves uniform, whole body irradiation, the chance that these effects will occur (but not their severity) is believed to be proportional to the equivalent dose. Risk may therefore be expressed as a singular equivalent value. Because uniform, whole-body irradiation seldom occurs and some organs and body tissues vary considerably in the absorbed dose received and their sensitivity to random radiation-induced responses, the International Commission on Radiological Protection (ICRP) introduced the **tissue weighting factor (W_T)** concept for the relative risk associated with irradiation of different body tissues (see Chapter 4). The weighting factor (Table 3-3) is a value that denotes the percentage of the summed stochastic (cancer plus genetic) risk stemming from irradiation of tissue (T) to the all-inclusive risk, when the entire body is irradiated in a uniform fashion. This factor assigns risks for potential biologic responses from various types of ionizing radiation on a common scale. The effective dose

Table 3-2

Quality Factors for Different Types of Ionizing Radiations

Type of ionizing radiation	Quality factor*
X-ray photons	1
Beta particles	1
Gamma photons	1
Thermal neutrons	5
Fast neutrons	20
High-energy external protons	1
Low-energy internal protons†	20
Alpha particles	20
Multiple charged particles of unknown energy	20

*Data from National Council of Radiation Protection and Measurements (NCRP): *Report No. 116, limitation of exposure to ionizing radiation,* Bethesda, Md, 1993, NCRP Publications.
†Protons produced as a result of neutrons interacting with the nuclei of tissue molecules.

Table 3-3
Organ or Tissue Weighting Factors (W$_T$)

Organ or tissue	Weighting factor (W$_T$)*
Gonads	0.20
Red bone marrow	0.12
Colon	0.12
Lung	0.12
Stomach	0.12
Bladder	0.05
Breast	0.05
Liver	0.05
Esophagus	0.05
Thyroid	0.05
Skin	0.01
Bone surface	0.01
Remainder	0.05

*Data from National Council on Radiation Protection and Measurements (NCRP): *Report #116, limitation of exposure to ionizing radiation,* Bethesda, Md, 1993, NCRP Publications.

equivalent (H$_E$) is the total of the products of the dose equivalent for each respective organ or tissue and the weighting factor for each. Thus for *n* organs or tissues that have been irradiated, the following equation holds true:

$$H_E = H_t = H_{t_1}W_1 + H_{t_2}W_2 + \ldots + H_{t_n}W_n$$

If population or group exposure to low doses of various sources of ionizing radiation must be described, the quantity **collective effective dose equivalent (S$_E$)** may be used. It is determined as the product of the dose equivalent for an individual belonging to the exposed population or group and the number of persons exposed. The radiation unit currently being used is *person-sievert*. This was previously referred to as *man-rem*.

Radiation Units

Coulomb per kilogram (SI unit of exposure)— roentgen (traditional unit)

The **coulomb (C)** is the basic unit of electrical charge. It represents the quantity of electrical charge flowing past a point in a circuit in 1 second when an electrical

current of 1 ampere* is used. In the SI the exposure unit is measured in **coulombs per kilogram (C/kg).** At the time of publication of this edition, no special name for this SI quantity has been assigned. This exposure unit is simply equal to an electrical charge of 1 coulomb produced in a kilogram of dry air by ionizing radiation. One roentgen (R), the traditional unit of radiation exposure, equals 2.58×10^{-4} C/kg. The roentgen is precisely defined as the photon (either x-ray or gamma ray) exposure that produces under standard conditions of pressure and temperature a total positive or negative ion charge of 2.58×10^{-4} C/kg of dry air. An expo-sure of 1 C/kg equals $1/2.58 \times 10^{-4}$ R, or 3.88×10^3 R. Therefore conversion of the roentgen, the tradi-tional unit of exposure, to coulombs per kilogram (C/kg), the SI unit, may be accomplished by multiplying by 2.58×10^{-4}.

Example: To convert 100 R to C/kg:

1. Set up the equation: $100 \text{ R} \times 2.58 \,(10)^{-4} \dfrac{\text{C/kg}}{\text{R}}$

2. Cancel R: $100 \text{ R} \times 2.58 \,(10)^{-4} \dfrac{\text{C/kg}}{\cancel{\text{R}}}$

3. Obtain answer: $258 \times 10^{-4} \dfrac{\text{C}}{\text{kg}}$

4. Write answer in standard scientific notation: 2.58×10^{-2} C/kg

Conversion of coulombs per kilogram (C/kg) to roentgen (R) may be accomplished by dividing by 2.58×10^{-4}.

Example: To convert 100 C/kg to R:

1. Set up the equation: $100 \text{C/kg} \div 2.58 \,(10)^{-4} \dfrac{\text{C/kg}}{\text{R}}$

2. Cancel C/kg: $100 \cancel{\text{C/kg}} \div 2.58 \,(10)^{-4} \dfrac{\cancel{\text{C/kg}}}{\text{R}}$

3. Obtain answer: 39×10^4 R

The coulomb per kilogram (roentgen) unit is used for x-ray equipment calibration because x-ray output is measured directly with an ionization chamber. It also

*The ampere is the SI unit of electrical current. One ampere represents the flow of electrons amounting to a charge of 1 coulomb crossing a unit area per second.

is used in the calibration of radiation-measuring instruments (refer to Chapter 9 for further information).

Gray (SI unit of absorbed dose)—rad (traditional unit)

The SI unit of absorbed dose is called a **gray (Gy)** and is defined as an energy absorption of 1 **joule (J)** per kilogram in the irradiated object. One gray (Gy) is therefore determined by the following simple equation:

$$1 \text{ Gy} = 1 \text{ J/kg}$$

(A joule [a unit of energy] may be defined as the work done or energy expended when a force of 1 newton acts on an object along a distance of 1 meter.)

Traditionally the rad has been used as the unit of absorbed dose. Rad stands for *radiation absorbed dose*. This unit indicates the amount of radiant energy transferred to an irradiated object by any type of ionizing radiation. The rad is equivalent to an energy transfer of 100 **erg** (a unit of energy and work) per gram of irradiated object. One rad may be expressed mathematically as follows:

$$1 \text{ rad} = 100 \text{ erg/g}$$

or

$$1 \text{ rad} = 1/100 \text{ J/kg}$$

Gray and rad are easily translated to compare absorbed dose values. If the absorbed dose is stated in rads, the equivalent number of gray may be determined by dividing by 100.

Example 1: number of rad divided by 100 = number of gray
5000 rads = 5000 divided by 100 rads per Gy = 50 Gy

Example 2: 5 rads = 5 divided by 100 rads per Gy = 0.05 Gy

If absorbed dose is stated in gray, the number of rads may be determined by multiplying by 100.

Example 1: number of gray multiplied by 100 = number of rad
15 gray = 15 × 100 rads per gray = 1500 rads

Example 2: 50 gray = 50 × 100 rads per gray = 5000 rads

SI subunits facilitate conversion from rad to gray. The milligray (mGy) equals $\frac{1}{1000}$ gray. This is a concept similar to a millirad (mrad), which equals $\frac{1}{1000}$ rad. In therapeutic radiology the centigray (cGy) is replacing the rad for recording of absorbed dose.

$$1 \text{ cGy } (\tfrac{1}{100} \text{ gray}) = 1 \text{ rad } (\tfrac{1}{100} \text{ Gy})$$

Example: number of centigray = 1 × number of rad; therefore if a patient receiving x-ray therapy treatment has received a total dosage of 5000 rad, the dosage can be recorded in SI subunits as 5000 × 1 cGy = 5000 cGy.

Sievert (SI unit of dose equivalent)—rem (traditional unit)

If a person receives exposure from various types of ionizing radiation, the dose equivalent for measuring biologic effects may be determined and expressed in the SI unit the **sievert (Sv).** This unit is used only for radiation protection purposes. It provides a common scale whereby varying degrees of biologic damage caused by equal absorbed doses of different types of ionizing radiation may be compared with the degree of biologic damage caused by the same amount of x-radiation or gamma radiation.

Dose equivalent stated in sievert is determined by multiplying the absorbed dose stated in gray times the quality or modifying factor of the radiation being used. This may be expressed in the following formula:

$$\begin{aligned} \text{DE} &= \text{Absorbed dose} \times \text{quality factor} \\ \text{(sievert)} &= \qquad \text{(gray)} \qquad \times \qquad \text{(QF)} \end{aligned}$$

Example (using gray and sievert): An individual received the following absorbed doses: 0.1 Gy of x-radiation, 0.05 Gy of fast neutrons, and 0.2 Gy of alpha particles; what is the *total* dose equivalent?

The formula for determining dose equivalent from n sources or types of radiation is as follows:

$$\text{DE} = (\text{absorbed dose} \times \text{quality factor})_1 + (\text{absorbed dose} \times \text{quality factor})_2 + \dots + (\text{absorbed dose} \times \text{quality factor})_n$$

(The quality factor for each of the radiations in question may be obtained from Table 3-2.)

Answer:

Radiation type	Absorbed dose	×	QF	=	Absorbed dose equivalent
X-radiation	0.1 Gy	×	1	=	0.1 Sv
Fast neutrons	0.05 Gy	×	20	=	1.0 Sv
Alpha particles	0.2 Gy	×	20	=	4.0 Sv
	Total dose equivalent			=	5.1 Sv

Traditionally the rem has been used as the unit of the quantity dose equivalent and was defined as the dose equivalent of any type of ionizing radiation that produces the same biologic effect as 1 rad of x-radiation. Hence 1 rad of x-rays represents a different dose equivalent in rem than does 1 rad of **alpha particles.** An absorbed dose stated in rad may be converted to a dose equivalent by use of the quality factor for the type of radiation being considered. *Rem* stands for *rad-equivalent-man.* The following example demonstrates the use of this traditional unit.

Example (using rad and rem): An individual received the following absorbed doses: 10 rad of x-radiation, 5 rad of fast neutrons, and 20 rad of alpha particles; what is the *total* dose equivalent?

The formula for determining dose equivalent is as follows:

$$DE = \text{absorbed dose} \times \text{quality factor}$$
$$(rem) = (rad) \times (QF)$$

(The quality factor for each of the radiations in question may be obtained from Table 3-2.)

Answer:

Radiation type	Absorbed dose	×	QF	=	Absorbed dose equivalent
X-radiation	10 rad	×	1	=	10 rem
Fast neutrons	5 rad	×	20	=	100 rem
Alpha particles	20 rad	×	20	=	400 rem
	Total dose equivalent			=	510 rem

Sievert and rem are easily compared. One sievert equals 100 rem (1 sievert (Sv) = 100 rem). Subunits

---

Box 3-1

SI and Traditional Unit Equivalents

1 SI exposure unit equals	1. $C/kg = \dfrac{1}{2.58 \times 10^{-4}} R$
1 coulomb equals	1. 1 ampere-second
1 coulomb per kilogram of air equals	1. 1 SI unit of exposure
	2. $\dfrac{1}{2.58 \times 10^{-4}} R$
1 gray equals	1. 1 J/kg
	2. 100 rad
	3. 100 cGy
	4. 1000 mGy
1 sievert equals	1. 1 J/kg (for x-radiation, QF = 1)
	2. 100 rem
	3. 100 cSv
	4. 1000 mSv
1 erg equals	1. 10^{-7} J
1 joule equals	1. 10^7 erg
	2. 1 newton-meter
	3. 6.24×10^{18} eV
1 roentgen (R) equals	1. 2.58×10^{-4} C/kg of air
1 milliroentgen (mR) equals	1. $^1/_{1000}$ R or 10^{-3} R
1 rad equals	1. 100 erg/g
	2. $^1/_{100}$ J/kg
	3. $^1/_{100}$ Gy
	4. 1 cGy
1 millirad equals	1. $^1/_{1000}$ rad
1 rem equals	1. $^1/_{100}$ J/kg (for x-radiation, QF = 1)
	2. $^1/_{100}$ Sv
	3. 1 centisievert (cSv)
	4. 10 mSv
1 millirem equals	1. $^1/_{1000}$ rem

---

also may be used to specify absorbed dose limits. One centisievert equals 1 rem (1 centisievert (cSv) = 1 rem). Ten millisievert equals 1 rem (10 millisievert (mSv) = 1 rem). If the dose equivalent is stated in sievert, the number of rem may be determined simply by multiplying by 100.

Example: 10 Sv = 10 × 100 rem per Sv = 1000 rem

Table 3-4					
Summary of Radiation Quantities and Units					
Type of radiation	Quantity	SI	Traditional unit	Measuring medium	Effect measured
X- or gamma	Exposure *(X)*	Coulomb per kilogram (C/kg)	Roentgen (R)	Air	Ionization of air
All ionizing radiations	Absorbed dose (D)	Gray (Gy)	Rad	Any object	Amount of energy per unit mass absorbed by object
All ionizing radiations	Dose equivalent (H)	Sievert (Sv)	Rem	Body tissue	Biologic effects

If the dose equivalent is stated in rem, the number of sievert may be determined by dividing the number of rem by 100.

Example: 500 rem = 500 ÷ 100 rem per Sv = 5 Sv

If the dose equivalent is stated in a subunit such as millisievert, the number of rem may be determined by dividing the number of millisievert by 10.

Example: 100 mSv = 100 ÷ 10 per rem = 10 rem

If the dose equivalent is stated in rem, the number of millisievert may be determined by multiplying the number of rem by 10.

Example: 100 rem = 100 × 10 millisievert (mSv) per rem = 1000 mSv

Box 3-1 and Table 3-4 provide a summary of radiation quantities, units, and equivalents.

Summary

The historical evolution of radiation quantities and units has been presented in this chapter. Standardized radiation quantities, expressed in both International System (SI) and traditional units for measuring ionizing radiation exposure *(X)*, absorbed dose (D), and dose equivalent (H), have been defined and described. For exposure in air only the unit coulomb per kilogram (C/kg), or roentgen (R), is used. The unit gray (Gy), or rad, is used for absorbed dose measurement. When all types of radiation must be considered, dose equivalent is used as the quantity of choice for measuring biologic effects. Sievert (Sv) or rem are the units used in these cases.

Two additional dosimetric quantities are used in radiation protection to describe internal and external dose measurements. As in diagnostic radiology, when radiation exposure is localized, the effective dose equivalent (H_E) is used to relate the absorbed dose to different body organs. If a population receives radiation exposure from different sources, the collective effective dose equivalent is used. The person-sievert (previously man-rem) is the radiation unit of choice.

The tissue weighting factor (W_T) concept for the relative risk associated with irradiation of different body tissues has been introduced and assigns risks for potential biologic responses from various type of ionizing radiations on a common scale. Formulas and calculations for determining exposure in air only, absorbed dose, and dose equivalent in terms of SI and traditional units have been described to enable the reader to perform mathematical computations.

Review Questions

1. Who was the first American to die from radiation-induced cancer (in 1904)?
   A. Thomas A. Edison
   B. Wilhelm C. Roentgen
   C. Clarence Dally
   D. Marie Curie

2. Which of the following was used as the first unit to measure exposure to ionizing radiations?
   A. Roentgen
   B. Skin erythema
   C. Sievert
   D. Rad

3. Which of the following effects must be measured to determine the *total* amount of radiation exposure in a specific volume of dry air under standard conditions of pressure and temperature?
   A. Energy absorption
   B. Biologic damage
   C. Cellular activity
   D. Quantity of ionization

4. Which of the following provides a method by which to calculate the effective absorbed dose for *all* types of ionizing radiations?
   A. Absorbed dose
   B. Dose equivalent
   C. Exposure
   D. Ionization of air

5. Which of the following are the ionizing radiations that produce virtually the *same* biologic effects for equal absorbed doses in body tissue?
   A. X-rays, beta particles, and gamma rays
   B. Alpha particles, beta particles, and gamma rays
   C. X-rays, neutrons, and gamma rays
   D. X-rays, alpha particles, and fast neutrons

6. Which of the following is the SI unit of exposure?
   A. Sievert
   B. Roentgen
   C. Gray
   D. Coulomb per kilogram

7. Which of the following statements is correct?
   A. 1 C/kg of dry air $= \dfrac{1}{258 \times 10^{-4}}$ gray
   B. 1 C/kg of dry air $= \dfrac{1}{2.58 \times 10^{-4}}$ roentgen
   C. 2.58×10^{-4} C/kg of dry air $= 10$ sievert
   D. 2.58×10^{-4} C/kg of dry air $= 50$ roentgen

8. If the absorbed dose is stated in rad, gray may be determined by performing which of the following equations?
   A. Multiplying by 100
   B. Adding 100
   C. Dividing by 100
   D. Subtracting 100

9. Which of the following terms describes the amount of energy per unit mass transferred from an x-ray beam to an object?
   A. Exposure
   B. Dose equivalent
   C. SI
   D. Absorbed dose

10. Which of the following terms describes the measurement of ionization produced by x-ray or gamma ray photons *in air only?*
    A. Exposure
    B. Absorbed dose
    C. Dose equivalent
    D. Skin erythema dose

11. In the diagnostic radiology energy range from 30 to 150 kVp, which of the following tissues possesses the *greatest* ability to absorb radiant energy through the process of photoelectric absorption?
    A. Muscle
    B. Bone
    C. Fat
    D. Air

12. Which of the following factors may be multiplied to determine dose equivalent?
    A. Rad $\times$ quality factor
    B. Rem $\times$ roentgen
    C. Gray $\times$ quality factor
    D. A and C only

13. In the SI, 1 J of energy absorbed from any type of ionizing radiation in 1 kg of any irradiated object equals which of the following?
    A. 10 Sv
    B. 5 C/kg
    C. 1 rad
    D. 1 Gy

14. If a patient receiving x-ray therapy treatment receives a total dosage of 6000 rad, the dosage may be recorded as _____ if SI is used.
    A. 12,000 Gy
    B. 6000 cGy
    C. 600 rad
    D. 60 R

15. 200 rem equals which of the following?
    A. 2 mSv
    B. 20 mSv
    C. 200 mSv
    D. 2000 mSv

16. Which of the following is used to adjust the absorbed dose value to measure biologic effects of different types of ionizing radiation?
    A. Exposure-absorbed dose ratio
    B. Ionization factor
    C. Quality factor
    D. Rate of linear energy transfer

17. A quality factor has been established for each of the following ionizing radiations: x-rays, fast neutrons, and alpha particles. What is the total dose equivalent in sievert for a person who has received the following exposures: 5 rad of x-rays, 2 rad of fast neutrons, and 4 rad of alpha particles?
    A. 1.25 Sv
    B. 10.5 Sv
    C. 125 Sv
    D. 1250 Sv

18. Which of the following units are *not* SI units?
    A. Roentgen
    B. Coulomb per kilogram, gray, sievert
    C. Rad and rem
    D. A and C only

19. Of the following equivalents, which equals 1 rad?
    1. 100 erg/g
    2. 1/100 J/kg
    3. 0.01 Gy
    A. 1 only
    B. 2 only
    C. 3 only
    D. 1, 2, and 3

20. To determine absorbed dose, the amount of energy absorbed by the irradiated object must be measured by which of the following methods?
    A. Determining the quantity of ionization in a specific volume of dry air at atmospheric pressure
    B. Calculating the dose equivalent
    C. Calculating the skin-entrance exposure of the object
    D. Determining the quantity of energy deposited per kilogram of the object

21. For x-ray and gamma ray photons with energies up to 3 MeV, which of the following quantities may be defined as the measure of the total electric charge per unit mass that these radiations generate in air *only?*
    A. Absorbed dose
    B. Dose equivalent
    C. Exposure
    D. Collective effective dose equivalent

22. As the intensity of x-ray exposure of air increases, the electrical resistance of the air will react in which of the following ways?
    A. Decrease
    B. Increase
    C. Remain the same

23. 10 C/kg equals _____ roentgen.
    A. 258×10^{-4}
    B. 25.8×10^{-4}
    C. 3.9×10^4
    D. 39×10^4

24. 1 millirem equals _____ rem.
    A. $\frac{1}{10}$
    B. $\frac{1}{100}$
    C. $\frac{1}{1000}$
    D. $\frac{1}{10,000}$

25. Which of the following radiation quantities is used to describe population or group exposures to low doses from various sources of ionizing radiation?
   A. Absorbed dose
   B. Dose equivalent
   C. Effective dose equivalent
   D. Collective effective dose equivalent

26. The concept of tissue weighting factors is used to do which of the following?
   A. Measure absorbed dose from all ionizing radiations
   B. Assign risks for potential biologic responses from various types of ionizing radiations on a common scale
   C. Modify the quality factor for various types of ionizing radiation
   D. Eliminate the use of the dose equivalent

27. 10^{-6} may be numerically expressed as which of the following?
   A. *
   B. G
   C. μ
   D. +

28. Which of the following is the unit of collective effective dose equivalent?
   A. Coulomb per kilogram-sievert
   B. Gray-sievert
   C. Person-sievert
   D. Rad-sievert

29. Which of the following is the radiation unit used for diagnostic x-ray equipment calibration performed with an ionization chamber?
   A. Sievert (rem)
   B. Gray (rad)
   C. Rem (rom)
   D. Coulomb per kilogram (roentgen)

30. 15 sievert equals _____ rem.
   A. 15
   B. 150
   C. 1500
   D. 15,000

31. 20 mSv equals _____ rem.
   A. 0.02
   B. 2
   C. 20
   D. 200

32. 30 rem equals _____ mSv.
   A. 3
   B. 30
   C. 300
   D. 3000

33. A quality factor has been established for each of the following ionizing radiations: x-rays, fast neutrons, and alpha particles. What is the *total* dose equivalent in sievert for a person who has received the following exposures: 0.9 Gy of x-rays, 0.03 Gy of fast neutrons, and 0.06 rad of alpha particles?
   A. 2.7 Sv
   B. 27 Sv
   C. 270 Sv
   D. 2700 Sv

Bibliography

Anderson R: New dose limits boggle the mind, *ASRT Scanner* (27)2:1, Dec 1994 and Jan 1995.

ASRT Scanner 27(1):15, Oct and Nov 1994.

ASRT Scanner 27(2):15 Dec 1994 and Jan 1995.

Ball JL, Moore AD: *Essential physics for radiographers,* London, 1980, Blackwell Scientific Publications.

Barnett MH: *The biological effects of ionizing radiation: an overview,* HEW Publication FDA 77-8004, Rockville, Md, 1976, US Department of Health, Education, and Welfare, Public Health Service, Food and Drug Administration, Bureau of Radiological Health.

Bushong S: *Radiologic science for technologists: physics, biology, and protection,* ed 6, St Louis, 1997, Mosby.

Carlton RR, Adler AM: *Principles of radiographic imaging: an art and a science,* Albany, NY, 1992, Delmar.

Christensen EE, Curry III TS, Dowdey JE: *An introduction to the physics of diagnostic radiology,* ed 2, Philadelphia, 1978, Lea & Febiger.

Curry III TS, Dowdey JE, Murry Jr RC: *Christensen's introduction to the physics of diagnostic radiology,* ed 3, Philadelphia, 1984, Lea & Febiger.

Early PJ, Sodee DB: *Principles and practice of nuclear medicine,* ed 2, St Louis, 1995, Mosby.

Frankel R: *Radiation protection for radiologic technologists,* New York, 1976, McGraw-Hill.

Fullerton GD et al, editors: *Biological risks of medical irradiation,* Medical Physics Monograph No. 5, New York, 1980, American Association of Physicists in Medicine.

Hall EJ: *Radiobiology for the radiologist,* ed 4, Philadelphia, 1994, JB Lippincott.

Hall EJ: Risk of cancer causation by diagnostic x-rays, *Cancer Prevention,* Mar 1990, p 1.

Hendee WR, Ritenour ER: *Medical imaging physics,* ed 3, St Louis, 1992, Mosby.

Hildreth R: *From x-ray martyrs to low level radiation,* Kalamazoo, 1981, Industrial Graphics Services.

International Commission on Radiation Units and Measurements (ICRU): *Radiation quantities and units,* ICRU Report No. 33, Washington, D.C., 1980, ICRU.

Johns HE, Cunningham JR: The physics of radiology, ed 3, Springfield, Ill, 1983, Charles C Thomas..

Malott JC, Fodor III J: *The art and science of medical radiography,* ed 7, St Louis, 1993, Mosby.

National Council of Radiation Protection and Measurements (NCRP): *Report #91, recommendations on limits for exposure to ionizing radiation,* Bethesda, Md, 1987, NCRP Publications.

National Council of Radiation Protection and Measurements (NCRP): *Report #93, ionizing radiation exposure of the population of the United States,* Bethesda, Md, 1987, NCRP Publications.

National Council of Radiation Protection and Measurements (NCRP): *Report #116, limitation of exposure to ionizing radiation,* Bethesda, Md, 1993, NCRP Publications.

Noz ME, Maguire Jr GQ: *Radiation protection in the radiologic and health sciences,* ed 2, Philadelphia, 1985, Lea & Febiger.

Ritenour ER: *Radiation protection and biology: a self-instructional multimedia learning series, instructor manual,* Denver, 1985, Multi-Media Publishing.

Scheele RV, Wakley J: *Elements of radiation protection,* Springfield, Ill, 1975, Charles C. Thomas.

Selman J: *The basic physics of radiation therapy,* ed 2, Springfield, Ill, 1973, Charles C. Thomas.

Selman J: *The fundamentals of x-ray and radium physics,* ed 7, Springfield, Ill, 1985, Charles C. Thomas.

Shapiro J: *Radiation protection: a guide for scientists and physicians,* ed 3, Cambridge, Mass, 1990, Harvard University Press.

Sinclair WK: Radiation protection recommendations on dose limits: the role of the NCRP and ICRP and future developments, *Rad Oncol Biol Phys* 31(2):387, 1995.

Thomas CL, editor: *Taber's cyclopedic medical dictionary,* ed 13, Philadelphia, 1973, FA Davis.

Thompson MA et al: *Principles of imaging science and protection,* Philadelphia, 1994, WB Saunders.

Watson E: Radiation dose limits lowered, *ASRT Scanner* 27(1):15, Oct and Nov 1994.

4

Limits for Exposure to Ionizing Radiation

ALARA concept

Center for Devices and Radiological Health (CDRH)

collective effective dose
equivalent (S_E)

Consumer-Patient Radiation
Health and Safety Act of
1981

cumulative whole-body ef-
fective dose equivalent
(EDE) limit

effective dose equivalent
(H_E)

effective dose equivalent
(EDE) limit (occupational
and nonoccupational)

effective dose
equivalent–limiting (EDE)
system

International Commission on
Radiological Protection
(ICRP)

National Academy of Sci-
ences/National Research
Council Committee on
the Biological Effects of
Ionizing Radiation
(NAS/NRC-BEIR)

National Council on Radiation Protection and Mea-
surements (NCRP)

negligible risk

nonstochastic (deterministic) effects

Nuclear Regulatory Commission (NRC)

organ weighing factor (W_T)

Radiation Control for Health
and Safety Act of 1968

radiation hormesis

radiation-induced malig-
nancy

radiation safety officer
(RSO)

risk

stochastic (probabilistic) effects

total effective dose (TED)

total effective dose equivalent (TEDE) limit

United Nations Scientific
Committee on the Ef-
fects of Atomic Radia-
tion (UNSCEAR)

United States Environmental
Protection Agency (EPA)

United States Food and Drug
Administration (FDA)

United States Occupational
Safety and Health Ad-
ministration (OSHA)

*After completing this chapter, the reader will be able
to perform the following:*

- List the four major organizations that share the responsibility for evaluating the relationship between
radiation dose equivalent and induced biologic effects.

- Recognize the United States regulatory agencies responsible for enforcing established radiation effective
dose equivalent–limiting standards.

- Discuss the role of the radiation safety officer and list
various responsibilities that he or she must fulfill.

- Define *effective dose equivalent (EDE) limits.*

- Explain the purpose of the Radiation Control for
Health and Safety Act of 1968.

- List the important provisions of the code of standards
for diagnostic x-ray equipment that began on August
1, 1974.

- Explain the ALARA concept.

- Explain the purpose of the Consumer-Patient Radiation Health and Safety Act of 1981 (Title IX of Public Law 97–35).

- Describe current radiation protection philosophy and
state the goal and objectives of radiation protection.

- Identify radiation-induced responses of serious concern for radiation protection programs.

- Define *risk* as it relates to the medical imaging industry.

- Identify the risks from exposure to ionizing radiation
at low absorbed doses.

- Explain the basis for the effective dose
equivalent–limiting (EDE) system.

- Explain the purpose of an organ weighting factor
(W_T).

- Discuss current National Council on Radiation Protection and Measurements (NCRP) recommendations.

- Given appropriate data, calculate the total cumulative whole-body effective dose equivalent (CEDE) for
a radiation worker.

- Define and explain *collective effective dose equivalent*
(S_E).

- Examine the concept of radiation hormesis.

Continued

53

Objectives—*cont'd*

- State, in terms of International System (SI) units and traditional units, the following:
  a. Total annual effective dose equivalent (TEDE) limit for whole-body occupational exposure excluding medical and natural background exposure, which are stochastic effects.
  b. Total annual occupational effective dose equivalent (TEDE) limits for tissues and organs; deterministic effects such as the crystalline lens of the eye; and all other tissues and organs, including reproductive cells, red bone marrow, breast, lung, localized areas of skin, and limbs.
  c. Occupational cumulative lifetime whole-body effective dose equivalent (EDE) limit.
  d. Annual effective dose equivalent (EDE) limit for continuous or frequent exposure of the general public from man-made sources other than medical irradiation.
  e. Annual effective dose equivalent (EDE) limit for infrequent exposure of the general public.
  f. Annual effective dose equivalent (EDE) limit for an occupationally exposed student 18 years or older.
  g. Occupational monthly effective dose equivalent (EDE) limit for the embryo and fetus after declaration of the pregnancy.

E xposure of the general public, patients, and radiation workers to ionizing radiation must be limited to minimize the risk of harmful biologic effects. Occupational and nonoccupational effective dose equivalent (EDE) limits have been developed by scientists to this end. This **effective dose equivalent–limiting (EDE) system** has been incorporated into Title 10 of the Code of Federal Regulations, Part 20. It supersedes the maximal permissible dose (MPD) system previously used.

The concept of radiation exposure and associated risk of **radiation-induced malignancy** is the basis of the EDE system. Information contained in NCRP Report No. 116 and ICRP Publication No. 60 serve as resources for the revised recommendations. Future radiation protection standards are expected to continue to be based on risk.

Because members of the medical radiography team share the responsibility for patient safety from radiation exposure and also are subject to such exposure in the performance of their professional duties, they must be familiar with previous, existing, and new guidelines. By staying abreast of these guidance vehicles, they will be better able to provide the radiation safety necessary for the protection of those concerned. Radiation workers may obtain the required knowledge by becoming familiar with the functions of the various advisory groups and regulatory agencies discussed in this chapter (Fig. 4-1).

Radiation Protection Standards Organizations

The discussion that follows concerns the four major organizations responsible for evaluating the relationship between radiation dose equivalent and induced

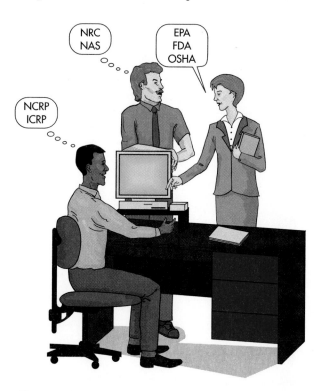

Fig. 4-1 The various advisory groups and regulatory agencies, usually referred to by their acronyms, may be extremely confusing.

biologic effects. In addition, the organizations are concerned with formulating risk estimates of somatic and genetic effects after irradiation. These four main groups are as follows:

1. International Commission on Radiological Protection (ICRP)
2. National Council on Radiation Protection and Measurements (NCRP)
3. United Nations Scientific Committee on the Effects of Atomic Radiation (UNSCEAR)
4. National Academy of Sciences/National Research Council Committee on the Biological Effects of Ionizing Radiation (NAS/NRC-BEIR)

A summary of radiation standards organizations is presented in Table 4-1.

Table 4-1
Summary of Radiation Protection Standards Organizations

Organization	Function
ICRP	Evaluates information on biologic effects of radiation and provides radiation protection guidance through general recommendations on occupational and public dose limits
NCRP	Reviews regulations formulated by the ICRP and decides ways to include those recommendations into U.S. radiation protection criteria
UNSCEAR	Evaluates human and environmental ionizing radiation exposure and derives radiation risk assessments from epidemiologic data and research conclusions; provides information to organizations such as the ICRP for evaluation
NAS/NRC-BEIR	Reviews studies of biologic effects of ionizing radiation and risk assessment and provides the information to organizations such as the ICRP for evaluation

International Commission on Radiological Protection (ICRP)

The **International Commission on Radiological Protection (ICRP)** is considered to be the international authority regarding the safe use of sources of ionizing radiation. Since its inception in 1928 the ICRP has been the leading international organization responsible for providing clear and consistent radiation protection guidance through its recommendations on occupational and public dose limits. These are published as reports in selective scholarly journals. The information on which the recommendations are based is supplied by organizations such as UNSCEAR and NAS/NRC-BEIR. The ICRP only makes recommendations; it does not function as an enforcement agency. Each nation must develop and enforce their own specific regulations.

National Council on Radiation Protection and Measurements (NCRP)

In the United States a nonprofit corporation known as the **National Council on Radiation Protection and Measurements (NCRP)** reviews the recommendations formulated by the ICRP. The NCRP determines the way ICRP recommendations are incorporated into U.S. radiation protection criteria. The Council accomplishes this task by formulating general recommendations and publishing them in the form of various NCRP Reports, which may be purchased from NCRP Publications in Bethesda, Maryland. Because NCRP is not an enforcement agency, implementation of its recommendations lies with federal and state agencies that have the power to enforce such standards after they have been established.

United Nations Scientific Committee on the Effects of Atomic Radiation (UNSCEAR)

The **United Nations Scientific Committee on the Effects of Atomic Radiation (UNSCEAR)** is another group that plays a prominent role in the formulation of radiation protection guidelines. This group evaluates human and environmental ionizing radiation exposures from a variety of sources, including radioactive materials, radiation-producing machines, and radiation accidents. UNSCEAR uses epidemiologic data (e.g., information from follow-up studies of Japanese atomic bomb survivors) and research conclusions to derive radiation risk assessments.

National Academy of Sciences/National Research Council Committee on the Biological Effects of Ionizing Radiation (NAS/NRC-BEIR)

The **National Academy of Sciences/National Research Council Committee on the Biological Effects of Ionizing Radiation (NAS/NRC-BEIR)** is another advisory group that reviews studies of biologic effects of ionizing radiation and risk assessment. This group formulated the 1990 BEIR V Report, *Health Effects of Exposure to Low Levels of Ionizing Radiation.* BEIR V supersedes four earlier BEIR reports that list studies of biologic effects and associated risk of groups of people who were either routinely or accidentally exposed to ionizing radiation. Such groups include early radiation workers, atomic bomb victims of Hiroshima and Nagasaki, and evacuees from the Chernobyl nuclear power station disaster.

As previously described, recommendations for EDE limits are made by the ICRP, NCRP, UNSCEAR, and NAS/NRC-BEIR. Based on these recommendations, limits on radiation exposure are established by congressional acts or state mandates. National and state agencies are charged with the responsibility of enforcing standards after they are established.

United States Regulatory Agencies

After radiation protection standards have been determined, responsible agencies must enforce them for the protection of the general public, patients, and occupationally exposed personnel.

Regulatory agencies include the following:
1. Nuclear Regulatory Commission (NRC)
2. Agreement states
3. Environmental Protection Agency (EPA)
4. Food and Drug Administration (FDA)
5. Occupational Safety and Health Administration (OSHA)

A summary of the United States regulatory agencies is presented in Table 4-2.

Nuclear Regulatory Commission (NRC)

The **Nuclear Regulatory Commission (NRC),** formerly known as the Atomic Energy Commission (AEC), is a federal agency. It has the power to enforce radiation protection standards. However, the NRC does not regulate or inspect diagnostic x-ray imaging facilities. The main function of the NRC is to oversee the nuclear energy industry. This agency reports on the design and working mechanics of nuclear power stations, the production of nuclear fuel, the handling of expended fuel, and the supervision of hazardous radioactive waste material. More specifically the NRC controls the manufacturing and use of radioactive substances formed in nuclear reactors and used in research, the healing arts (e.g., nuclear medicine procedures, radiation therapy treatment), and industry.

The NRC publishes rules and regulations in Title 10 of the United States Code of Federal Regulations. The United States Office of the Federal Register prepares and distributes this document. Fundamental ra-

Table 4-2
Summary of United States Regulatory Agencies

Agency	Function
NRC	Oversees the nuclear energy industry, enforces radiation protection standards, and publishes its rules and regulations in Title 10 of the United States Code of Federal Regulations
Agreement states	Enforce radiation protection regulations through their respective health departments
EPA	Facilitates the development and enforcement of regulations pertaining to the control of radiation in the environment
FDA	Conducts an ongoing product radiation control program, regulating the design and manufacture of electronic products, including x-ray equipment
OSHA	Functions as a monitoring agency in places of employment, predominantly in industry

diation protection standards governing occupational radiation exposure may be found in Part 20 of Title 10. Therefore the abbreviation 10CFR20 is used.

Agreement states

The majority of states in the United States have entered into agreements with the NRC to assume the responsibility of enforcing radiation protection regulations through their respective health departments. These states are known as **agreement states.** In nonagreement states, both the state and the NRC enforce radiation protection regulations by sending agents to health care facilities. Hospitals that use x-rays and radioactive materials are evaluated to determine whether they are in compliance with existing radiation safety regulations. Individual states also may legislate their own regulations regarding radiation safety. Inspection of nuclear reactors and assurance of adherence to federal radiation safety regulations in agreement or nonagreement states fall solely under the jurisdiction of the NRC.

Environmental Protection Agency (EPA)

The **United States Environmental Protection Agency (EPA)** facilitates the development and enforcement of regulations pertaining to the control of radiation in the environment. It provides direction to federal agencies, oversees the general area of environmental monitoring, and has the authority for specific areas such as determination of the action level for radon.

Food and Drug Administration (FDA)

Under Public Law 90-602, the Radiation Control for Health and Safety Act of 1968, the **United States Food and Drug Administration (FDA)** conducts an ongoing products radiation control program, regulating the design and manufacture of electronic products, including diagnostic x-ray equipment. A more detailed explanation of the Radiation Control for Health and Safety Act of 1968 is given later in this chapter.

To determine the level of compliance with standards in a given x-ray facility, the FDA conducts on-site inspections of x-ray equipment. Compliance with FDA standards ensures protection of occupationally and nonoccupationally exposed persons from faulty manufacturing.

Occupational Safety and Health Administration (OSHA)

The **United States Occupational Safety and Health Administration (OSHA)** functions as a monitoring agency in places of employment, predominantly in industry. OSHA regulates occupational exposure to radiation through Part 1910 of Title 29 of the United States Code of Federal Regulations (29 CFR 1910). It is responsible for regulations concerning the "right to know" of employees with regard to hazards that may be present in the workplace. OSHA also oversees regulations concerning the need for training programs in the workplace.

Radiation Safety Officer (RSO)

A **radiation safety officer (RSO)** is a person such as a medical physicist, health physicist, or radiologist designated by an institution and approved by the Nuclear Regulatory Commission and the state to ensure that internationally accepted guidelines for radiation protection are followed by the institution. The RSO is responsible for developing an appropriate radiation safety program for the institution and maintaining radiation monitoring records for all personnel.

Effective Dose Equivalent–Limiting (EDE) System

At the time of this publication the effective dose equivalent–limiting (EDE) system is the current method for assessing radiation exposure and associated risk of biologic damage to radiation workers and the general public (Fig. 4-2). **Effective dose equivalent (EDE) limit** concerns the upper boundary dose of ionizing radiation that results in a negligible risk of bodily injury or genetic damage. The sum of both external and internal whole-body exposures is considered when EDE limits are established. These upper limits are designed to minimize the risk to humans in terms of nonstochastic (deterministic) and stochastic (probabilistic) effects. These effects are discussed later in this chapter and in Chapter 6.

Upper boundary radiation exposure limits are designed to ensure that risks to which occupationally exposed persons are subjected are similar to those encountered by employees in other safe industries.

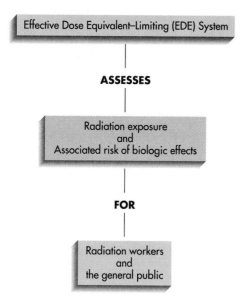

Fig. 4-2 Effective dose equivalent–limiting system.

Radiation risks should be derived from the complete injury caused by radiation exposure. The risk of terminal cancer, genetic imperfections induced by reproductive cell mutations, relative span of life lost, and the contribution of nonterminal cancer to a poorer quality of life must be taken into account.

Radiation Control for Health and Safety Act of 1968 (Public Law 90-602)

In 1968 the United States Congress passed the **Radiation Control for Health and Safety Act** (Public Law 90-602) to protect the public from the hazards of unnecessary radiation exposure resulting from electronic products such as microwave ovens and color televisions. Diagnostic x-ray equipment also was included. The act permitted the establishment of the **Center for Devices and Radiological Health (CDRH).** Until 1982 this organization was known as the Bureau of Radiological Health (BRH). The CDRH falls under the jurisdiction of the FDA. Essentially, it is responsible for conducting an ongoing electronic product radiation control program. This includes setting up standards for the manufacture, installation, assembly, and maintenance of machines used for radiologic procedures.

Further responsibilities include assessing the biologic effects of ionizing radiation, evaluating radiation emissions from electronic products in general, and conducting research to reduce radiation exposure.

The code of standards for diagnostic x-ray equipment went into effect on August 1, 1974. This code applies to complete systems and major components manufactured after that date. Equipment in use before August 1, 1974, does not need to be modified or discarded. Some important provisions of the standards for diagnostic x-ray equipment include the following:

1. Automatic limitation of the radiographic beam to the image receptor regardless of image receptor size, a condition known as positive beam limitation
2. Appropriate minimal permanent filtration of the x-ray beam to ensure an acceptable level of beam quality. Filtration provides significant reduction in the intensity of very "soft" x-rays that contribute only to added patient absorbed dose.
3. Ability of x-ray units to duplicate certain radiation exposures for any given combination of kilovolts at peak value (kVp), milliamperes (mA), and time to ensure both exposure reproducibility and linearity. *Reproducibility* is defined as consistency in output in radiation intensity for identical generator settings from one individual exposure to other subsequent exposures.* A variance of 5% or less is acceptable. *Exposure linearity* is defined as consistency in output radiation intensity at a selected kVp setting when changing from one milliamperage and time combination to another. *Linearity,* which is defined as the ratio of the difference in mR/mAs values between two successive generator stations to the sum of those mR/mAs values, must be less than 0.1.
4. Inclusion of beam limitation devices for spot films taken during fluoroscopy. Such devices should be located between the x-ray source and the patient.
5. Presence of "beam on" indicators to give visible warnings when x-ray exposures are in progress and

---

*Mathematically, reproducibility is described by the coefficient of variation "C," which is equal to the standard deviation of at least five successive output measurements employing the same technique factors divided by the average or mean value of those measurements. The regulation requires that C must not exceed 0.05.

both visual and audible signals when exposure has terminated.

6. Inclusion of manual backup timers for automatic (photo-timed) exposure control to ensure the termination of the exposure if the automatic timer fails.

Public Law 90-602 does not regulate the diagnostic x-ray user. It is strictly an equipment performance standard.

ALARA Concept

In 1954 the National Committee on Radiation Protection (later to be known as the National Council on Radiation Protection and Measurements) put forth the principle that radiation exposures should be kept "as low as reasonably achievable" with consideration for economic and social factors. This principle, known as the **ALARA concept,** is accepted by all regulatory agencies. It also may be referred to as *optimization* in accordance with ICRP Publication No. 37 and Publication No. 55. Medical radiographers and radiologists share the responsibility to keep occupational and nonoccupational dose equivalents as low as possible. In practice this translates into dose equivalents well below maximal allowable levels. This goal can usually be achieved simply through the employment of proper safety procedures performed by qualified personnel. Such procedures should be clearly described in the imaging center's radiation safety program.

The ALARA concept presents an extremely conservative model with respect to the relationship between ionizing radiation dose and potential risk. The relationship is assumed to be completely linear (i.e., biologic effect and radiation dose are directly proportional) and without any threshold (Fig. 4-3). In the interest of safety, risk of injury should be overestimated rather than underestimated.

Consumer-Patient Radiation Health and Safety Act of 1981 (Title IX of Public Law 97-35)

The **Consumer-Patient Radiation Health and Safety Act of 1981** (see Appendix F) provides federal legislation requiring the establishment of minimal standards for the accreditation of education programs for

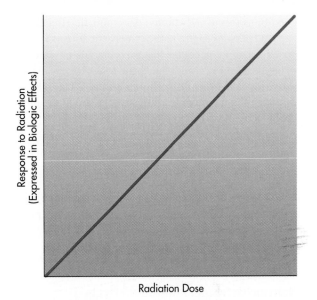

Fig. 4-3 Hypothetical linear (straight-line), nonthreshold curve for radiation dose–response relationship. The straight-line curve passing through the origin in this graph indicates both that the response to radiation (in terms of biologic effects) is directly proportional to the dose of radiation and no known level of radiation dose exists below which absolutely no chance of sustaining biologic damage is evident.

persons who administer radiologic procedures and the certification of such persons. The purpose of this federal act, which is under the directorship of the Secretary of Health and Human Services, is to ensure that medical and dental radiologic procedures are consistent with rigorous safety precautions and standards. Individual states are encouraged to enact similar statutes and administer certification and accreditation programs based on the standards established therein. Because no legal penalty exists for noncompliance, many states, unfortunately, have not responded with appropriate legislation.

Goal for Radiation Protection

NCRP Report No. 116, *Limitation of Exposure to Ionizing Radiation,* provides the most recent guidance on radiation protection. This report enunciates the goal of radiation protection, which reads as follows: "to prevent the occurrence of serious radiation-induced conditions (acute and chronic deterministic effects) in exposed persons and to reduce stochastic effects in exposed persons to a degree that is acceptable in relation to the benefits to the individual and to society from the activities that generate such exposures."[1] The whole essence of radiation protection is contained in the preceding statement.

Radiation-Induced Responses of Concern in Radiation Protection

Two all-inclusive categories encompass the radiation-induced responses of serious concern in radiation protection programs. These categories are as follows:

1. Nonstochastic (deterministic) effects
2. Stochastic (probabilistic) effects

Nonstochastic (deterministic) effects

Nonstochastic or deterministic effects are biologic somatic effects of ionizing radiation that exhibit a threshold dose below which the effect does not normally occur and above which the severity of the biologic damage increases as the dose increases. The biologic damage escalates because greater numbers of cells are injured at higher radiation doses. In general, nonstochastic effects occur only after large doses of radiation. Such radiation doses are much greater than those typically encountered by a patient in diagnostic radiology.* These deterministic effects may be early, such as (1) erythema, or diffused redness over an area of skin after irradiation; (2) a decrease in the white blood cell count; and (3) epilation, or loss of hair. Other, more serious early consequences of radiation sickness also may occur, such as (1) the hematopoietic syndrome, (2) gastrointestinal syndrome, and (3) cerebrovascular syndrome. These may occur within a few hours or days after high-level radiation exposure. The aforementioned syndromes are collectively referred to as the *acute radiation syndrome.* (The radiation syndromes are discussed in detail in Chapter 6.) Deter-

ministic somatic effects also may occur months or years after high-level radiation exposure. They are classified as late effects and include cataract formation, fibrosis, organ atrophy, loss of parenchymal cells, reduced fertility, and sterility caused by a decrease in reproductive cells.

Early deterministic somatic effects such as erythema and late deterministic somatic effects such as cataract formation have a high probability of occurring with radiation doses in excess of 2 Gy (200 rad). The frequency of occurrence of high-dose deterministic effects is not proportional to dose. Hence, they exhibit a non–straight-line dose-effect curve that is sigmoidal with a threshold (see Fig. 6-16, B).

Stochastic (probabilistic) effects

Stochastic (probabilistic) effects are nonthreshold, randomly occurring biologic somatic changes in which the chance of occurrence of the effect rather than the severity of the effect is proportional to the dose of ionizing radiation. Examples of these are cancer and genetic alterations. Stochastic effects may be demonstrated with the use of both the linear (see Fig. 6-16, *A*, Chapter 6) and linear-quadratic dose-response curves (see Fig. 6-18, Chapter 6). A stochastic event is an all-or-none response. This means that ionizing radiation can cause a disease process event such as cancer to occur within the general large population. Because these effects are random, determining which members of an exposed population will develop cancer is not possible before the radiation dose. Injury may result from exposure of a single cell or from damage in a sensitive substructure such as a gene. The assumption is that no minimal safe dose exists. The probability of an occurrence in a population, however, does increase in proportion to the absorbed dose of ionizing radiation delivered to the entire population. Therefore the net effect on a population group depends on the number of individuals irradiated as well as the mean dose that each individual receives.

The probability of causing radiation-induced cancer increases with absorbed dose when somatic cells are exposed to ionizing radiation. However, the severity of the disease is not dose related. For example, if a cancer induced by 2 Gy (200 rad) of ionizing radiation

---

*A significant exception to this is high–dose ratio fluoroscopic procedures. For these studies, entrance exposure rates as high as 20 roentgens per minute are not uncommon. Fluoroscopic exposure of 15 minutes amounts to a patient entrance dose of approximately 3 gray (Gy) (300 rad). This represents a therapeutic dose level.

and a cancer induced by 0.2 Gy (20 rads) of ionizing radiation are compared, the cancer induced by the larger absorbed dose is no worse than the cancer induced by the smaller absorbed dose. However, the chance of cancer induction from the larger dose is greater.

When ionizing radiation damages reproductive cells, mutations may develop that could bring about injurious consequences in subsequent generations. These may include birth defects induced by irradiation of the unborn child in utero (teratogenesis) and birth defects caused by irradiation of reproductive cells (sperm and ova) before conception (mutagenesis). Although epidemiologic studies analyzing groups such as the Japanese atomic bomb survivors have provided sufficient evidence of the induction of cancers in humans from high-radiation absorbed doses, no conclusive epidemiologic evidence suggests that low-level ionizing radiation exposures, such as those used in the most commonly performed diagnostic imaging procedures, can cause malignancies in humans. The sample sizes of the human population necessary to perform statistically valid studies to determine the carcinogenic potential of low absorbed doses of sparsely ionizing radiation are impracticable. Because the potential risk of low-level radiation exposure to the general population is a concern, radiation protection procedures must always be employed during diagnostic examinations. Currently the potential risk for cancer induction from low absorbed doses of ionizing radiation can only be estimated by extrapolating from high-dose data, using either a linear or linear-quadratic model (see Figures 6-17 and 6-18 in Chapter 6). With each model the calculated risk from low-dose radiation is small compared with the risk for cancer, birth defects, and genetic mutations under normal circumstances. The fact that the latter occurs in considerable proportions in human populations makes the obtaining of precise estimates of the role of ionizing radiation alone in producing stochastic effects extraordinarily difficult. Therefore identifying any stochastic occurrence increase in the general population exposed to small amounts of ionizing radiation is subject to considerable doubt. A summary of both stochastic (probabilistic) and nonstochastic (deterministic) effects is presented in Box 4-1.

Box 4-1

Summary of Serious Radiation-Induced Responses of Concern

Nonstochastic effects	Stochastic effects
Early effects	Cancer
Erythema (diffused redness over an area of skin after irradiation)	
Blood changes (decrease of lymphocytes and platelets)	*Genetic effects*
	Teratogenesis (irradiation of the fetus in utero)
Epilation (loss of hair)	Mutagenesis (irradiation of the reproductive cells before conception)
Acute radiation syndrome	
Hematopoietic syndrome	
Gastrointestinal syndrome	
Cerebrovascular syndrome	

Late effects
Cataract formation
Fibrosis
Organ atrophy
Loss of parenchymal cells
Reduced fertility
Sterility

Objectives of Radiation Protection

Radiation protection has two explicit objectives:
1. To prevent any clinically important radiation-induced nonstochastic (deterministic) effect from occurring by adhering to absorbed dose limits that are beneath the threshold levels
2. To limit the risk of stochastic responses to a conservative level as weighted against societal needs, values, benefits acquired, and economic considerations

Current Radiation Protection Philosophy

Both genetic and somatic responses to ionizing radiation were considered in developing the present effective dose equivalent–limiting recommendations. Current radiation protection philosophy is based on the assumption that a linear, nonthreshold relationship exists between radiation dose and biologic response. This means that the chance of biologic damage and the amount of damage sustained are directly proportional to the amount of radiation absorbed and no known level of radiation dose exists below which the probability of biologic damage is zero (see Fig. 4-3). Consequently, even the most minuscule dose of radiation has the potential to cause some harm. The current philosophy also accepts the premise that ionizing radiation possesses a beneficial as well as a destructive potential. It proposes that, when employed in the healing arts for the welfare of the patient, the potential benefits of exposing the patient to ionizing radiation must far outweigh the potential risks involved (Fig. 4-4).

Risk

In general terms, *risk* may be defined as the probability of injury, ailment, or death resulting from an activity. In the medical imaging industry, **risk** is viewed as the possibility of inducing a radiogenic cancer or genetic defect after irradiation. The way people look at probability and severity affects the perception of risk. No conclusive proof exists that low-level ionizing radiation causes a statistically significant increase in the threat of a malignancy. Although this risk may in fact be negligible, the subject is still

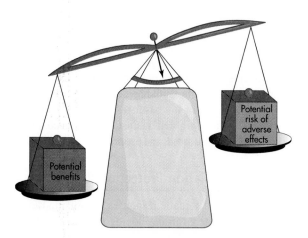

Potential benefits vs. potential risk of adverse effects

Fig. 4-4 The potential benefits of exposing the patient to ionizing radiation must outweigh the potential risk of adverse effects.

highly controversial. (A discussion of risk estimates for both stochastic and nonstochastic effects is presented in Chapter 6.)

Revised concepts of radiation exposure and risk have brought about the recent changes in NCRP recommendations for limits on exposure to ionizing radiation. Because many conflicting views exist on assessing the risk of cancer induction from low-level radiation exposure, the trend has been to create more rigorous radiation protection standards. The adoption of the effective dose equivalent–limiting system is a direct consequence of this conservatism. The benefit obtained from any diagnostic radiologic procedure must always be weighed against the risk that is taken. (Methods for assessing risk estimates for cancer induction are discussed in Chapter 6.)

Occupational risk associated with radiation exposure may be equated with occupational risk in other so-called safe industries (refer to Chapter 8, page 191). That risk is generally estimated to be a 2.5% chance of fatal accident over an entire career. The lifetime fatal risk in hazardous occupations such as logging and deep-sea fishing is many times greater.

To ensure that the hazard to radiation workers is no greater than the hazard to the general working public, the NCRP proposes that radiation protection programs for radiation workers should be designed to prevent individual workers from having total external plus internal cumulative dose equivalents in excess of their age in years times 10 mSv (1 rem).[1] Consider the following situation: A worker at age 40 has been employed at a nuclear power plant for 10 years. He had previously been employed as a radiation worker in another industry, during the course of which he received a cumulative dose equivalent of 100 millisievert (mSv) (10 rem). Therefore the radiation protection program for his current position should be such that he has not accumulated a total dose equivalent greater than 300 mSv (30 rem) during 10 years of employment.

The embryo-fetus in utero is particularly sensitive to radiation exposure. Epidemiologic studies of atomic bomb survivors exposed in utero has provided conclusive evidence of a dose-dependent increase in the incidence of severe mental retardation for fetal doses greater than approximately 0.4 sievert (Sv) (40 rem). The greatest risk for radiation-induced mental retardation occurred when the embryo-fetus was exposed 8 to 15 weeks after conception.

Basis for the Effective Dose Equivalent–Limiting System

The essential concept underlying radiation protection is that any organ in the human body is vulnerable to damage from exposure to ionizing radiation. Therefore every organ is essentially at risk because of the assumed stochastic (probabilistic) nature of somatic or genetic radiation-induced effects.

The EDE-limiting system includes, for the determination of **effective dose equivalent (H_E),** all radiation-vulnerable human organs that can contribute to potential risk, rather than only those human organs considered to be critical. In earlier recommendations such as NCRP Report No. 39 (released in 1971), crucial organs such as the gonads, blood-forming organs such as red bone marrow, and lung tissue were identified.[2]

The EDE system is an attempt to equate the various risks of cancer and genetic effects to the tissues or organs that were exposed to radiation. Because various tissues and organs do not have the same degree of sensitivity to these effects, the system employed must compensate for the differences in risk from one organ to another. Therefore an **organ weighting factor (W_T)** is used. This factor "indicates the ratio of the risk of stochastic effects attributable to irradiation of a given organ or tissue *(T)* to the total risk when the whole body is uniformly irradiated."[3] Weighting factors recommended by the ICRP in Report No. 60 (released in 1991) and adopted by the NCRP in Report No. 116 (released in 1993) are reproduced in Box 4-2.

Current NCRP Recommendations

The NCRP reiterates and updates its position on radiation protection standards and publishes recommendations on these standards in the form of reports. Recommendations contained in NCRP Report No. 116 now supersede those contained in NCRP Reports No. 91 and No. 39. A summary of some important issues and changes follows.

An annual **total effective dose equivalent (TEDE) limit** of 50 mSv (5 rem) has been established, with an added recommendation that the lifetime **total effective dose (TED)** in mSv should not exceed 10 times the occupationally exposed person's age in years. A radiation worker's lifetime effective dose must be limited to his or her age in years times 10 mSv (years times 1 rem). This is called the **cumulative whole-body effective dose equivalent (EDE) limit.** Adhering to this limit ensures that the lifetime risk for these workers remains acceptable. EDE limits, however, do not include radiation exposure from natural background radiation or exposure acquired as

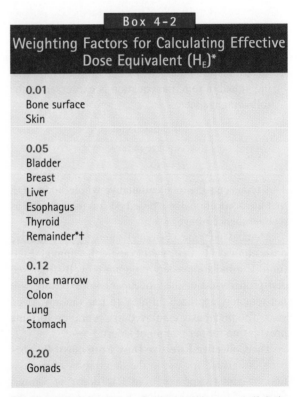

Box 4-2

Weighting Factors for Calculating Effective Dose Equivalent (H_E)*

0.01
Bone surface
Skin

0.05
Bladder
Breast
Liver
Esophagus
Thyroid
Remainder*†

0.12
Bone marrow
Colon
Lung
Stomach

0.20
Gonads

From National Council on Radiation Protection and Measurements: *Limitation of exposure to ionizing radiation,* NCRP Report No. 116, Bethesda, Md, 1993, NCRP.
*The remainder takes into account the following additional tissues and organs: adrenals, brain, small intestine, large intestine, kidney, muscle, pancreas, spleen, thymus, and uterus.
†In extraordinary circumstances in which one of the remainder tissues or organs receives a dose equivalent in excess of the highest dose in any of the 12 organs for which a weighting factor is specified, a weighting factor of 0.025 should be applied to that tissue or organ and a weighting factor of 0.025 to the average dose in the other remainder tissues or organs

a consequence of a worker undergoing medical imaging procedures. The limits do include the possibility of both internal and external exposure. The EDE is therefore the sum or total of both internal and external equivalent dose.

The following example demonstrates the application of the cumulative whole-body EDE limit. In the example, H represents the EDE.

Example: Determine the cumulative EDE limit to the whole body of an occupationally exposed person who is 30 years old.

Answer: In International System (SI) units:

$$H = 10 \text{ mSv} \times \text{age (in years)}$$
$$H = 10 \text{ mSv} \times 30$$
$$H = 300 \text{ mSv}$$

To determine the cumulative EDE limit of the same individual in rem, the equation is expressed in the following manner:

In traditional units:

$$H = \text{age in rem}$$
$$H = 30$$

This represents the total cumulative whole-body EDE that the occupationally exposed person may receive as a consequence of age.

Medical imaging personnel almost never receive dose equivalents that are close to the annual EDE limit. If a radiation safety program is well structured and properly maintained, occupational exposure will not remotely approach 50 mSv (5 rem) in any given year. The previously employed age proration formula provides no further margin of safety.

The **Collective Effective Dose Equivalent (S_E)** has been designated for use in the description of population or group exposure from low doses of various sources of ionizing radiation. S_E is determined as the product of the dose equivalent for an individual belonging to the exposed population or group and the number of persons exposed. The person-sievert (man-rem) is the unit of choice to express this quantity. For example, if 1000 people during the course of a year each receive a low-level dose equivalent of 0.5 mSv (50 mrem), the S_E is 500 person-sievert (50 man-rem).

The ICRP and NCRP are still considering the possibility of reducing exposure standards because of (1) revised risk estimates derived from recent reevaluations of dosimetric studies on the atomic bomb survivors of Hiroshima and Nagasaki[4] and (2) the appearance, as a result of longer follow-up time, of increased numbers of solid tumors in the survivor population. According to recent studies, ionizing radiation was estimated to be three times more damaging than previously thought. Levels of ionizing radiation formerly considered acceptable have been revised downward.

In the future the annual EDE limit for occupationally exposed persons may be limited to 10 or 20 mSv (1 or 2 rem) per year.[a] Of course, such a change will necessitate further evaluation of actual risk for persons employed in radiation industries. Lowering of the current limits is the responsibility of the NRC, individual states, and the FDA.

An annual EDE limit for whole-body occupational exposure has been set at a maximum of 50 mSv (5 rem) by the NCRP.[1] A limit also has been set for individual members of the general public not occupationally exposed. The NCRP-recommended annual EDE limit is 1 mSv (0.1 rem) for continuous or frequent exposures from artificial sources other than medical irradiation and a limit of 5 mSv (0.5 rem) annually for infrequent exposure.[1]

To reduce exposure for pregnant female members of the medical radiography team, the NCRP now recommends a monthly EDE not exceeding 0.5 mSv (0.05 rem) to the embryo-fetus after declaration of the pregnancy. This EDE excludes both medical and natural background radiation[1] and is designed to restrict significantly the total lifetime risk of leukemia and other malignancies in persons exposed in utero. Deterministic effects such as small head size and mental retardation are expected to be negligible if the EDEs remain below the established limit.

Students of radiography should not exceed an EDE of 1 mSv (0.1 rem) exposure annually. Below the age of 18, students should receive no occupational exposure. However, occasional exposure for the purposes of education and training are permitted, provided that special care is taken to ensure that the annual EDE limit of 1 mSv (0.1 rem) is not exceeded.

Nonstochastic limits for tissues and organs have been set to prevent excessive doses to specific regions of the body. They include the following: 150 mSv (15 rem) to the crystalline lens of the eyes and 500 mSv (50 rem) to all other tissues and organs, including the red bone marrow, breast, lung, reproductive cells, limbs, and localized areas of skin.[1]

To provide a low-exposure cut-off level so that regulatory agencies may dismiss a level of individual risk as negligible, an annual Negligible Individual Dose of 0.01 mSv (0.001 rem) has been set. This means that below this effective dose level a reduction of individual exposure is unnecessary.

Radiation Hormesis (Immunity!)

In Report No. 5 of the National Academy of Science on the Biological Effects of Ionizing Radiation (BEIR V), conclusions regarding the adverse effects on health from low levels of ionizing radiation are based on extrapolations from radiation dose equivalents greater than 0.5 Sv (50 rem). Such radiation levels are significantly greater than ordinary background radiation levels (3.5 mSv or 350 mrem per year). BEIR V espouses the linear "no threshold" view of the Japanese atomic bomb lifetime survival study (LSS) data. However, recent studies from the Radiation Effects Research Council in Hiroshima indicate an apparent threshold dosage in the atomic bomb LSS data that is approximately between 0.2 and 0.5 Sv (20 to 50 rem). This lower value corresponds to the amount of natural radiation that average U.S. residents receive in their lifetimes. What is curious is that the lifetime survival data appear to indicate that Japanese atomic bomb survivors with moderate radiation exposure of 5 mSv to 50 mSv, or 0.5 rem to 5 rem, the equivalent to 1.5 to 15 years of natural radiation, have a reduced cancer death rate compared with a normally exposed control population. These data contradict the predictions of the BEIR V report and, if substantiated, seem to cast doubt on the BEIR V conclusion that any amount of radiation is potentially harmful. The reverse might actually be true, at least for moderate amounts

of radiation exposure. More specifically, in seven Western states having background radiation levels higher than other states by about 1 mSv per year (100 mrem per year), residents experience about 15% fewer cancer deaths per 1000 individuals than the U.S. average. A study was conducted in China from 1972 to 1975 of two stable populations of about 70,000 persons, each of whose annual background radiation levels differed by about 2 mSv (200 mrem). This study disclosed a cancer rate in the more exposed population of only about 50% of that of the other group. Other intriguing studies exist. These suggest a potential **radiation hormesis** effect, which is a beneficial consequence of radiation for populations continuously exposed to moderately high levels of radiation. During the course of humankind's long progress up the evolutionary ladder, advantageous genetic mutations caused by radiation exposure may have occurred, resembling those that allow lower animals today to demonstrate radiation hormesis. Therefore to assume risk from very small amounts of radiation exposure (two or three times normal background levels) may be incorrect.

Occupational and Nonoccupational Dose Equivalent Limits

For the protection of radiation workers and the population as a whole, EDE limits (Box 4-3) have been established as guides. All medical imaging personnel should be familiar with current NCRP recommendations. For this group the most important item is the 50 mSv (5 rem) per year whole-body occupational EDE limit. This annual upper boundary on the monitoring-badge reading is designed to limit stochastic (probabilistic) effects of radiation. It takes into account the dose equivalent in all radiation-sensitive organs found in the body.

Because the tissue weighting factors (Box 4-2) used for calculating effective dose are so small for some organs, a single organ may receive an unreasonably large dose while the effective dose remains within the total effective dose limit. Therefore special limits are set for the crystalline lens of the eye, red bone marrow, breast, lung, reproductive organs, limbs,

Box 4-3

Summary of NCRP Recommendations*† (NCRP Report No. 116)

A. Occupational exposures‡
  1. EDE limits
    a. Annual   50 mSv   (5 rem)
    b. Cumulative   10 mSv × age   1 rem × age
  2. Equivalent dose annual limits for tissues and organs
    a. Lens of eye   150 mSv   (15 rem)
    b. All others (e.g., red bone marrow, breast, lung, gonads, skin, extremities)   500 mSv   (50 rem)
B. Guidance for emergency occupational exposure‡ (see Section 14, NCRP #116)
C. Public exposures (annual)
  1. EDE limit, continuous or frequent exposure‡   1 mSv   (0.1 rem)
  2. EDE limit, infrequent exposure‡   5 mSv   (0.5 rem)
  3. Equivalent dose limits for tissues and organs‡
    a. Lens of eye   15 mSv   (1.5 rem)
    b. Skin, hands and feet   50 mSv   (5 rem)
  4. Remedial action for natural sources:
    a. EDE (excluding radon)   >5 mSv   (>0.5 rem)
    b. Exposure to radon and its decay products§   >0.007Jhm^{-3} (>2 WLM)
D. Education and training exposures (annual)‡
  1. EDE limit   1 mSv   (0.1 rem)
  2. Equivalent dose limit for tissues and organs
    a. Lens of eye   15 mSv   (1.5 rem)
    b. Skin, hands and feet   50 mSv   (5 rem)
E. Embryo-fetus exposures‡ (monthly)
  Equivalent dose limit   0.5 mSv   (0.05 rem)
F. Negligible individual dose (annual)‡   0.01 mSv   (0.001 rem)

*Excluding medical exposures.
†See Tables 4.2 and 5.1 in NCRP Report #116 for recommendations on W_R and W_T, respectively.
‡Sum of external and internal exposures, excluding doses from natural sources.
§*WLM* stands for *working level month* and refers to a cumulative exposure for a working month (170 hours). As applied to radon and its daughter products, 1 WLM represents the cumulative exposure experienced in a 170-hour period due to a radon concentration of 100 pCi/L. The occupational limit for miners is 4 WLM per year, which results in a dose equivalent of approximately 0.15 Sv (15 rem) per year.

and localized areas of skin to prevent nonstochastic effects.

Summary

The concept of occupational and nonoccupational EDE limits has been described in this chapter. Adherence to these limits minimizes the possibility of harmful biologic effects. Box 4-3 provides a summary of EDE limits in terms of both SI and traditional radiation units. The concept of radiation exposure and associated risk of radiation-induced malignancy is the basis of the EDE system. The sum of both external and internal whole-body exposures is considered when establishing EDE limits. Accounting for tissue weighting factors is of vital importance because various tissues and organs do not have the same degree of sensitivity. For example, the dose to bone marrow is more of a threat than the dose to the tissues of the hand. The EDE limiting system must compensate for such differences. It also must take into consideration the different biologic threats posed by different types of ionizing radiation even when absorbed dose is the same. The EDE system has been incorporated into Title 10 of the Code of Federal Regulations, Part 20.

The ICRP, NCRP, UNSCEAR, and NAS/NRC-BEIR are major organizations that share the responsibility for evaluating the relationship between radiation dose equivalent and induced biologic effects. These organizations also are concerned with formulating risk estimates of somatic and genetic effects after irradiation. UNSCEAR and NAS/NRC-BEIR supply information to the ICRP, which makes recommendations on occupational and public dose limits. In the United States the NCRP reviews the recommendations formulated by the ICRP. The NCRP devises ways to include ICRP recommendations into U.S. radiation protection criteria by formulating their own general recommendations. Federal agencies such as the NRC and state agencies that have entered into agreements with the NRC implement NCRP recommendations. Functioning as the watchdog of the nuclear energy industry, the NRC controls the manufacture and use of radioactive substances formed in nuclear reactors and used in research, medicine, and industry. Rules and regulations of the NRC are published in Title 10 of the United States Code of Federal Regulations. Fundamental radiation protection standards governing occupational radiation exposure may be found in Part 20 of Title 10. Other United States regulatory agencies include the EPA, FDA, and OSHA. The EPA facilitates the development and enforcement of regulations pertaining to the control of radiation in the environment. Under the Radiation Control for Health and Safety Act of 1968 the FDA conducts an ongoing electronic product radiation control program to regulate product design and manufacture. Diagnostic x-ray equipment is included with electronic products. To determine compliance with x-ray equipment standards, the FDA conducts on-site inspections of such equipment in individual institutions. OSHA functions as a monitoring agency in the workplace. This agency regulates occupational exposure to radiation through Part 1910 of Title 29 of the United States Code of Federal Regulations. OSHA is responsible for regulations concerning the right to know of employees with regard to hazards that may be present in places of employment. OSHA also oversees regulations concerning the need for training programs in the workplace.

To ensure that internationally accepted guidelines for radiation protection are followed, individual health care facilities generally have a designated radiation safety officer (RSO). This individual is responsible for developing an appropriate radiation safety program for the institution. The RSO also maintains personnel radiation-monitoring records.

Radiation exposure should be kept "as low as reasonably achievable" with consideration for economic and social factors. This principle is known as the ALARA concept. It also is referred to as optimization.

Minimal standards for the accreditation of education programs for persons who administer radiologic procedures and certification of such persons are incorporated into the Consumer-Patient Radiation Health and Safety Act of 1981.

Serious radiation-induced responses may be classified as either nonstochastic (deterministic) or stochastic (probabilistic) effects. Biologic somatic effects of ionizing radiation that exhibit a threshold dose below which the effect does not normally occur and above which the severity of the biologic damage increases as the dose increases are called nonstochastic effects. These effects may occur early and are not typically encountered by patients undergoing diagnostic radiologic procedures. Stochastic effects are nonthreshold, randomly occurring biologic somatic changes in which the chance of occurrence of the effect rather than the severity of the effect is proportional to the dose of ionizing radiation. Cancer and genetic defects are examples of such effects. Box 4-1 summarizes nonstochastic and stochastic effects.

The NCRP has established an annual TEDE limit of 50 mSv (5 rem), with an added recommendation that the lifetime TEDE in mSv should not exceed 10 times the occupationally exposed person's age in years. A radiation worker's lifetime effective dose, or EDE limit, must be limited to his or her age in years times 10 mSv (years times 1 rem). In the description or population or group exposure from low doses of various sources of ionizing radiation, S_E may be used. The person-sievert (man-rem) unit is used for this quantity.

Some studies suggest the possibility of a radiation hormesis effect for certain populations continuously exposed to moderately high levels of radiation. This type of effect is a beneficial consequence of radiation (e.g., an advantageous genetic mutation). Therefore to assume risk from very small amounts of radiation exposure (which are two to three times normal background levels) may be incorrect.

Review Questions

1. Which of the following agencies is responsible for enforcing radiation safety standards?
   A. ICRP
   B. NRC
   C. NCRP
   D. UNSCEAR

2. Which of the following terms means random in nature?
   A. Deterministic
   B. Epidemiologic
   C. Nonstochastic
   D. Stochastic

3. Determine the cumulative effective dose equivalent to the whole body of an occupationally exposed person who is 27 years old.
   A. 2700 mSv
   B. 270 mSv
   C. 27 mSv
   D. 2.7 mSv

4. Biologic effects such as cataracts that result from exposure to ionizing radiation appear to have which of the following:
   A. Sigmoid dose-response nonthreshold relationship
   B. Circular dose-response threshold relationship
   C. Curvilinear threshold dose pattern
   D. Linear, nonthreshold dose pattern

5. Which of the following defines the upper boundary dose of ionizing radiation that will result in a *negligible risk* of bodily injury or genetic damage?
   A. Maximal permissible dose
   B. Dose limits
   C. Collective effective dose
   D. Effective dose equivalent

6. Which of the following groups have provided sufficient evidence of the induction of stochastic effects in human beings resulting from high radiation absorbed doses?
   A. Japanese atomic bomb survivors
   B. General population of the United States
   C. Population of occupationally exposed radiographers in the United States
   D. The 2 million people living within 50 miles of the Three Mile Island nuclear power plant after the accident on March 28, 1979.

7. The NCRP recommends that radiation exposure should be kept at which of the following levels?
   A. As low as reasonably achievable
   B. At threshold levels
   C. Slightly above upper boundary limits
   D. At 0.01 mSv/yr

8. Which of the following annual total whole-body occupational radiation effective dose equivalent limits applies to the radiographer during routine operations?
   A. 5 mSv (0.5 rem)
   B. 50 mSv (5 rem)
   C. 250 mSv (25 rem)
   D. 750 mSv (75 rem)

9. To reduce exposure of pregnant female members of the medical radiography team, the NCRP currently recommends a monthly effective dose equivalent not exceeding _____ to the embryo-fetus after declaration of a pregnancy.
   A. 0.5 mSv (0.05 rem)
   B. 5 mSv (0.5 rem)
   C. 150 mSv (15 rem)
   D. 250 mSv (250 rem)

10. For members of the general public not occupationally exposed, the NCRP recommends an annual effective dose equivalent limit of _____ for continuous or frequent exposures from artificial sources of ionizing radiation other than medical irradiation and a limit of _____ for infrequent annual exposure.
    A. 1 mSv (0.1 rem), 5 mSv (0.5 rem)
    B. 3 mSv (0.3 rem), 8 mSv (0.8 rem)
    C. 10 mSv (1 rem), 20 mSv (2 rem)
    D. 50 mSv (5 rem), 75 mSv (7.5 rem)

11. When exposed as part of their educational experience, 18-year-old students should *not* exceed an effective dose equivalent limit of _____ annually.
    A. 0.5 mSv (0.05 rem)
    B. 1 mSv (0.1 rem)
    C. 5 mSv (0.5 rem)
    D. 50 mSv (5 rem)

12. The NCRP recommends a cumulative whole-body occupational effective dose equivalent limit of a person's age in years multiplied by which of the following?
    A. 1 mSv (0.1 rem)
    B. 10 mSv (1 rem)
    C. 100 mSv (10 rem)
    D. 1000 mSv (100 rem)

13. When whole-body occupational exposure is controlled by keeping the effective dose equivalent well below the upper boundary limit, the possibility of inducing stochastic effects of radiation is _____ .
    A. Increased
    B. Maintained at an acceptable level
    C. Minimized
    D. None of the above

14. In 1968 the Radiation Control for Health and Safety Act (Public Law 90-602) was passed by the U.S. Congress to protect the public from the hazards of unnecessary radiation exposure resulting from which of the following?
    A. Diagnostic x-ray equipment only
    B. Therapeutic x-ray equipment only
    C. Electronic products excluding diagnostic x-ray equipment
    D. Electronic products including diagnostic x-ray equipment

15. For radiation workers, such as medical imaging personnel, occupational risk may be equated with occupational risk in which of the following?
    A. Other safe industries
    B. Somewhat hazardous industries
    C. Hazardous industries
    D. Extremely hazardous industries

16. What is the term applied to a beneficial consequence of radiation for populations continuously exposed to low levels of radiation above background?
    A. Nonoccupational dose equivalent effect
    B. Radiation negligible risk level effect
    C. Radiation hormesis effect
    D. Radiation benevolent effect

17. Which of the following is the unit of choice to express the collective effective dose equivalent?
    A. Group-gray (group-rad)
    B. Person-coulomb per kilogram (person-roentgen)
    C. Person-sievert (man-rem)
    D. Group-coulomb (group-roentgen)

18. Which of the following concepts is behind the establishment of the effective dose equivalent-limiting system?
    A. Negligible risk
    B. Organ radiosensitivity
    C. Radiation hormesis
    D. Radiation exposure and associated risk of possible radiation-induced malignancy

19. Which of the following groups are radiation protection standards organizations?
    1. ICRP
    2. NCRP
    3. UNSCEAR
    A. 1 and 2 only
    B. 1 and 3 only
    C. 2 and 3 only
    D. 1, 2, and 3

20. Somatic effects of ionizing radiation that exhibit a threshold dose below which the effect does not normally occur and above which the severity of the biologic damage increases as the dose increases are classified as which of the following?
    A. Deterministic effects
    B. Epidemiologic effects
    C. Probabilistic effects
    D. Stochastic effects

21. The term *teratogenesis* refers to which of the following?
    A. Birth defects caused by irradiation of reproductive cells before conception
    B. Birth defects induced by irradiation of the unborn child in utero
    C. Cancer caused by ionizing radiation exposure
    D. Somatic effects of ionizing radiation caused by low-level exposure

22. Revised estimates derived from recent reevaluations of dosimetric studies on the atomic bomb survivors of Hiroshima and Nagasaki indicate which of the following?
    A. A decrease in the number of solid tumors in the survivor population
    B. An increase in the number of solid tumors in the survivor population
    C. That low-level radiation causes cancer
    D. That the risk of radiation-induced cancer is nonexistent

23. Which of the following agencies was previously known as the Atomic Energy Commission?
    A. FDA
    B. ICRP
    C. NCRP
    D. NRC

24. Fundamental radiation protection standards governing occupational radiation exposure may be found in which of the following documents?
    A. 5CFR10
    B. 10CFR20
    C. The ALARA manual
    D. Public Law 90-602

25. Which of the following are classified as *late* deterministic somatic effects?
    1. Cataract formation
    2. Organ atrophy
    3. Radiation-induced malignancy
    A. 1 and 2 only
    B. 1 and 3 only
    C. 2 and 3 only
    D. 1, 2, and 3

Endnotes

a. Manual 60 of the ICRP (Oxford, 1991, Pergamon Press) contains a recommendation for lowering the allowable occupational level of exposure to ionizing radiation from 50 mSv per year (5 rem per year) to 20 mSv per year (2 rem per year) averaged over defined periods of 5 years. This lower limit is not enforced in the United States.

References

1. National Council on Radiation Protection and Measurements: *NCRP Report #116, limitation of exposure to ionizing radiation,* Bethesda, Md, 1993, NCRP Publications.
2. National Council on Radiation Protection and Measurements: *NCRP Report #39, basic radiation protection criteria,* Washington, DC, 1971, NCRP Publications.
3. National Council on Radiation Protection and Measurements: *NCRP Report #91, recommendations on limits for exposure to ionizing radiation,* Bethesda, Md, 1987, NCRP Publications.
4. Committee on Biological Effects of Ionizing Radiation, National Research Council, Commission of Life Sciences, Board of Radiation Research: *Health effects of exposure to low levels of ionizing radiation (BEIR V Report),* Washington, DC, 1989, National Academy Press.

Bibliography

Anderson R: New dose limits boggle the mind, *ASRT Scanner* 27(2):1, Dec 1994 and Jan 1995.
Ballinger PW: *Merrill's atlas of radiographic positions and radiologic procedures,* ed 8, vol 1, St Louis, 1995, Mosby.
Bushong S: *Radiologic science for technologists: physics, biology and protection,* ed 6, St Louis, 1997, Mosby.
Carneron JR: Radiation hormesis, *Physics Today* 45(3):13, 1992 (letter).
Christensen EE, Curry III TS, Dowdey JE: *An introduction to the physics of diagnostic radiology,* ed 2, Philadelphia, 1978, Lea & Febiger.
Committee on the Biological Effects of Ionizing Radiations (BEIR V): *Health effects of exposure to low levels of ionizing radiation,* Washington, D.C., 1990, National Academy Press.
Curry III TS, Dowdey JE, Murry Jr RC: *Christensen's introduction to the physics of diagnostic radiology,* ed 3, Philadelphia, 1984, Lea & Febiger.
Dowd SB: *Practical protection and applied radiobiology,* Philadelphia, 1994, WB Saunders.
Early PJ, Sodee DB: *Principles and practice of nuclear medicine,* ed 2, St Louis, 1995, Mosby.
Frankel R: *Radiation protection for radiologic technologists,* New York, 1976, McGraw-Hill.
Fullerton GD et al, editors: *Medical Physics Monograph No 5,* New York, 1980, published for the American Association of Physicists in Medicine by the American Institute of Physics.
Hagler M: Radiation protection update, *RT Image* 3(20):10, 1990.

Hall EJ: *Radiobiology for the radiologist,* ed 4, Philadelphia, 1994, Lippincott.

Hall EJ: *Radiobiology for the radiologist,* ed 3, Philadelphia, 1988, Lippincott.

Hendee WR, editor: *Health effects of low-level radiation,* Norwalk, Conn, 1984, Appleton-Century-Crofts.

Hendee WR, Ibbott GS: *Radiation therapy physics,* ed 2, St Louis, 1996, Mosby.

Hendee WR, Ritenour ER: *Medical imaging physics,* ed 3, St Louis, 1992, Mosby.

International Commission on Radiation Units and Measurements (ICRU): *Radiation quantities and units,* ICRU Report No. 33, Washington, D.C., 1980, ICRU.

International Commission on Radiological Protection: *Cost-benefit analysis in the optimization of radiation protection,* ICRP Publication No. 37, Elmsford, NY, 1983, Pergamon.

International Commission on Radiological Protection: *Optimization and decision-making in radiological protection,* ICRP Publication No. 55, Elmsford, NY, 1989, Pergamon.

International Commission on Radiological Protection: *Recommendations,* Report No. 60, New York, 1991, Pergamon.

International Commission on Radiological Protection: *Recommendations of the ICRP,* ICRP Publication No. 26, Elmsford, NY, 1977, Pergamon.

Land CE: Estimating cancer risks from low doses of ionizing radiation, *Science* 209:1197, 1981.

Loudin A: The radiation debate continues, *RT Image* 3(51):10, 1990.

National Council on Radiation Protection and Measurements (NCRP): *Report #39, basic radiation protection criteria,* Washington, D.C., 1971, NCRP Publications.

National Council on Radiation Protection and Measurements (NCRP): *Report #43, review of the current state of radiation protection philosophy,* Washington, D.C., 1975, NCRP Publications.

National Council on Radiation Protection and Measurements (NCRP): *Report #91, recommendations on limits for exposure to ionizing radiation,* Bethesda, Md, 1987, NCRP Publications.

National Council on Radiation Protection and Measurements (NCRP): *Report #93, ionizing radiation exposure of the population of the United States,* Bethesda, Md, 1987, NCRP Publications.

National Council on Radiation Protection and Measurements (NCRP): *Report #107, implementation of the principle of as low as reasonably achievable (ALARA) for medical and dental personnel,* Bethesda, Md, 1990, NCRP Publications.

National Council on Radiation Protection and Measurements (NCRP): *Report #116, limitation of exposure to ionizing radiation,* Bethesda, Md, 1993, NCRP Publications.

Noz ME, Maguire Jr GQ: *Radiation protection in radiologic and health sciences,* ed 2, Philadelphia, 1985, Lea & Febiger.

Noz ME, Maguire Jr GQ: *Radiation protection in the radiologic and health sciences,* Philadelphia, 1979, Lea & Febiger.

Reimenschneider J: ICRP recommends lower maximum dose, *RT Image* 3(28):22, 1990.

Reimenschneider J: Rethinking radiation protection standards, *RT Image* 3(6):6, 1990.

Scheele RV, Wakley J: *Elements of radiation protection,* Springfield, Ill, 1975, Charles C. Thomas.

Seeram E: *Radiation protection,* Philadelphia, 1997, Lippincott-Raven.

Selman J: *The fundamentals of x-ray and radium physics,* ed 7, Springfield, Ill, 1985, Charles C. Thomas.

Selman J: *The fundamentals of x-ray and radium physics,* ed 6, Springfield, Ill, 1978, Charles C. Thomas.

Sevcik J: Putting the radiation risk into perspective, *RT Image* 2(12):1, 1989.

Sinclair WK: Radiation protection recommendations on dose limits: the role of the NCRP and ICRP and future developments, *Radiation Oncology Biol Phys* 31(2):387, 1995.

Thompson MA et al: *Principles of imaging science and protection,* Philadelphia, 1994, WB Saunders.

Travis EL: *Primer of medical radiobiology,* ed 2, St Louis, 1989, Mosby.

US Department of Health, Education, and Welfare (HEW), Public Health Service, Food and Drug Administration, Bureau of Radiological Health, Division of Compliance (HFX-400): *A practitioner's guide to the diagnostic x-ray equipment standard,* Publication (FDA) 78-8050, Rockville, Md, 1978, HEW.

US Department of Health, Education, and Welfare (HEW), Public Health Service, Food and Drug Administration, Bureau of Radiological Health, Division of Compliance X-Ray Products Branch: *Assembler's guide to diagnostic x-ray equipment,* HEW Publication (FDA) 76-8002, Rockville, Md, 1975, HEW.

Watson E: Radiation Dose Limits Lowered, *ASRT Scanner* 27(1):15, Oct and Nov 1994.

Webster EW et al: *A primer on low-level ionizing radiation and its biological effects,* American Association of Physicists in Medicine (AAPM) Report No. 18, New York, 1986, American Institute of Physics (published for the AAPM).

5

Overview of Cell Biology

Chapter Outline

acid-base balance

adenine (A)

adenosine triphosphate
  (ATP)

amino acids

anaphase

antibodies

carbohydrates (saccharides)

cell division

cell membrane

cellular life cycle

chromatids

chromosomes

cytoplasm

cytoplasmic organelles

cytosine (C)

deoxyribonucleic acid (DNA)

endoplasmic reticulum (ER)

enzymatic proteins

genes

glucose

guanine (G)

hormones

hydrogen bonds

inorganic compounds

lipids (fats)

macromolecules

meiosis

messenger RNA (mRNA)

metabolism

metaphase

mitochondria

mitosis (M)

mitotic spindle

nitrogenous organic bases

nucleic acids

nucleotides

nucleus

organic compounds

osmosis

peptide bond

prophase

proteins

protein synthesis

protoplasm

purines

pyrimidines

reduction division

repair enzymes

ribonucleic acid (RNA)

somatic cells

structural proteins

sugar-phosphate chains

telophase

thymine (T)

transfer RNA (tRNA)

uracil (U)

After completing this chapter, the reader will be able to perform the following:

- Explain the need for a basic knowledge of cell structure, composition, and function as a foundation for radiation biology.

- Identify and describe some important functions of the major classes of organic and inorganic compounds that exist in the cell.

- Describe the molecular structure of DNA and explain the way it functions in the cell.

- List the various cellular components and identify their physical characteristics and functions.

- Distinguish between the two types of cell division, mitosis and meiosis, and describe each process.

Biology is a science that explores living things and life processes. Cells are the basic units of all living matter and are essential for life. The cell is the fundamental component of structure, development, growth, and life processes. Before imaging professionals can develop an understanding of the effects of ionizing radiation on a living system such as the human body, which is composed of large numbers of various types of cells, they must acquire a basic knowledge of cell structure, composition, and function. This chapter provides the reader with an overview of cell biology as a foundation for radiation biology.

The Cell

Cells exist in many different forms and perform many different functions. Some cells function as free-moving, independent units, some belong to loosely organized communities that wander, and some remain fixed in one position and function as part of the tissues of larger organisms throughout their lifetimes. Every mature human cell is highly specialized and has predetermined tasks to perform in support of the body. Cells move, grow, react, protect themselves, regulate life processes, and reproduce. To ensure efficient cell operation, the body must provide food as a source of raw material for the release of energy, oxygen to help break down the food, and water to transport inorganic substances (compounds that do not contain carbon) such as calcium and sodium into and out of the cell. In turn, normal cellular functioning enables the body to maintain homeostasis or equilibrium, allowing it to return to and maintain normal functioning despite the changes it undergoes as a result of influences to which it is subjected.

Cells are engaged in an ongoing process of obtaining energy and converting it to their own special purposes. They absorb molecular nutrients through the cell membrane and use these nutrients in the production of energy and synthesis of molecules. If exposure to ionizing radiation damages the components involved in molecular synthesis beyond repair, cells function abnormally or die.

Cell Chemical Composition

Protoplasm

Cells are made of **protoplasm,** the building material for all living things. This substance carries on the complex process of **metabolism** (chemical reactions that modify foods for cellular use), the reception and processing of food and oxygen and elimination of waste products, which enable the cell to perform the vital functions of synthesizing proteins and producing energy.

Protoplasm consists of organic (carbon-containing compounds such as those found in nature or produced artificially) and inorganic materials, either dissolved or suspended in water. The biomolecules that compose protoplasm are formed from 24 elements, the four primary elements involved being carbon, hydrogen, oxygen, and nitrogen. When combined with phosphorus and sulfur, they compose the essential major organic compounds: proteins, carbohydrates, lipids, and nucleic acids. These compounds are discussed in detail later in this chapter.

The most important inorganic substances are water and mineral salts. Water aids in sustaining life and is the most abundant inorganic compound in the body. Depending on cell type, water normally accounts for 80% to 85% of protoplasm. Mineral salts exist in smaller quantities and also are of vital importance.

Organic compounds

The four major classes of **organic compounds** (proteins, carbohydrates, lipids [fats], and nucleic acids) all contain carbon (Box 5-1). Carbon is the basic constituent of all organic matter. By combining with hydrogen, nitrogen, and oxygen, it makes life possible. Of all the organic compounds, protein contains the most carbon.

Box 5-1

Major Classes of Organic Compounds that Compose the Cell

Proteins
Carbohydrates
Lipids (fats)
Nucleic acids

Proteins

Proteins comprise about 15% of cell content. They are essential for growth, the construction of new body tissue (including acellular tissue such as hair and nails), and the repair of injured or debilitated tissue. Proteins are formed by combining **amino acids** (the structural units of protein) into long chainlike molecular complexes. In these complexes, a chemical link called a **peptide bond** connects each amino acid. Protein production, or **protein synthesis,** involves 22 different amino acids. The order of arrangement of these amino acids determines the precise function of each protein molecule, and the type of protein molecules that any given cell contains determines the characteristics of that cell. Chromosomes and genes organize the amino acids into the proper sequences to form specific structural and enzymatic proteins (Fig. 5-1).

Structural proteins such as those found in muscle provide the body with its shape and form and are a source of heat and energy. By functioning as catalysts (agents that affect the speed of chemical reactions without being altered themselves), **enzymatic proteins** (enzymes) control the cell's various physiologic activities. Enzymes cause an increase in cellular activ-

ity that in turn causes biochemical reactions to occur more rapidly to meet the needs of the cell. Hence proper cell functioning depends on enzymes.

In addition to providing structure and support for the body, proteins also may function as hormones and antibodies. **Hormones** are chemical secretions manufactured by various endocrine glands and carried by the bloodstream to influence the activities of other parts of the body. They regulate body functions such as growth and development. **Antibodies** are molecules produced by specialized cells in the bone marrow called B lymphocytes. Lymphocytes are white blood cells involved in the body's immune reactions. Antibodies are produced when other lymphocytes in the body, known as T lymphocytes, detect the presence of molecules that do not belong to the body. These foreign objects (e.g., bacteria, flu viruses) are called *antigens.* The antibodies chemically attack the antigens and thereby constitute the body's primary defense mechanism against infection and disease.

Carbohydrates

Carbohydrates, which also are referred to as **saccharides,** make up about 1% of cell content. They include starches and various sugars. Carbohydrates range from simple to complex compounds, even though they are composed of only carbon, hydrogen, and oxygen. Simple sugars such as glucose, fructose, and galactose have six carbon atoms and six molecules of water (e.g., glucose has the chemical formula $C_6H_{12}O_6$). **Glucose** is the primary energy source for the cell. Because it is a simple sugar, it is called a *monosaccharide.* Disaccharides also are sugars. These have two units of a simple sugar or two monosaccharides linked together. Sucrose (cane sugar) is an example of a disaccharide. Both monosaccharides and disaccharides have relatively small molecules. Polysaccharides contain several or many molecules of simple sugar. Plant starches and animal glycogen are the two most important polysaccharides.

Carbohydrates, simply described as chains of sugar molecules, function as short-term energy storers for the body. Their primary purpose is to provide fuel for cell metabolism. They also are important structural parts of cell walls and intercellular materials.

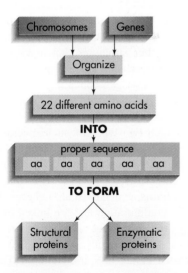

Fig. 5-1 Chromosomes and genes organize the 22 different amino acids into proper sequences to form the different structural and enzymatic proteins.

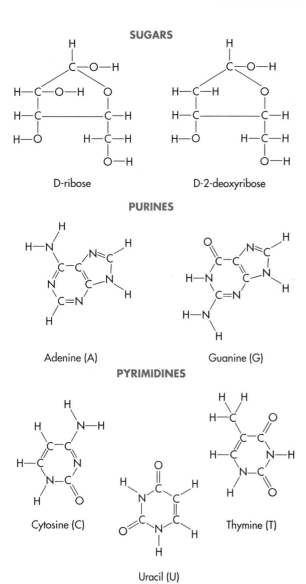

Fig. 5-2 The components of nucleic acid (*H* = hydrogen, *C* = carbon, *N* = nitrogen, *O* = oxygen). Sugars are strung together with phosphate groups, and a base is attached to each sugar. DNA uses D-2-deoxyribose sugar, and RNA uses D-ribose. Both nucleic acids use the same two purines, but thymine *(T)* in DNA is replaced by uracil *(U)* in RNA. (From Cherfas J, *Man-made life*, New York, 1982, Pantheon.)

Lipids

Lipids, which also are referred to as **fats** or fatlike substances, constitute about 2% of cell content. They are made up of a molecule of glycerine (a sweet, colorless, odorless, syrupy liquid) and three molecules of fatty acid. When glucose is broken down in the body during respiration, fats are among the generated intermediate products. When some of these fats combine with an acidic group of atoms (e.g., the carboxyl group, COOH), a fatty acid is formed. An example of a fatty acid is CH_3COOH, which is commonly known as acetic acid. Fatty acids are constituents of amino acids from which proteins are built. Lipids are water-insoluble organic **macromolecules** (large molecules built from smaller chemical structures) that consist of carbon, hydrogen, and oxygen. They are the structural parts of cell membranes. Lipids are present in all body tissues and perform a variety of functions for the cell. They act as reservoirs for the long-term storage of energy, insulate and guard the body against the environment, support and protect organs such as the eyes and kidneys, provide essential substances necessary for growth and development, and assist in the digestive process.

Nucleic acids

Nucleic acids, which compose about 1% of the cell, are very large, complex macromolecules (Fig. 5-2). The much smaller structures that make up nucleic acids are called **nucleotides.** Each nucleotide is a unit formed from a nitrogen-containing organic base, a five-carbon sugar molecule (deoxyribose), and a phosphate molecule.

Cells contain two types of nucleic acids that are important to human metabolism: **deoxyribonucleic acid (DNA)** and **ribonucleic acid (RNA).** The DNA macromolecule is composed of two long **sugar-phosphate chains,** which twist around each other in a double helix configuration and are linked by pairs of **nitrogenous organic bases** at the sugar molecules of the chains to form a tightly coiled structure resembling a twisted ladder or spiral staircase. The sugar-phosphate compounds are the rails, and the pairs of nitrogenous organic bases, which consist of complimentary chemicals, are the steps or rungs of the DNA ladderlike structure (Fig. 5-3). **Hydrogen bonds** attach the bases to each other, joining the two side rails of the DNA ladder.

The four nitrogenous organic bases in DNA macromolecules are **adenine (A), cytosine (C), guanine (G),** and **thymine (T).** Adenine and guanine are compounds called **purines,** and the compounds cytosine and thymine are classified as **pyrimidines.** A significant characteristic of the organic bases is that purines always link only with pyrimidines in certain specific combinations; more precisely, adenine always bonds only with thymine and cytosine bonds only with guanine. This characteristic is the reason the two strands of DNA are described as complementary. Nitrogenous organic base-bonding unions other than adenine-thymine combinations and cytosine-guanine combinations cannot occur.

DNA, the master chemical, contains all the information the cell needs to function. It carries the genetic information necessary for cell replication and regulates all cellular activity to direct protein synthesis. DNA determines the characteristics of a person by regulating the sequences of amino acids in the person's constituent proteins during the synthesis of these proteins; these sequences of amino acids are determined by the order of adenine-thymine and cytosine-guanine base pairs in the DNA macromolecules (which constitute the genetic codes of the macromolecules). Different sequences of amino acids produce proteins with different functions. Protein characteristics determine cell characteristics, and cell characteristics ultimately determine the characteristics of the entire individual. All the information necessary to construct and maintain a living organism is written in the "book" of DNA—the letters, words, and sentences are composed of the nitrogenous organic bases.

Because DNA is found mostly in the cell nucleus, it cannot directly influence cellular activity such as growth and differentiation, which occur in the cytoplasm (the part of the cell that lies outside the nucleus). Instead, DNA regulates cellular activity indirectly, transmitting its genetic information outside the cell nucleus by reproducing itself in the form of **messenger RNA (mRNA),** the substance responsible for making proteins out of amino acids.

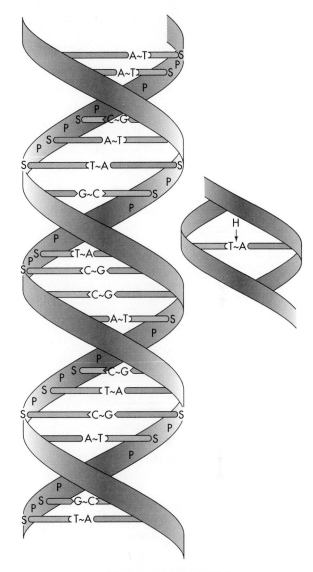

Fig. 5-3 Diagram of a DNA macromolecule that illustrates its twisted ladderlike or spiral-staircase–like configuration. Alternating sugar and phosphate molecules form the side rails of the ladder, and the nitrogenous organic bases, which consist of the complimentary chemicals adenine *(A)*, thymine *(T)*, guanine *(G)*, and cytosine *(C)*, form the rungs or steps. A hydrogen bond joins the bases together.

DNA serves as a prototype for mRNA, which is identical to DNA except that it contains the five-carbon sugar molecule ribose rather than deoxyribose, and **uracil (U),** a pyrimidine base found *only* in RNA, replaces thymine as the nitrogenous organic base. An mRNA macromolecule resembles one half of a DNA macromolecule. It appears as a single strand of the DNA ladderlike configuration, the ladder being severed in half lengthwise (Fig. 5-4).

Macromolecules of mRNA carry their genetic codes (in their sequences of nitrogenous organic bases—e.g., U, U, C, C, A, U, G) from the cell nucleus through the endoplasmic reticulum (the network of sacs and canals that winds through the cytoplasm) to the ribosomes where proteins are manufactured. Here the mRNA transfers its genetic codes to another kind of RNA molecule called **transfer RNA (tRNA).** This tRNA combines with and transports individual amino acids from different areas of the cell to the ribosomes, where the amino acids are arranged and attached in specific orders to form chainlike protein molecules. Each tRNA molecule is coded for a particular amino acid; because each of the 22 different amino acids has a tRNA, at least 22 different types of tRNA exist. The cell's "protein factories," the ribosomes, travel along the mRNA, linking tRNA and its corresponding amino acids in the correct order so that the proteins necessary to provide for the needs of the cell are produced (Fig. 5-5).

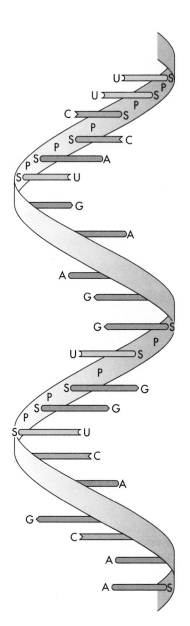

Fig. 5-4 Messenger RNA *(mRNA)* resembles one half of a DNA macromolecule. It appears as a single strand (one side rail) of the DNA ladderlike configuration, the ladder being severed in half lengthwise. Uracil *(U)* replaces thymine *(T)* as one of the nitrogenous organic bases in the mRNA molecule.

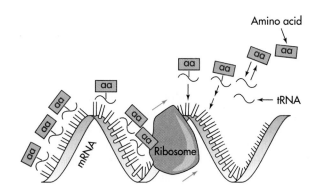

Fig. 5-5 Ribosomes, the cell's protein factories, travel along the mRNA rails linking tRNA and its corresponding amino acids in the proper sequences to produce the proteins appropriate for the needs of the cell.

Many of the proteins produced in the ribosomes are enzymes, which cause vital chemical reactions to take place within the cell at the appropriate time. Some of the enzymes produced are called **repair enzymes.** These enzymes can mend damaged molecules and are therefore capable of helping the cell to recover from a small amount of radiation-induced damage. Both the catalytic and repair capabilities of enzymes are of vital importance to the survival of the cell.

Chromosomes are tiny rod-shaped bodies, which under a microscope appear to be long threadlike structures. Chromosomes are composed of DNA. A normal human being has 46 different chromosomes. The DNA that makes up each chromosome is divided into hundreds of segments called genes. Each segment contains information responsible for directing cytoplasmic activities, controlling growth and development of the cell, and transmitting hereditary information. Thus **genes** are the basic units of heredity (Fig. 5-6). They control the formation of proteins in every cell through the intricate process of genetic coding.

Inorganic compounds

Inorganic compounds are compounds that do not contain carbon. The inorganic compounds found in the body occur in nature independent of living things; they are acids (hydrogen-containing compounds that can attack and dissolve metal such as HNO_3, nitric acid), bases (alkali or alkaline earth OH compounds that can neutralize acids such as $Mg(OH)_2$, otherwise known as milk of magnesia), and salts (chemical compounds resulting from the action of an acid and a base on one another). Salts are sometimes referred to as electrolytes. Water is the primary inorganic substance contained in the human body; it comprises approximately 80% to 85% of the body's weight. Within the cell, water is indispensable for metabolic activities because it is the medium in which the chemical reactions that are the basis of these activities occur; it also functions as a solvent by dissolving chemical substances within the cell. Outside the cell, water functions as a transport vehicle for materials the cell uses or eliminates. In addition, water acts as the medium in which acids, bases, and salts are dissolved. After they are dissolved in solution, their concentration may be regulated. Water also is responsible for maintaining a constant body temperature of 98.6° F (37° C).

Mineral salts exist in smaller quantities to maintain the correct proportion of water in the cell. These salts are necessary for proper cell function, creation of energy, and conduction of impulses along nerves. The constituents of salts exist as ions (particles carrying a positive or negative electric charge) in the cell. These ions cause materials to be altered, broken down, and recombined to form new substances. Potassium (K) constitutes most of the positive ions (cations) present in cells, whereas phosphate (P) constitutes the majority of negative ions (anions). Potassium is of primary importance in maintaining adequate amounts of intracellular fluid. Water tends to move across cell surfaces or membranes into areas in which a high concentration of ions is present. This motion is referred to as **osmosis.** Thus by balancing the concentration of potassium ions (as well as sodium [Na] and chloride [Cl] ions), the cell regulates the amount of fluid it contains. Potassium also aids in maintaining **acid-base balance** (a state of equilibrium or stability between acids and bases).

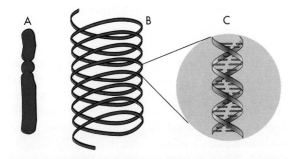

Fig. 5-6 A chromosome viewed under a microscope appears rod-shaped *(A);* when further magnified, a chromosome appears as a tightly wound spiral structure *(B)* composed of hundreds of genes, which is a segment of the DNA macromolecule *(C).*

Cell Structure

The normal cell (Fig. 5-7) has a number of components:
1. Cell membrane
2. Cytoplasm

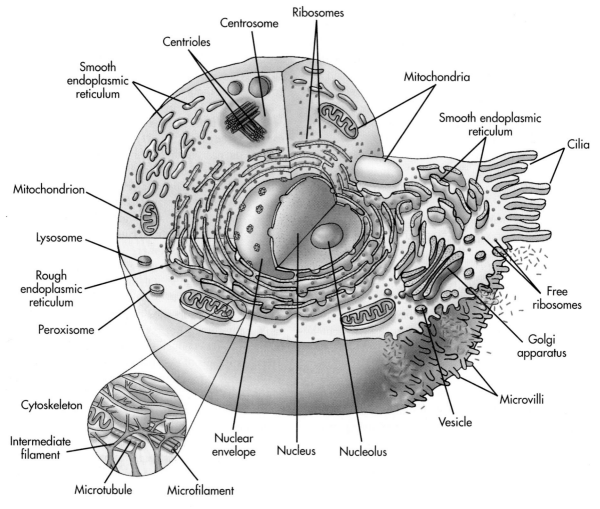

Fig. 5-7 Diagram of a typical cell, demonstrating its basic components. (From Thibodeau A, *Anatomy and physiology*, ed 3, St Louis, 1996, Mosby.)

3. Cytoplasmic organelles
   a. Endoplasmic reticulum
   b. Golgi apparatus
   c. Mitochondria
   d. Lysosomes
   e. Ribosomes
   f. Centrosomes
4. Nucleus

Cell membrane

The **cell membrane** is a frail structure encasing and surrounding the cell. It functions as a barricade to protect cellular contents from their environment and controls the passage of water and other materials into and out of the cell. Because the cell membrane allows penetration only by certain types of substances and regulates the speed at which these substances travel within the cell, it plays a primary role in the cell's transport system. When a substance moves through the cell membrane by osmosis, the transport system is classified as passive because the movement depends more on the concentrations of particles in fluid than it does on the cell membrane. When the movement of a substance across a cell membrane is controlled more by the properties and powers of the cell membrane than it is by the relative concentrations of particles in fluid, the transport system is classified as active. In active transport the cell must expend energy to pump substances into and out of itself.

Cytoplasm

Cytoplasm is the protoplasm that exists outside the cell's nucleus. It makes up the majority of the cell and contains large amounts of all the cell's molecular components with the exception of DNA. All cellular metabolic functions occur in the cytoplasm. Functioning like a factory, it performs the following major functions:

1. Accepting unrefined materials and assembling from these materials new substances such as carbohydrates, lipids, and proteins
2. Breaking down materials to produce energy
3. Packaging substances for distribution to other areas of the cell or to various sites in the body through the circulation
4. Eliminating waste products

Cytoplasmic organelles

The cytoplasm contains all the miniature cellular components. These little organs of the cell are referred to as **cytoplasmic organelles.** They consist of tiny tubules (small tubes), vesicles (small cavities or sacs containing liquid), granules (small insoluble nonmembranous particles found in cytoplasm), and fibrils (minute fibers or strands that are frequently part of a compound fiber). Together these structures perform the various functions of the cell in a systematized way. DNA, which is located outside of the cytoplasm, determines the function of each cytoplasmic organelle, and RNA carries the instructions into the cytoplasm.

Endoplasmic reticulum

The **endoplasmic reticulum (ER)** is a vast irregular network of tubules and vesicles spreading and interconnecting in all directions throughout the cytoplasm. It enables the cell to communicate with the extracellular environment and transfer food from one part of the cell to another. Thus the ER functions as the highway system of the cell. For example, mRNA travels from the nucleus to different locations in the cytoplasm through the endoplasmic reticulum.

Cells have two types of ER: rough surfaced (granular) and smooth (agranular). If ribosomes (small, spherical organelles that attach to the ER) are present on the surface of the endoplasmic reticulum, the surface is rough or granular. If they are not present, the surface is smooth or agranular. This observation can be made on viewing various types of cells through an electron microscope. The cell type determines the type of ER. For example, cells that actively manufacture proteins for export such as the pancreatic cells, which produce insulin, have a lot of rough or granular ER. A lesser amount of rough or granular ER is found in cells that synthesize proteins mainly for their own use.

Golgi apparatus or complex

The Golgi apparatus or complex extends from the nucleus to the cell membrane and consists of tubes and tiny sacs located near the nucleus. It unites large carbohydrate molecules and then combines them with proteins to form glycoproteins. When the cell manufactures enzymes and hormones, the Golgi apparatus concentrates, packages, and transports them through the cell membrane so that they can exit the cell, enter the bloodstream, and be carried to the areas of the body at which they are required.

Mitochondria

Large, bean-shaped structures called **mitochondria** function as the "powerhouses" of the cell. They contain highly organized enzymes in their inner membranes that produce energy for cellular activity by breaking down nutrients through a process of oxidation. Oxidation is the combining of a substance with oxygen. The oxidation of iron produces iron oxide, commonly known as rust. The definition of oxidation, however, has been broadened to include reactions in which electrons are lost by an atom. Some of the enzymes combined in the mitochondria are essential in the production of **adenosine triphosphate (ATP),** a high-energy–releasing phosphate compound essential for sustaining life. This compound plays a role in active transport within the cell. In active transport, molecules are moved through cell membranes regardless of the relative concentrations of particles. This requires energy, which is supplied by ATP.

The number of mitochondria in cells varies from a few hundred to several thousand. The greatest number are found in cells exhibiting the greatest activity.

Lysosomes

Lysosomes are small pealike sacs that are of great importance for digestion within the cytoplasm. They contain a group of different enzymes, and their primary function appears to be the breaking down of large molecules that either penetrate into the cell through microscopic channels or are drawn in by the cell membrane itself. If lysosomes fail in their cellular "garbage disposal" tasks, the resulting accumulation of large molecules may lead to obstruction of normal functions in organs. Lysosomes are sometimes referred to as "suicide bags," because the enzymes they contain can break down and digest not only proteins and certain carbohydrates, but also the cell itself when the lysosome's surrounding membrane breaks. Exposure to radiation may induce such a rupture. When this occurs, the cell dies.

Ribosomes

Ribosomes are small spherical organelles that attach to the endoplasmic reticulum. They consist of two thirds RNA and one third protein. Ribosomes are commonly referred to as the cell's "protein factories" because their job is to manufacture (synthesize) the various proteins that cells require using the blueprints provided by mRNA.

Centrosomes

Centrosomes are located in the center of the cell near the nucleus. They contain the centrioles, which are pairs of small, hollow, cylindrical structures believed to play a part in the formation of the mitotic spindle during cell division. Cell division is discussed later in this chapter.

Nucleus

Separated from the other parts of the cell by a double-walled membrane (nuclear envelope), the **nucleus** forms the heart of the cell. It is a spherical mass of protoplasm containing the genetic material, DNA. The nucleus also contains a rounded body called the nucleolus, which holds a large amount of RNA. The nucleus controls cell division and multiplication and the biochemical reactions that occur within the cell. By directing protein synthesis, the nucleus plays an essential role in active transport, metabolism, growth, and heredity. A summary of cell components may be found in Table 5-1.

Cell Division

Cell division is the multiplication process whereby one cell divides to form two or more cells. Mitosis and meiosis are the two types of cell division that occur in the body. When **somatic cells** (all cells in the human body except the germ cells) divide, they undergo mitosis. Genetic cells (the oogonium, or the female germ cell, and the spermatogonium, or the male germ cell) undergo meiosis.

Mitosis (M)

Through the process of **mitosis (M)** (Fig. 5-8), a parent cell divides to form two daughter cells identical to the parent cell. This process results in an approximately equal distribution of all cellular material between the two daughter cells. The **cellular life cycle** may be pictured as in Fig. 5-9. Different phases of cell growth, maturation, and division occur in each cell cycle. Four distinct phases of the cellular life cycle are identifiable: M, G_1, S, and G_2. Additionally, mitosis can be divided into four subphases: prophase, metaphase, anaphase, and telophase.

Mitosis is the division phase of the cellular life cycle. It is actually the last phase of the cycle. After it has commenced, it takes only about 1 hour to complete in all cells. Interphase, the period of cell growth that occurs before actual mitosis, consists of three phases: G_1, S, and G_2. G_1, the earliest phase, is the phase between reproductive events. It is the gap or interval in the growth of the cell that occurs between mitosis and DNA synthesis. Depending on the type of cells involved, this phase may take just a few minutes or it may take several hours. G_1 is designated as the pre-DNA–synthesis phase. During G_1 a form of RNA is synthesized in the cells that are to reproduce. This RNA is needed before actual DNA synthesis can efficiently begin. S is the actual DNA synthesis phase. While this phase is taking place, each DNA molecule

Table 5-1		
Summary of Cell Components		
Title	Site	Activity
Cell membrane	Cytoplasm	Functions as a barricade to protect cellular contents from their environment and controls the passage of water and other materials into and out of the cell; performs many additional functions such as elimination of wastes and refining of material for energy through breakdown of the materials
Endoplasmic reticulum	Cytoplasm	Enables the cell to communicate with the extracellular environment and transfers food from one part of the cell to another
Golgi apparatus	Cytoplasm	Unites large carbohydrate molecules and combines them with proteins to form glycoproteins and transports enzymes and hormones through the cell membrane so that they can exit the cell, enter the bloodstream, and be carried to areas of the body in which they are required
Mitochondria	Cytoplasm	Produce energy for cellular activity by breaking down nutrients through a process of oxidation
Lysosomes	Cytoplasm	Dispose of large particles such as bacteria and food as well as smaller particles; also contain hydrolytic enzymes that can break down and digest proteins, certain carbohydrates, and the cell itself if the lysosome's surrounding membrane breaks
Ribosomes	Cytoplasm	Manufacture the various proteins that cells require
Centrosomes	Cytoplasm	Believed to play some part in the formation of the mitotic spindle during cell division
DNA	Nucleus	Contains the genetic material, controls cell division and multiplication and also biochemical reactions that occur within the cell
Nucleolus	Nucleus	Holds a large amount of RNA

is copied and then divided (replicated) into corresponding daughter DNA molecules. The chromosome changes in shape from a figure with two **chromatids** (highly coiled duplicate strands of DNA) connected to a centromere (region on a chromosome serving as a junction point) to a figure with four chromatids connected to a centromere (Fig. 5-10). Two pairs of chromatids having exactly the same DNA substance and form result. When compared with phases G_1 and G_2, the S phase is relatively long. It takes a maximum of 15 hours. G_2 is the post-DNA–manufacturing interval in the cellular life cycle. It is a relatively short period occupying approximately 1 to 5 hours of the whole cycle. During this phase, cells manufacture certain proteins and RNA molecules needed to enter and complete the next mitosis. When G_2 is complete, cells enter the first phase of mitosis, the prophase, and the process of division commences.

Interphase

Interphase is the period of cell growth that occurs before actual mitosis. As previously stated, G_1, S, and G_2 are the phases of the cell cycle that compose interphase. Cells are not yet undergoing division during this phase. If a cell is viewed through a microscope during interphase, the nucleus looks somewhat odd. DNA may be visualized by using a specific stain designed to make it visible; it appears as clumps of material shaped in different patterns. These patterns are seen throughout the nucleus. Individual chromosomes are not visible during interphase. During the synthesis portion of interphase (S), each chromosome reproduces itself and splits longitudinally, forming two chromatids attached to each other at the centromere. Hence the cell's DNA molecules have duplicated in preparation for cell division. Genetic information also is transcribed into different kinds of RNA molecules

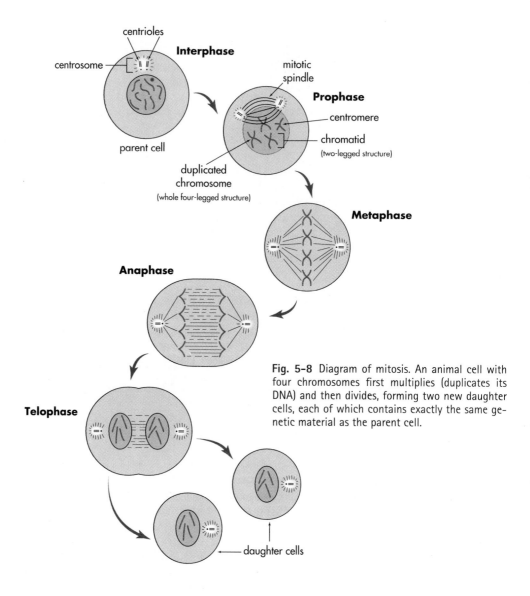

Fig. 5-8 Diagram of mitosis. An animal cell with four chromosomes first multiplies (duplicates its DNA) and then divides, forming two new daughter cells, each of which contains exactly the same genetic material as the parent cell.

such as mRNA and tRNA, which, after passing into the cytoplasm, translate the genetic information by promoting the synthesis of specific proteins.

Prophase

During **prophase** the nucleus enlarges, the DNA complex (the chromatid network of threads) coils up more tightly, and the chromatids become more visible on stained microscopic slides. Chromosomes enlarge, and the DNA begins to take structural form. The nuclear membrane disappears, and the centrioles (small hollow cylindrical structures) migrate to opposite sides of the cell and begin to regulate the formation of the **mitotic spindle,** the delicate fibers that are attached to the centrioles and extend from one side of the cell to the other.

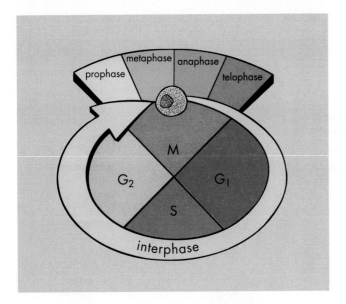

Fig. 5-9 The cellular life cycle may be pictured as four distinct, identifiable phases: M, G₁, S, and G₂. M may be divided into four subphases: prophase, metaphase, anaphase, and telophase. (From Bushong SC, *Radiologic science for technologists: physics, biology and protection*, ed 6, St Louis, 1997, Mosby.)

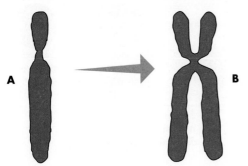

Fig. 5-10 While the S phase is taking place, the chromosome changes in shape from a figure with two chromatids connected to a centromere to a figure with four chromatids connected to a centromere. **A,** Two-chromatid figure. **B,** Four-chromatid figure.

Metaphase

As **metaphase** begins, the fibers collectively referred to as the mitotic spindle form between the centrioles. Each chromosome (which now consists of two chromatids) lines up in the center of the cell attached by its centromere to the mitotic spindle. This forms the equatorial plate. The centromeres then duplicate and each chromatid attaches itself individually to the spindle. At the end of metaphase the chromatids are strung out along the mitotic spindle much like laundry hung on a clothesline. During

metaphase, cell division can be stopped and chromosomes can be examined under a microscope. Chromosome damage caused by radiation can then be evaluated.

Anaphase

During **anaphase** the duplicate centromeres migrate in opposite directions along the mitotic spindle, carrying the chromatids to opposite sides of the cell.

Telophase

During **telophase** the chromatids undergo changes in appearance by uncoiling and becoming long, loosely spiraled threads. Simultaneously the nuclear membrane reforms and two nuclei (one for each new daughter cell) appear. The cytoplasm also divides near the equator of the cell to surround each new nucleus. After the completion of this cell division, each daughter cell contains exactly the same amount of genetic material (46 chromosomes) as the parent cell.

Meiosis

Meiosis (Fig. 5-11) is a special type of cell division that reduces the number of chromosomes in each daughter cell to half the number of chromosomes in the parent cell. Male and female germ cells, or sperm and ova, each begin meiosis with 46 chromosomes.

MEIOSES

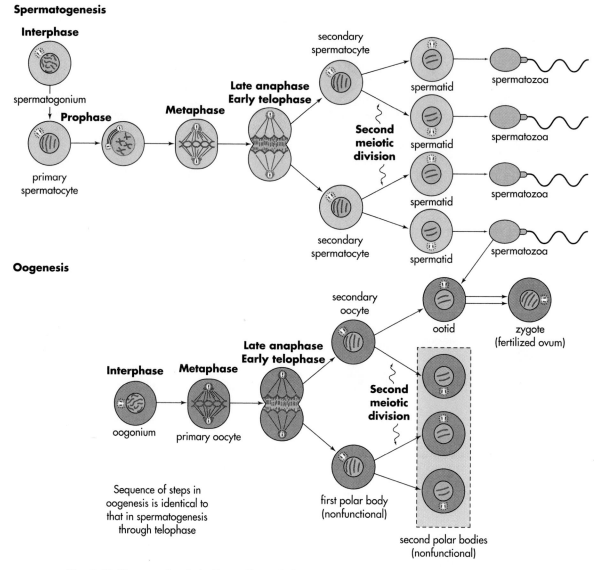

Fig. 5-11 Diagram of meiosis. Four cells result from one germ cell. In spermatogenesis, four spermatids become mature spermatozoa. In oogenesis, one ootid may be fertilized, and three second polar bodies remain nonfunctional.

However, before the male and female germ cells unite to produce a new organism, the number of chromosomes in each must be reduced by one half to ensure that the daughter cells (zygotes) formed when they unite will contain only the normal number of 46 chromosomes. Hence meiosis is really a process of **reduction division** (Fig. 5-12).

Paradoxically, meiosis begins with a doubling of the amount of genetic material; as in mitosis, DNA replication occurs during interphase. As a result of

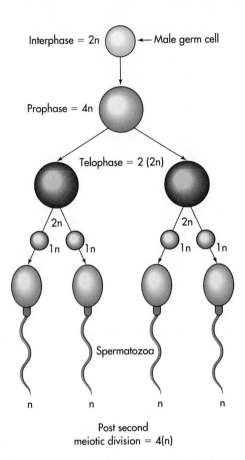

Interphase = 2n ← Male germ cell

Prophase = 4n

Telophase = 2 (2n)

2n   2n

1n   1n   1n   1n

Spermatozoa

n   n   n   n

Post second
meiotic division = 4(n)

Fig. 5-12 Meiosis is a process of reduction division. If *n* represents the number of chromosomes in a germ cell that is capable of uniting with another germ cell to produce a new organism, then *n* = 23 for a human being. Before meiosis the germ cell contains 2*n*, or 46, chromosomes.

DNA replication, each one-chromatid chromosome duplicates, forming a two-chromatid chromosome. This means that sperm and egg cells begin meiosis with twice the amount of genetic material as the original parent germ cell. Thus at the beginning of meiosis, the number of chromosomes increases from 2*n* to 4*n* (*n* = 23).

The various phases of meiosis are similar to those occurring in mitosis. The major difference between the two types of cell division begins at the end of the telophase. In meiosis, after the parent germ cell has formed two daughter cells, each of which (in hu-

man beings) contains 46 chromosomes, the daughter cells divide without DNA replication; chromosome duplication does not occur at this phase of division. These two successive divisions result in the formation of four granddaughter cells, each of which contains only 23 chromosomes. This means that the proper number of 46 chromosomes will be produced when a female ovum containing 23 chromosomes is fertilized by a male sperm containing 23 chromosomes.

During meiosis, the sister chromatids exchange some chromosomal material (genes). This process, called crossing over, results in changes in genetic composition and traits that can be passed on to future generations.

Summary

This chapter reviewed the fundamentals of cell biology. Cells, the basic units of all living matter, are the primary components of structure, growth, and life processes. They exist in many different forms and perform widely diverse functions to support the entire body. On the other hand the body must provide food, energy, and water to ensure efficient cell operation. When cellular function is normal, the body maintains homeostasis.

Cells are made of protoplasm, which consists of carbon-containing organic compounds, including proteins, carbohydrates, lipids (fats), and nucleic acids, and inorganic materials such as water and mineral salts. Proteins are essential for growth, the construction of new body tissue, and repair of injured or debilitated tissue. Characteristics carried by each individual cell are determined by the type of protein it contains. Specific structural and enzymatic proteins are formed when chromosomes and genes organize amino acids into proper sequences. Structural proteins provide the body with its shape and form and serve as a source of heat and energy. Enzymatic proteins control the cell's various physiologic activities. Proteins also may function as hormones and antibodies. As hormones they regulate body functions such as growth and development. As antibodies they function as the body's primary defense mechanism by attacking antigens such as bacteria and flu viruses.

Carbohydrates, or saccharides, include starches and various sugars. They function as short-term energy storers for the body. Their primary purpose is to provide fuel for cell metabolism. Lipids, or fats, are present in all body tissues. They act as reservoirs for the long-term storage of energy, insulate and guard the body against the environment, support and protect organs such as the eyes and kidneys, provide substances necessary for growth and development, and assist in the digestive process. The nucleic acids are deoxyribonucleic acid (DNA) and ribonucleic acid (RNA). The DNA macromolecule is formed by two long sugar-phosphate chains twisted around each other in a double helix configuration and linked by pairs of nitrogenous bases composed of adenine (A), cytosine (C), guanine (G), and thymine (T) at the sugar molecule. DNA contains all the information the cell needs to function. This master chemical carries the genetic information necessary for cell replication and regulates cellular activity to direct protein synthesis. It determines the characteristics of a person by regulating the sequence of amino acids while they are being manufactured. DNA regulates cellular activity such as growth and differentiation indirectly by reproducing itself in the form of messenger RNA (mRNA) to transmit its genetic information outside the cell nucleus. In turn, mRNA makes proteins from amino acids. The mRNA macromolecules carry their genetic codes from the cell nucleus to the ribosomes, where proteins are manufactured. Here they transfer their genetic codes to another kind of RNA molecule called transfer RNA (tRNA), which combines and transports individual amino acids from different areas of the cell to the ribosome, where the amino acids are arranged and attached in specific order to form chainlike protein molecules to meet the needs of the cells. Some proteins produced in the ribosomes are enzymes that initiate necessary reactions within the cell at the appropriate time. Repair enzymes mend damaged molecules, which can help cells recover from a small amount of radiation-induced damage.

Tiny DNA-containing rod-shaped bodies called chromosomes contain genes, the basic units of heredity. Genes control protein formation in every cell through the intricate process of genetic coding.

Water is the primary inorganic compound in the human body. It comprises approximately 80% to 85% of the body's weight. Chemical reactions that support metabolic activity occur in water. Water also dissolves chemical substances within the cell. Outside the cell, it serves as a transport vehicle for material the cell uses or eliminates. Water maintains body temperature at 98.6° F (37° C). Smaller quantities of mineral salts maintain the correct proportion of water in the cell. They support proper cell function, creation of energy, and conduction of impulses along nerves.

The normal cell has several components. The cell membrane encases and surrounds the cell, functions as a barricade to protect cellular contents from their environment, and controls the passage of water and other materials into and out of the cell. Cytoplasm is the portion of the cell outside the nucleus in which all metabolic activity occurs. The endoplasmic reticulum enables the cell to communicate with the extracellular environment and transport food from one part of the cell to another through its irregular network of tubules and vesicles throughout the cytoplasm. The Golgi apparatus or complex unites large carbohydrate molecules and then combines them with proteins to form glycoproteins. The powerhouses of the cell, the mitochondria, contain highly organized enzymes that produce energy for cellular activity. Lysosomes, which contain different enzymes important for digestion within the cytoplasm, break down large molecules. They function as cellular garbage disposals, but when exposed to radiation, they may rupture, resulting in cell death. Ribosomes are the cell's protein factories, synthesizing the various proteins that cells require. The nucleus forms the heart of the cell. A spherical mass of protoplasm containing DNA, it controls cell division and multiplication and biochemical reactions that occur within the cell.

Somatic cells divide through mitosis (M), a process whereby a parent cell divides to form two daughter cells identical to the parent cell. Genetic cells divide through the process of meiosis, a special type of cell division that reduces the number of chromosomes in each daughter cell to half the number of chromosomes in the parent cell. The cellular life cycle has four distinct phases: M, the division phase; G_1, the phase between reproductive events; S, the actual DNA synthesis phase; and G_2, the post-DNA manufacturing interval. Mitosis (M) may be divided into four subphases: prophase, the phase in which DNA begins to take structural form and the mitotic spindle begins to form; metaphase, the phase when the chromatids are strung out along the mitotic spindle; anaphase, the phase when the chromatids migrate to opposite sides of the cell; and telophase, the phase when the chromatids undergo changes in appearance and become new complete chromosomes. The various phases of meiosis are similar to those occurring in mitosis. The major difference between them occurs at the end of telophase. No DNA replication occurs. The next two successive divisions result in the formation of four granddaughter cells, each containing only half the number of chromosomes.

The reader should now be prepared to learn the ways in which cell structure, composition, and function may be adversely affected by exposure to ionizing radiation. Chapter 6 describes these adverse effects.

Review Questions

1. In a DNA macromolecule, the sequence of _____ determines the characteristics of every living thing.
   A. Sugars
   B. Phosphates
   C. Nitrogenous organic bases
   D. Hydrogen bonds

2. In the human cell, protein synthesis occurs in which of the following locations?
   A. Nucleus
   B. Mitochondria
   C. Ribosomes
   D. Endoplasmic reticulum

3. DNA regulates cellular activity indirectly by reproducing itself in the form of _____ to carry genetic information from the cell nucleus to ribosomes located in the cytoplasm.
   A. Messenger DNA
   B. Messenger RNA
   C. Messenger REM
   D. Transfer RNA

4. Which of the following is a process of reduction cell division?
   A. Mitosis
   B. Meiosis
   C. Molecular synthesis
   D. Amniocentesis

5. Human cells contain which four major organic compounds:
   A. Nucleic acids, water, protein, and mineral salts
   B. Mineral salts, carbohydrates, lipids, and proteins
   C. Carbohydrates, lipids, nucleic acids, and water
   D. Proteins, carbohydrates, lipids, and nucleic acids

6. Interphase consists of which of the following phases?
   A. M, G_1, and S
   B. G_1, S, and G_2
   C. S, G_2, and M
   D. G_2, M, and G

7. Radiation-induced chromosome damage may be evaluated during which of the following processes?
   A. Prophase
   B. Metaphase
   C. Anaphase
   D. Telophase

8. Which human cell component controls cell division and multiplication as well as biochemical reactions that occur within the cell?
   A. Endoplasmic reticulum
   B. Mitochondria
   C. Lysosomes
   D. Nucleus

9. Antibodies are produced by which of the following?
   A. Erythrocytes
   B. Lymphocytes
   C. Thrombocytes
   D. Platelets

10. Carbohydrates also may be referred to as which of the following?
    A. Lipids
    B. Nucleic acids
    C. Hormones
    D. Saccharides

11. Which of the following must the human body provide to ensure efficient cell operation?
    1. Food as a source of raw material for the release of energy
    2. Oxygen to help break down food
    3. Water to transport inorganic substances into and out of the cell
    A. 1 and 2 only
    B. 1 and 3 only
    C. 2 and 3 only
    D. 1, 2, and 3

12. Which of the following cellular organelles function as cellular garbage disposals?
    A. Endoplasmic reticulum
    B. Mitochondria
    C. Lysosomes
    D. Ribosomes

13. Which of the following are activities of the cell membrane?
    1. Protection of the cellular contents from their environment
    2. Control of the passage of water and other materials into and out of the cell
    3. Acceptance and processing of unrefined material
    A. 1 and 2 only
    B. 1 and 3 only
    C. 2 and 3 only
    D. 1, 2, and 3

14. The nuclear envelope that separates the nucleus from other parts of the cell is which of the following?
    A. A single membrane
    B. A double-walled membrane
    C. A triple-walled membrane
    D. A quadruple-walled membrane

15. The nucleolus contains which of the following?
    A. Centrosomes
    B. Ribonucleic acid
    C. Ribosomes
    D. Lysosomes

Bibliography

Anthony CP: *The textbook of anatomy and physiology,* ed 6, St Louis, 1963, Mosby.

Anthony CP, Thibodeau GA: *Textbook of anatomy and physiology,* ed 13, St Louis, 1989, Mosby.

Bovd W: *A textbook of pathology structure and function in disease,* ed 8, Philadelphia, 1970, Lea & Febiger.

Burke SR: *Human anatomy and physiology for the health sciences,* New York, 1980, John Wiley & Sons.

Bushong SC: *Radiologic science for technologists: physics, biology and protection,* ed 6, St Louis, 1997, Mosby.

Casarett AP: *Radiation biology,* Englewood Cliffs, NJ, 1968, Prentice-Hall.

Chabner DE: *The language of medicine,* Philadelphia, 1976, W.B. Saunders.

Crouch JE: *Functional human anatomy,* ed 4, Philadelphia, 1985, Lea & Febiger.

Crouch JE, McClintic JR: *Human anatomy and physiology,* ed 2, New York, 1976, John Wiley & Sons.

DeRobertis EDP, DeRobertis EMF: *Cell and molecular biology,* ed 8, Philadelphia, 1987, Lea & Febiger.

Frankel R: *Radiation protection for radiologic technologists,* New York, 1976, McGraw-Hill.

Hegner B: *Pathophysiology,* Long Beach, Calif, 1980, Elot.

Jacob SW, Francone CA, Lossow WJ: *Structure and function in man,* ed 4, Philadelphia, 1978, W.B. Saunders.

Mallett M: *A handbook of anatomy and physiology for students of medical radiation technology,* ed 3, Mankato, Minn, 1979, Burnell.

Memmler RL, Wood DL: *The human body in health and disease,* ed 4, Philadelphia, 1977, J.B. Lippincott.

Memmler RL, Wood DL: *Structure and function of the human body,* ed 2, Philadelphia, 1977, J.B. Lippincott.

Nourse AE, the editors of *Time-Life Books: The body,* Life Science Library, New York, 1968, Time-Life Books.

Pfeiffer J, the editors of *Time-Life Books: The cell,* Life Science Library, New York, 1964, Time-Life Books.

Ritenour ER: *Radiation protection and biology: a self-instructional multi-media learning series,* Denver, 1985, Multi-Media Publishing.

Selman J: *Elements of radiobiology,* Springfield, Ill, 1983, Charles C. Thomas.

Thomas CL, editor: *Taber's cyclopedic medical dictionary,* ed 13, Philadelphia, 1977, F.A. Davis.

Thompson MA et al: *Principles of imaging science and protection,* Philadelphia, 1994, W.B. Saunders.

Travis EL: *Primer of medical radiobiology,* ed 2, Chicago, 1989, Mosby.

6

Radiation Biology

Chapter Outline

aberrations (lesion or
    anomaly)
absolute risk
acute radiation syndrome
    (ARS)
apoptosis
biologic damage
biologic dosimetry
carcinogenesis
cell survival curve
chromosome breakage
desquamation
direct action
double-strand break
doubling dose
early (acute) somatic effects
epidemiologic studies
epilation
erythema
free radical
genetic effects
germ (reproductive) cells
hematopoietic syndrome
high-LET radiation
hypoxic cells
indirect effect
ionizing radiation

late somatic effects
LD 50/30
linear energy transfer (LET)
low-LET radiation
lymphocytes
mutagens
mutation
nonspecific life span short-
    ening
nonthreshold
oxygen enhancement ratio
    (OER)
point mutation
radiation biology
radiation dose-response
    relationship
radiosensitivity
relative biologic effective-
    ness (RBE)
relative risk
single-strand break
somatic cells
somatic effects
syndrome
target theory
threshold

*After completing this chapter, the reader will be able
to perform the following:*

- Define *radiation biology* and explain its relevance to radiation protection.
- Describe the way ionizing radiation damages living systems.
- List the three radiation energy transfer determinants and explain their individual concepts.
- Differentiate between the three levels of biologic damage that may occur in living systems as a result of exposure to ionizing radiation.
- Describe the process of direct and indirect action of ionizing radiation on the molecular structure of living systems.
- Draw a diagram to illustrate the various effects of ionizing radiation on a DNA macromolecule.
- Describe the effects of ionizing radiation on chromosomes.
- Explain the target theory.
- Describe the effects of ionizing radiation on the cell.
- Explain the purpose for and function of survival curves for mammalian cells.
- List the factors that affect cell radiosensitivity.
- State and describe the law of Bergonié and Tribondeau.
- Describe the effects of ionizing radiation on various types of cells.
- Explain the significance of organic damage resulting from exposure of living systems to ionizing radiation.
- Draw diagrams demonstrating the various radiation dose–response relationships.
- Identify the factors on which somatic and genetic damage depend.
- List and describe the various early (acute) somatic effects of ionizing radiation on living systems.
- Identify and describe the stages of acute radiation syndrome.
- Recall the LD 50/30 for human adults and explain its significance.
- Identify and describe the various late somatic effects of ionizing radiation on living systems.

Continued

Radiation biology is the branch of biology concerned with the effects of ionizing radiation on living systems. Areas of study included in this science are the sequence of events occurring after the absorption of energy from ionizing radiation, the action of the living system to make up for the consequences of this energy assimilation, and the injury to the living system that may be produced.

The human body is a living system composed of large numbers of various types of cells, most of which may be damaged by radiation. Because the potential harmful effects of ionizing radiation on living systems occur primarily on the cellular level, those who administer ionizing radiation to human beings for medical purposes should have a basic understanding of cell structure, composition, and function and the adverse effects on these of ionizing radiation. This chapter provides the reader with a basic knowledge of aspects of radiation biology relevant to the subject of radiation protection.

Ionizing Radiation

Ionizing radiation damages living systems by ionizing (removing electrons from) the atoms composing the molecular structures of these systems. X-ray and gamma-ray photons can impart energy to orbital electrons in atoms if the photons happen to pass near the electrons. High-energy charged particles such as alpha and beta particles and protons also may ionize atoms by interacting electromagnetically with orbital elec-

trons. The alpha particle, which is composed of two protons and two neutrons and therefore carries an electric charge of plus two, strongly attracts the negatively charged electron as it passes by.

Biologic damage, then, begins with the ionizations produced by various types of radiation. An ionized atom will not bond properly with the molecules necessary for the normal functioning of an organism.

Radiation Energy Transfer Determinants

Characteristics of ionizing radiation such as charge, mass, and energy vary among the different types of radiation. These attributes determine the extent to which different radiation modalities transfer energy into biologic tissue. To understand the way ionizing radiation causes injury or changes the severity of injury in biologic tissue, three important concepts must be studied:

1. Linear energy transfer (LET)
2. Relative biologic effectiveness (RBE)
3. Oxygen enhancement ratio (OER)

Linear energy transfer (LET)

When passing through a medium, ionizing radiation may interact with it during its passage and as a result deposit energy along its path. The average energy deposited per unit of path length is called **linear energy transfer (LET)**. LET is generally described in units of kiloelectron volts (keV) per micron (1 micron (μm) = 10^{-6} m). Because the amount of ionization produced in an irradiated object corresponds to the amount of energy it absorbs and because both chemical and biologic effects in tissue coincide with the degree of ionization experienced by the tissue, LET is an important factor in assessing potential tissue and organ damage from exposure to ionizing radiation.

LET radiations may be divided into two general categories: (1) low and (2) high. **Low-LET radiations** are external electromagnetic radiations such as x-rays and gamma rays (short-wavelength, high-energy waves emitted by the nuclei of radioactive substances) that have neither mass nor charge. These penetrating electromagnetic radiations are sparsely ionizing and interact randomly along their path length. They do not relinquish all their energy quickly. When these low-LET radiations interact with biologic tissues, they

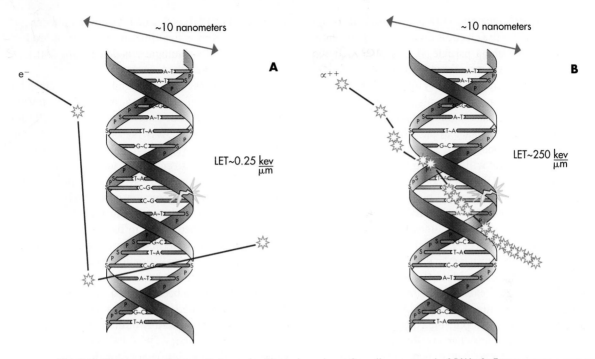

Fig. 6-1 Electron and alpha particle passing through nucleus of a cell near strand of DNA. **A,** For an electron, several interactions may occur in the vicinity of a DNA strand, creating a risk for damage to the DNA. **B,** Because so many interactions may occur in the vicinity of a DNA strand, some damage is likely.

cause damage primarily through an indirect action that involves the production of free radicals. Also, but much less likely, the radiation may directly induce single-strand breaks in the ladderlike deoxyribonucleic acid (DNA) structure. (These topics are discussed in detail later in this chapter.) Because low-LET radiation generally causes sublethal damage to DNA, repair enzymes can usually reverse the cellular damage.

High-LET radiation includes particles that possess substantial mass and charge. Some typical examples are alpha particles, ions of heavier nuclei, and charged particles released from interactions between neutrons and atoms. Low-energy neutrons, which carry no electrical charge, also are a form of high-LET radiation. All these lose energy more rapidly than low-LET radiations because they produce much more ionization per unit distance traveled. As a result, they exhaust their energy in a shorter path length and therefore cannot travel or penetrate as far.

Figure 6-1 shows an electon and an alpha particle passing through the nucleus of a cell in the vicinity of a strand of DNA. The size of the entire area is only about 10 nanometers (10 billionths of a meter, or 10 millionths of a millimeter). The electron represents either a Compton scattered electron or a photoelectron resulting from the interaction of a photon from a diagnostic x-ray beam. The alpha particle represents one of the particles ejected from the nucleus of an atom after radioactive decay of an element such as radon.

The parameter that describes the average energy deposited over small distances in the material is the LET. The presence of many more alpha particle interactions in the small region shown is reflected in the fact that the LET for the alpha particles shown in this example is 1000 times the LET of the electron. Each time the particle interacts, it loses some energy and slows down in the cell. When enough interactions have occurred, the particle comes to a stop and no further interactions take place. Thus because it does not interact as often, the electron may travel significantly farther than the alpha particle. A Compton scattered electron or photoelectron set in motion in a patient exposed to diagnostic x-rays may travel through thousands of cells (interacting in only some of them) with a low probability that a significant number of interactions will occur by chance in the DNA. An alpha particle such as the one shown may travel through only one or two cells but will have a high probability of interacting with the DNA of a cell it encounters.

For radiation protection, high-LET radiation is of greatest concern when internal contamination is possible—that is, when a radionuclide has been implanted, ingested, injected, or inhaled. Then the potential exists for irreparable damage because, with high-LET radiation, multiple-strand breaks in DNA are possible. For example, with a double-strand break in the same rung, of the DNA ladderlike structure, complete chromosome breakage occurs (see Figure 6-6, **A,** later in this chapter). Repair enzymes cannot undo this damage, and hence cell death will probably occur.

Relative biologic effectiveness (RBE)

Biologic damage produced by radiation escalates as the LET of radiation increases so that identical doses of radiations of various LETs do not render the same biologic effect. The **relative biologic effect (RBE)** describes the relative capability of radiations with differing LETs to produce a particular biologic reaction. RBE is the ratio of the dose of a reference radiation quality (conventionally 250 kVp x-rays) that is necessary to produce the same biologic reaction in a given experiment. The reaction is produced by a dose of the test radiation delivered under the same conditions. This is expressed as follows:

$$RBE = \frac{\text{Dose in Gy from 250 kVp x-rays (reference radiation)}}{\text{Dose in Gy of test radiation}}$$

Example: A biologic reaction is produced by 2 Gy of a test radiation. It takes 10 Gy of 250 kVp x-rays to produce the same biologic reaction. What is the RBE of the test radiation?

$$\frac{10}{2} = 5$$

The RBE is 5, which means that the test radiation is five times as effective in producing this biologic reaction as are 250 kVp x-rays.

Many researchers have determined RBE values for the various types of radiation, and their efforts toward this extremely difficult goal continue. The RBE for neutrons, in particular, has presented a special challenge. Because the various types of radiation differ in their biologic effectiveness per unit quantity of absorbed dose, the concept of RBE is not practical for specifying radiation protection dose levels. To overcome this limitation, the quality factor (QF), or modifying factor, has been used in the calculation of the dose equivalent to determine the ability of a dose of any kind of ionizing radiation to cause biologic damage. Quality factors are basically a measure of RBE. Typically, they have been selected conscientiously on the basis of measured values of the RBE of the radiation in question for a variety of biologic effects at low doses. In general a large QF is associated with a large value of RBE. (Quality factors for different types of ionizing radiations are listed in Table 3-1 of this text.)

Oxygen enhancement ratio (OER)

The **oxygen enhancement ratio (OER)** is the ratio of the radiation dose required to cause a particular biologic response of cells or organisms in an oxygen-deprived environment to the radiation dose required to cause an identical response under normally oxygenated conditions. This may be expressed as follows:

$$OER = \frac{\text{Radiation dose required to cause biologic response without } O_2}{\text{Radiation dose required to cause biologic response with } O_2}$$

The amount of cellular injury (e.g., lethality) for a species of ionizing radiation may be obtained by using this comparative measure.

In general, x-rays and gamma rays, which are low-LET radiations, have an OER of about 3.0 when the radiation dose is high. The OER may be less (about 2.0) when radiation doses are below 2 Gy (200 rads). Because high-LET radiations such as alpha particles produce their biologic effects from direct action—namely, direct ionization and disruption of biomolecules—the presence or absence of oxygen is of no consequence. Therefore the OER of high-LET radiation is approximately equal to 1. For low-LET radiation a significant fraction of bioeffects are caused by indirect actions in which a chemical species called a **free radical** (a solitary atom or usually a combination of atoms that behaves as an extremely reactive single entity) is formed. The free radicals dramatically increase the amount of biologic damage. (Both the direct and indirect action of radiation are discussed in detail later in this chapter.) However, the presence of oxygen in biologic tissues makes the damage produced by these free radicals permanent because oxygen reacts with free radicals to produce organic peroxide compounds, which represent nonrestorable changes in the chemical composition of the target material. Without oxygen, damage produced by the indirect action of radiation on a biologic molecule may be repaired, but when damage occurs through an oxygen-mediated process, the end result is permanent, or fixed. This phenomenon has been called *the oxygen fixation hypothesis.*

Molecular Effects of Irradiation

In living systems, **biologic damage** resulting from exposure to ionizing radiation may be observed on three levels: molecular, cellular, and organic. Any visible radiation-induced injuries to living systems at the cellular or organic level always begin with damage at the molecular level. Molecular damage results in the formation of structurally changed molecules that may impair cellular functioning.

Cells of the human body are highly specialized, with each cell having a predetermined task to perform; each cell's function is determined and defined by the structures of its constituent molecules. Because exposure to ionizing radiation can alter these structures, such exposure may disturb the cell's chemical balance and ultimately the way it operates. When this occurs, the cell no longer performs its normal tasks. If a sufficient quantity of **somatic cells** (*soma* is the Greek word for body; hence *somatic cells* refers to all cells in the body except the female and male germ cells) are affected, entire body processes may be disrupted. On the other hand, if radiation damages the **germ (reproductive) cells,** the damage may be passed on to future generations in the form of genetic mutations (changes in the genes). (More information pertaining to somatic and genetic effects are presented later in this chapter.)

When ionizing radiation interacts with a cell, ionizations and excitations (the addition of energy to a molecular system, which transforms it from a calm to an excited state) are produced in either vital biologic macromolecules (such as DNA) or water (H_2O), the medium in which the cellular organelles are suspended. Based on the site of the interaction the action of radiation on the cell is classified as either direct or indirect. For **direct action,** biologic damage occurs as a result of ionization of atoms on master, or key, molecules (DNA), which causes these molecules to become inactive or functionally altered. **Indirect action** involves the effects of reactive free radicals created by the interaction of radiation with water (H_2O) molecules. These agents can cause substantial disruption to master molecules, resulting in cell death.

Direct action may result after exposure to any type of radiation. However, direct action is much more likely to happen after exposure to high-LET radiations such as alpha particles, which produce countless ionizations in a very short distance of travel, rather than after exposure to low-LET radiations such as x-rays, which are sparsely ionizing.

Direct action

When ionizing particles interact directly with vital biologic macromolecules such as DNA, ribonucleic acid (RNA), proteins, and enzymes, damage to these molecules occurs from absorption of energy through photoelectric and Compton interactions. The ionization or excitation of the atoms of the biologic macromolecules results in breakage of the macromolecules' chemical bonds, causing them to become abnormal structures, which may in turn lead to inappropriate chemical reactions. When enzyme molecules are damaged by interaction with ionizing particles, essential biochemical processes may not occur in the cell at the appropriate time. For example, if an enzyme is inactivated, it will fail to elicit the appropriate biochemical reaction. Should this occur during the synthesis of a particular protein, the protein will not be manufactured, and if this protein was intended to perform a specific function, its nonexistence will hinder or prevent that function. In the event that other cell operations depend on the suppressed function, these operations sustain some type of damage as well. Thus a biologic chain reaction essentially occurs.

Radiolysis of water (interaction of radiation with H_2O)

X-ray photons may interact with and ionize water molecules contained within the human body. Such an interaction between an x-ray photon and a water molecule creates an ion pair consisting of a water molecule with a positive charge (HOH^+) and an electron (e^-). After the original ionization of the water molecule, several reactions may occur. One is that the positively charged water molecule (HOH^+) may recombine with the electron (e^-) to reform a stable water molecule ($HOH^+ + e^- = H_2O$). If this happens, no damage occurs. Alternately the electron (the negative ion) may join with another water molecule, producing a negative water ion ($H_2O + e^- = HOH^-$).

The positive water molecule (HOH^+) and the negative water molecule (HOH^-) are basically unstable. Hence they can break apart into smaller molecules. HOH^+ becomes a hydrogen ion (H^+) and a hydroxyl radical (OH^*), whereas HOH^- becomes a hydroxyl ion (OH^-) and a hydrogen radical (H^*). The asterisk symbolizes a free radical. A free radical is a configuration of either one or more atoms having no net electrical charge. This object is highly reactive because one of its constituents has an unpaired electron in the valence or outermost electron shell. Hence the interaction of radiation with water results in the formation of an ion pair, H^+ and OH^- (hydrogen ion and hydroxyl ion), and two free radicals, H^* and OH^* (a hydrogen radical and a hydroxyl radical) (Fig. 6-2).

Because the hydrogen and hydroxyl ions usually recombine to form a normal water molecule, the existence of these ions as free agents within the human body is insignificant in terms of biologic damage. The presence of hydrogen and hydroxyl free radicals, however, is not insignificant. As molecules containing an unpaired electron in their outer shell, they are chemically unstable and very reactive. They can produce undesirable chemical reactions and cause biologic damage by transferring their excess energy to other molecules, thereby either breaking these molecules' chemical bonds or at the very least creating point lesions (i.e., altered areas caused by the breaking of a single chemical bond) in the molecules. Approxi-

mately two thirds of all radiation-induced damage is believed to be ultimately caused by the hydroxyl free radical (OH^*). In addition, because free radicals have excess energy and can travel through the cell, they are capable of destructively interacting with other molecules located at some distance from their place of origin.

Hydrogen and hydroxyl radicals are not the only destructive substances that may be produced during the radiolysis of water. A hydroxyl radical (OH^*) may bond with another hydroxyl radical (OH^*) and form hydrogen peroxide ($OH^* + OH^* = H_2O_2$), a substance that is poisonous to the cell. Also, a hydroperoxyl radical (HO_2^*) is formed when a hydrogen free radical (H^*) combines with molecular oxygen (O_2). This radical and hydrogen peroxide are believed to be among the primary substances that produce biologic damage directly after the interaction of radiation with water.

Absorption of radiation also can cause a normal organic molecule (for simplicity, let us call it *RH*, where "H" stands for hydrogen and "R" can be some combination of other atoms) to form the free radicals, R* (an organic neutral free radical) and H*. Without oxygen or a force to attract an electron, these radicals can react with one another to reform the original organic molecule (RH). When oxygen is present, however, R* and H* may react with the oxygen to form the radicals RO_2^* and HO_2^*. Hence the organic molecule (RH) is destroyed. Moreover, the radicals RO_2^* and HO_2^* can react with other organic molecules to cause biologic damage. Thus a small-scale chain reaction of destructive events occurs that results from radiation depositing energy within tissue.

Indirect action

When free radicals previously produced by the interaction of radiation with water molecules act on a vital molecule such as DNA, the damaging action of ionizing radiation on the vital biologic macromolecule is indirect in the sense that the radiation is not the immediate cause of injury to the crucial biologic macromolecule. The byproducts of the radiation, the free radicals, are the immediate cause of this damage. Because water constitutes approximately 80% to 85% of the body's total weight, much more destructive chemical change results from indirect than from direct ac-

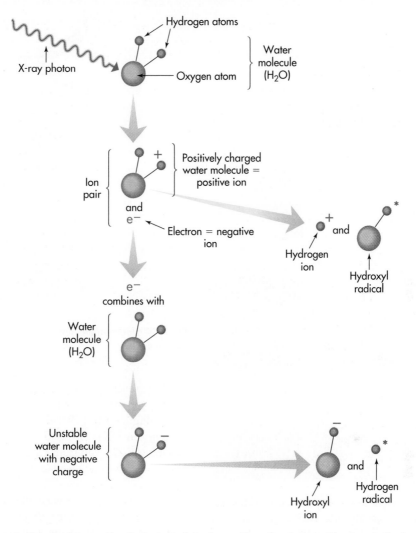

Fig. 6-2 Radiolysis of water. The final result of the interaction of radiation with water is the formation of an ion pair (H^+ and OH^-) and two free radicals (H^* and OH^*).

tion of ordinary ionizing radiation. In fact, about 95% of the effects of x-radiation and gamma radiation in macromolecules of living systems (in vivo) occur as a result of indirect action.

In summary the process of indirect action (Fig. 6-3) involves the breakdown of a water molecule into smaller molecules, producing both ions and free radicals in the process. As we have seen, the free radicals produced can recombine to form hydrogen peroxide, a cellular poison, and a hydroperoxyl radical, another

toxic substance. Both these agents are highly reactive and produce biologic damage. By themselves, free radicals may transfer excess energy to other molecules, thereby breaking their chemical bonds.

Effects of ionizing radiation on DNA macromolecules

If ionizing radiation interacts with a DNA macromolecule, the energy that can be transferred to that crucial macromolecule can rupture one of its chemical bonds,

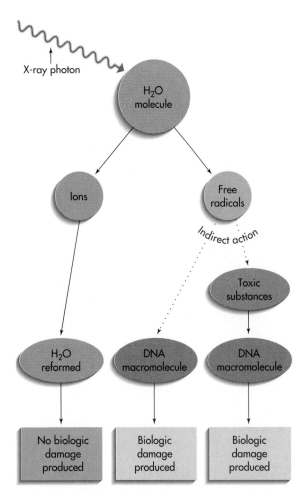

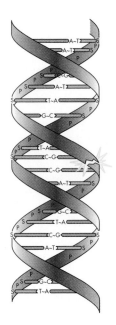

Fig. 6-4 Single-strand break in ladderlike DNA molecular structure.

Fig. 6-3 Indirect action of ionizing radiation on biologic molecules. X-ray photon interacts directly with a water (H_2O) molecule. The H_2O molecule breaks down into ions and free radicals. The ions can recombine to form a water molecule, thereby creating no biologic damage. The free radicals can migrate to another molecule, such as a DNA molecule located at some distance from the site of the initial ionization, and destructively interact with it by ionizing it or rupturing some chemical bonds. This creates molecular or point lesions in the DNA macromolecule. Free radicals can spread biologic damage by combining with other molecules to form toxic substances that also can migrate to distant DNA molecules and destructively interact.

possibly severing one of the sugar-phosphate chain siderails or strands of the ladderlike molecular structure **(single-strand break)** (Fig. 6-4). This type of injury to DNA is called a **point mutation.** Gene mutations may result from a single alteration along the sequence of nitrogenous bases. Point mutations commonly occur with low-LET radiations. Repair enzymes, however, may reverse this damage.

Further exposure of the affected DNA macromolecule to ionizing radiation may result in additional breaks in the sugar-phosphate molecular chain(s). These breaks also may be repaired, but **double-strand breaks** (one or more breaks in each of the two sugar-phosphate chains) (Fig. 6-5) are not repaired as easily as single-strand breaks. If repair does not take place, further separation may occur in the DNA chains, threatening the life of the cell. Double-strand breaks occur more commonly with densely ionizing (high-LET) radiations and often are associated with the loss or gain of one or more nitrogenous bases. When high-LET radiation interacts with DNA molecules, the ionization interactions may be so closely spaced that, by chance, both strands of the DNA chain are broken. If

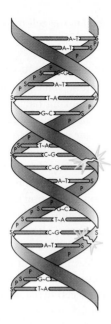

Fig. 6-5 A widely spaced double-strand break in the ladder-like DNA molecular structure.

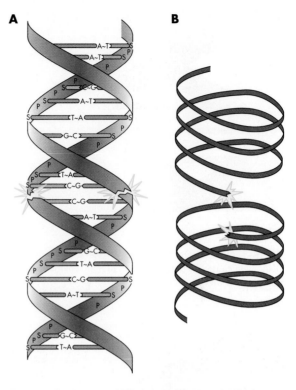

Fig. 6-6 Double-strand break in same rung of DNA ladder-like molecular structure **(A)** causes complete chromosome breakage, resulting in a cleaved or broken chromosome **(B).**

both strands are broken at the same nitrogenous base "rung," the result is the same as if both side rails of a ladder were cut at the same step or rung—the ladder would be cut into two pieces. If the DNA is cut into two pieces, the chromosome, which is composed of a long chain of twisted strands of DNA ladders, is itself broken. Thus some types of chromosomal damage that are particularly associated with high-LET radiation are related to double-strand breaks of DNA. Because the chance of repairing this damage is much slighter, the possibility of inducing a lethal alteration of nitrogenous bases within the genetic sequence is far greater.

When two interactions (hits), one on each of the two sugar-phosphate chains, occur within the same rung of the DNA ladderlike configuration (Fig. 6-6, A), the result is a cleaved or broken chromosome (Fig. 6-6, B), with each new portion containing an unequal amount of genetic material. If this damaged chromosome divides, each new daughter cell will receive an incorrect amount of genetic material. This will culminate in the death or impaired functioning of the new daughter cells.

In general, the interaction of high-energy radiation with a DNA molecule causes either a loss of or change in a nitrogenous base on the DNA chain. The direct consequence of this damage is an alteration of the base sequence (Fig. 6-7). Because the genetic information to be passed on to future generations is contained in the strict sequence of these bases, the loss or change of a base in the DNA chain is a **mutation.** It may not be reversible and may cause acute consequences for the cell, but more importantly, if the cell remains viable, incorrect genetic information will be transferred to one of the two daughter cells when the cell divides.

Covalent cross-links (chemical union created between atoms by the sharing of one or more pairs of electrons) involving DNA are another effect initiated by high-energy radiation. At low energies, however, covalent cross-links are probably caused by the

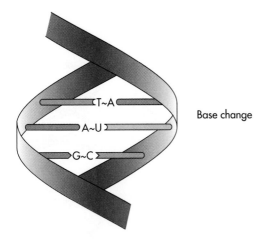

Fig. 6-7 Alteration of the nitrogen base sequence on the DNA chain caused by the interaction of high-energy radiation directly on a DNA molecule.

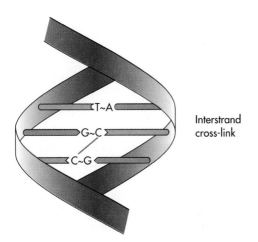

Fig. 6-8 Interstrand covalent cross-link produced by high-energy radiation interacting directly on a DNA molecule.

process of indirect action. A cross-link can form between two places on the same DNA strand. This joining is termed an *intrastrand cross-link*. Cross-linking also may occur between complementary DNA strands (Fig. 6-8) or between entirely different DNA molecules. These joinings are termed *interstrand cross-links*. Finally, DNA molecules also may become covalently linked to a protein molecule.[1] All these linkages

are potentially fatal to the cell if they are not properly repaired.

Effects of ionizing radiation on chromosomes

Large-scale structural changes in a chromosome brought about by ionizing radiation may be as grave for the cell as are radiation-induced changes in DNA. When changes occur in the DNA molecule, the chromosome exhibits the alteration. Because DNA modifications are discrete, they do not inevitably result in observable structural chromosome alterations.

After irradiation and during cell division, some radiation-induced chromosome breaks may be viewed microscopically. These alterations manifest themselves during the metaphase and anaphase of the cell division cycle, when the length of the chromosomes are visible. Because the events that have happened before these phases of cell division are not visible, they can only be assumed to have occurred. What can be seen, however, is the effect of these events, the gross or visible alterations in the structure of the chromosome. Both somatic cells and reproductive cells are subject to chromosome breaks induced by radiation.

After chromosome breakage, two or more chromosomal fragments are produced. Each of these fragments has a fractured extremity. These broken ends appear "sticky" and have the ability to adhere to another such sticky end. The broken fragments may rejoin in their original configuration, fail to rejoin and create an **aberration (lesion or anomaly),** or rejoin other broken ends and create new chromosomes that may not look structurally altered compared with the chromosome before irradiation.

Two types of chromosome anomalies have been observed at metaphase. They are called (1) chromosome aberrations and (2) chromatid aberrations. Chromosome aberrations happen when irradiation occurs early in interphase, before DNA synthesis takes place. In this situation the break caused by ionizing radiation is in a single strand of chromatin; during the DNA synthesis that follows, the resultant break is replicated when this strand of chromatin lays down an identical strand adjacent to itself, if repair is not completed before the start of DNA synthesis. Hence this leads to a chromosome aberration in which both chromatids exhibit the break. This break is visible at the next mitosis. Each daughter cell generated will have inherited a

A   B   C

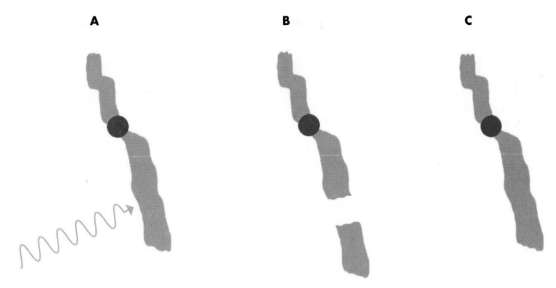

Fig. 6-9 The process of restitution, whereby the breaks rejoin in the original configuration with no visible damage. **A,** Chromosome break occurs because of a photon interaction. **B,** Fragment is fully separated from the rest of the chromosome. **C,** Broken fragment has reattached in its original location through the action of repair enzymes.

damaged chromatid as a consequence of a failure in the repair mechanism. Chromatid aberrations, on the other hand, result when irradiation of individual chromatids occurs later in interphase, after DNA synthesis has taken place. In this situation, only one chromatid of a pair might suffer a radiation-induced break. Therefore only one daughter cell is affected.

Ionizing radiation interacts randomly with matter. Because of this phenomenon, exposure to radiation produces a variety of structural changes in biologic tissue.

Some of these changes are as follows:
- A single-strand break in one chromosome
- A strand break in one chromatid
- A single-strand break in separate chromosomes
- A strand break in separate chromatids
- More than one break in the same chromosome
- More than one break in the same chromatid
- Chromosome stickiness, or clumping together

These structural changes may result in one of the following consequences to the cell:

1. Restitution, whereby the breaks rejoin in their original configuration with no visible damage (Fig. 6-9, *A-C*). In this case no damage to the cell occurs because the chromosome has been restored to the condition it was in before irradiation. The process of healing by restitution is believed to be the way in which 95% of single-chromosome breaks mend.[1]

2. Deletion, whereby a part of the chromosome or chromatid is lost at the next cell division, creating an aberration known as an acentric fragment (Fig. 6-10, *A-C*).

3. Broken-end rearrangement, whereby a grossly misshapen chromosome may be produced. Ring chromosomes, dicentric chromosomes, and anaphase bridges are examples of such distorted chromosomes (Fig. 6-11, *A-G*).

4. Broken-end rearrangement without visible damage to the chromosome, whereby the chromosome's genetic material has been rearranged even though the chromosome appears normal. Translocations are an example of such rearrangements (Fig. 6-12, *A* and *B*). Changes such as these inevitably result in mutation because the position of the genes on the chromosomes have been rearranged, thus altering the heritable characteristics of the cell.

A   **B**   **C**

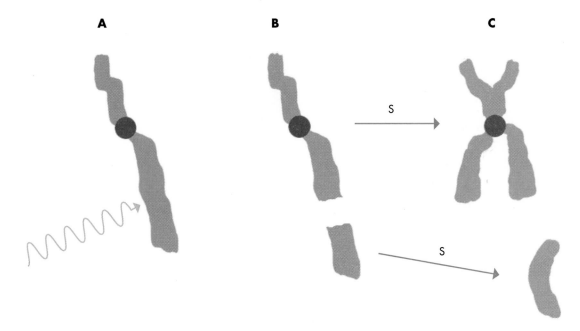

Fig. 6-10 The process of deletion, in which a part of a chromosome is lost at the next cell division, creating an acentric fragment. **A,** Chromosome break results from a photon interaction. **B,** Fragment is fully separated from the rest of the chromosome. **C,** After the next DNA synthesis phase of the cell cycle (labeled *S*), the remainder of the chromosome has been replicated normally but with fragments missing from the two arms of the chromosome. The replicated fragment is acentric, a section of genetic material without a centromere.

Target theory

Amid the many different types of molecules that lie within the cell, a master, or key, molecule that maintains normal cell function also is believed to be present. This master molecule is necessary for the survival of the cell. Because this molecule is unique in any given cell, no similar molecules in the cell are available to replace it; if the master molecule is inactivated by exposure to radiation, the cell will die (Fig. 6-13, *A* and *B*). Experimental data strongly support this concept and indicate that DNA is the irreplaceable master, or key, molecule that serves as the vital target.

Destruction of some of the molecules that are plentiful in the cell does not result in cell death. The reason for this is simply that cells have an abundance of similar molecules to take over and perform necessary functions for them in the event of their demise. If only a few nonDNA cell molecules are destroyed by radia-

tion exposure, the cell will probably not show any evidence of injury after irradiation.

In its passage through the molecular structures of living systems, radiation does not seek out master molecules in cells to destroy them; it interacts with these key molecules only by chance. The fundamental reason the cell is so sensitive to inactivation of its master molecule by radiation is that this molecule plays an absolutely essential role in directing the life support mechanisms of the cell. The **target theory** may be used to explain cell death and nonfatal cell abnormalities caused by radiation exposure.

Interactions between ionizing radiation and molecular targets such as DNA occur through both direct and indirect action. Determining which of the two types of effects or actions has been at work in any given case of cell death is virtually impossible, however.

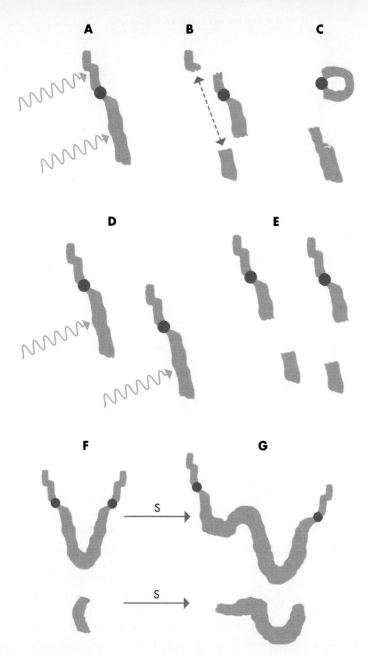

Fig. 6-11 The process of broken-end rearrangement may result in grossly misshapen chromosomes. **A,** Two chromosome breaks occur in a single chromosome as a result of the interactions of two photons. **B,** The fragments from opposite ends unite before DNA synthesis phase. **C,** The ends of the chromosome that are still attached to the centromere also unite, forming a "ring" chromosome. **D,** Chromosome breaks occur in two different chromosomes. **E,** The fragments are fully separated from the rest of their respective chromosomes. **F,** The ends of the chromosomes and the ends of the fragments have joined before DNA synthesis, forming a dicentric (two centromeres) and an acentric (no centromere) fragment. **G,** After DNA synthesis (labeled *S*), the chromosome is elongated but cannot split in two. The two centromeres are "bridged." This type of chromosomal damage leads to reproductive death of the cell (i.e., it cannot replicate or divide into two cells).

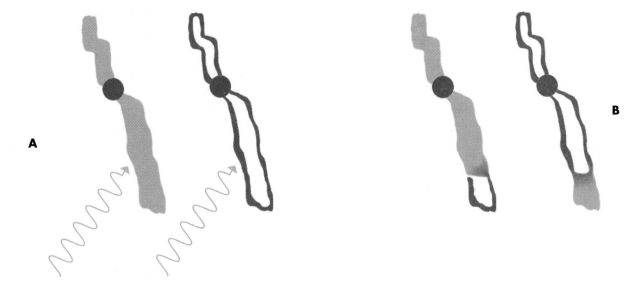

Fig. 6-12 The process of broken-end rearrangement may result in no visible damage to the chromosome, although the chromosome's genetic material has been rearranged—a result that will drastically alter its function within the cell, probably leading to cell death or failure to replicate.

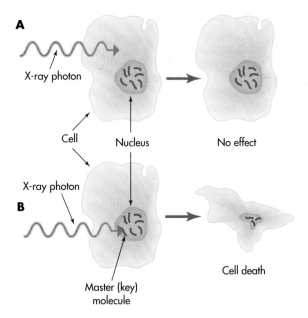

Fig. 6-13 The target theory holds that the cell will die after exposure to ionizing radiation only if the master, or key, molecule (DNA) is inactivated in the process. **A,** X-ray photon passes through the cell without interacting with the master molecule, which is located in the cell nucleus; no measurable effect results. **B,** X-ray photon enters the nucleus and interacts with and inactivates the master molecule; the cell dies as a result.

Cellular Effects of Irradiation

Ionizing radiation can adversely affect the cell. Damage to the cell's nucleus reveals itself in one of the following ways:

1. Instant death
2. Reproductive death
3. Apoptosis, or programmed cell death (interphase death)
4. Mitotic, or genetic, death
5. Mitotic delay
6. Interference of function
7. Chromosome breakage

Instant death

Instant death of large numbers of cells occurs when a volume is irradiated with an x-ray or gamma-ray dose of about 1000 Gy (100,000 rad) in a period of seconds or a few minutes. This large influx of energy causes gross disruption of cellular form and structure and severe changes in chemical machinery. As a result of receiving such a massive dose of ionizing radiation, a cell's DNA macromolecule breaks up and cellular proteins rapidly coagulate. Radiation doses high enough to cause this type of damage are vastly greater than those used for diagnostic examinations or even therapeutic treatments.

Reproductive death

Reproductive death generally results from exposure of cells to moderate doses of ionizing radiation (1 to 10 Gy or 100 to 1000 rad). Although the cell does not die when reproductive death occurs, it permanently loses its ability to procreate. Even though the cell has lost its reproductive capacity, it continues to metabolize and synthesize nucleic acids and proteins. The termination of cells' reproductive abilities does, however, prevent the transmission of damage to future generations of cells.

Apoptosis, or programmed cell death (interphase death)

A nonmitotic, or nondivision, form of cell death that occurs when cells die without attempting division during the interphase portion of the cell life cycle is termed *apoptosis*, or *programmed cell death*. This was formerly called *interphase death*. Apoptosis occurs spontaneously in both normal tissue and tumors in human beings and other vertebrate animals and amphibians, in the embryo and in the adult. An example of this process is the sequence of events during embryonic development whereby tadpoles lose their tails.

Certain types of programmed cell death are integral to the development and maintenance of organisms. Many types of cells are destined to die for the good of the organism. Tadpoles lose their tails and human beings lose webbing between their digits during embryonic development. All through life, human skin cells die and form the protective outer coating we usually refer to as *skin*. In apoptosis the cell shrinks and produces tiny membrane-enclosed structures called *blebs*. The cell nucleus and then the cell itself break up, and its fragments are usually ingested by other neighboring cells.

Researchers believe apoptosis may be instigated by radiation under some circumstances. The mechanisms of apoptosis and its relationship to radiosensitivity are areas of active research in radiobiology as of this writing. A new type of radiation therapy may involve activation of the genes that regulate apoptosis so that the occurrence of apoptosis becomes much more likely after irradiation in a tumor.

Radiosensitivity of the individual cell governs the dose required to cause apoptosis; the more radiosensitive the cell, the smaller the dose required to cause apoptotic death during interphase. A few hundred centigray (rad) can kill very sensitive cells such as lymphocytes or spermatogonia. Programmed cell death of less radiosensitive cells such as those in bone may require radiation doses of several thousand centigray (rad).

Mitotic, or genetic, death

Ionizing radiation can adversely affect cell division. It may retard the mitotic process or permanently inhibit it; cell death follows permanent inhibition. Mitotic, or genetic, death occurs when a cell dies after one or more divisions. Even relatively small doses of radiation can cause this type of cell death. The radiation dose required to produce mitotic death is less than the dose needed to produce interphase death in slowly dividing cells or nondividing cells.

Mitotic delay

Exposing a cell to as little as 0.01 Gy (1 rad) of ionizing radiation just before it begins dividing can cause mitotic delay, the failure of the cell to start dividing on time. After this delay the cell may resume its normal mitotic function. The underlying cause of this phenomenon is not known. Possible reasons for the delay may be (1) irradiation causing a chemical involved in mitosis to be altered, (2) proteins required for cell division not being synthesized, and (3) a change in the rate of DNA synthesis after irradiation.

Interference of function

Permanent or temporary interference of cellular function independent of the cell's ability to divide can be brought about by exposure to ionizing radiation. If repair enzymes are able to fix the damage, the cell can recover and continue to function.

Chromosome breakage

Chromosome breakage is a potential outcome when ionizing radiation interacts with a DNA macromolecule. These breaks may occur in one or both strands (sugar-phosphate chains) of the DNA ladderlike structure and have been discussed previously (see "Direct action").

If cells are irradiated during mitosis and chromosome breakage occurs, permanent chromosome abnormalities will be evident in future mitotic cycles. Because chromosome breakage results in a loss of genetic material, this may lead to genetic mutations in succeeding generations.

Survival Curves for Mammalian Cells

Cells vary in their radiosensitivity. This fact is particularly important in determining the types of cancer cells that will respond to radiation therapy. A classic method of displaying the sensitivity of a particular type of cell to radiation is the **cell survival curve.**[2] Some examples of cell survival curves are shown in Fig. 6-14. A cell survival curve is constructed from

data obtained by a series of experiments. First the cells are made to grow "in culture," meaning in a laboratory environment such as a petri dish. Then the cells are exposed to a specified dose of radiation. After radiation exposure the ability of the cells to divide, or form new "colonies" of cells, is measured. The fraction of cells that are able to form new colonies through cell division is then reported as the fraction of cells that have survived irradiation. The process is repeated for a range of radiation doses, and the results are graphed with the log of the surviving fraction on the vertical axis and the dose on the horizontal axis. Fig. 6-14 shows two curves, one for high-LET radiation and one for low-LET radiation. The curve for low-LET radiation shows very little change in survival at low doses, followed by a linear portion in which survival decreases in regular proportions at higher doses. This indicates that at low doses the cell is able to find and repair some of the damage. At higher doses the repair mechanism is overwhelmed. For the high-LET cell survival curve, no shoulder exists. If damage occurs, it is usually so extensive as to be irreparable.

Cell Radiosensitivity

The human body is composed of different types of cells and tissues, which vary in their degree of **radiosensitivity.** Immature cells are nonspecialized (undifferentiated) and undergo rapid cell division, whereas more mature cells are specialized in their function (highly differentiated) and divide at a slower rate or else do not divide. These factors affect the cells' degree of radiosensitivity. Examples of radiosensitive cells include basal cells of the skin, intestinal crypt cells, and reproductive cells. Radioinsensitive cells include brain, muscle, and nerve cells. Because combinations of both immature and mature cells in various ratios form the different body tissues and organs, radiosensitivity varies from one tissue and organ to another.

When ionizing radiation interacts with cell atoms and molecules, the amount of radiation energy transferred (absorbed in the tissue) plays a major role in determining the amount of the biologic response. As LET increases (as the radiation transfers more energy per unit length of travel), the ability of the radiation to

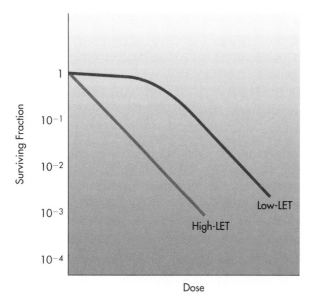

Fig. 6-14 Cell survival curves for the same cell line irradiated with both low- and high-LET radiation. For low-LET radiation a "shoulder" to the curve at lower doses indicates the cell's ability to repair some damage at low doses. High-LET radiation typically has no shoulder, indicating that little or no repair takes place.

cause biologic effects also generally increases until it reaches a maximal value. Hence LET affects cell radiosensitivity.

As addressed earlier in this chapter, oxygen enhances the effects of ionizing radiation on biologic tissue by increasing tissue radiosensitivity. If oxygen is present when a tissue is irradiated, more free radicals (which possess the ability to attack and damage organic molecules) are formed in the tissue; this increases the indirect damage potential of the radiation.

During diagnostic radiologic procedures, fully oxygenated human tissues are exposed to x-radiation. However, diagnostic radiologic and nuclear medicine procedures employ low doses of radiations (x-rays and/or gamma rays) that also are low in LET. Consequently, very few cells are killed by the radiations used in these procedures.

In radiotherapy the presence of oxygen plays a significant role in radiosensitivity. When radiation is used to treat certain types of cancerous tumors, high-pressure (hyperbaric) oxygen has sometimes been used in conjunction with it to increase tumor radiosensitivity. Cancerous tumors often contain **hypoxic cells** (cells that lack an adequate amount of oxygen) in addition to normally aerated cells. These hypoxic cells severely inhibit the indirect mechanism of radiation interaction with cells and therefore are radioresistant (particularly to low-LET radiations); hence they are more difficult to destroy than normally oxygenated cells. When oxygen tensions in capillaries are increased by hyperbaric oxygenation, hypoxic cells may reoxygenate and become sensitive to radiation; consequently, their chances of being destroyed by therapeutic radiation increase. Radiosensitization also may be accomplished with chemical enhancing agents such as misonidazole.[3]

Law of Bergonié and Tribondeau

In 1906, two French scientists, J. Bergonié and L. Tribondeau, established the following law: "The radiosensitivity of cells is directly proportional to their reproductive activity and inversely proportional to their degree of differentiation." This means that the most pronounced radiation effects occur in cells having the least maturity and specialization or differentiation, the greatest reproductive activity, and the longest mitotic phases. This law is true for all types of cells in the human body. Consequently, within the realm of diagnostic radiology, the embryo-fetus, which contains a large number of immature, nonspecialized cells, is more susceptible to radiation damage than is the child or the adult.

Effects of ionizing radiation on various types of cells

Equal doses of ionizing radiation produce different degrees of damage in different kinds of human cells because of differences in cell radiosensitivity. The more mature and specialized in performing specific functions a cell is, the less sensitive it is to radiation. In the following sections the radiation response of some of the most important cell groups is examined in detail.

Blood cells

Ionizing radiation adversely affects blood cells by depressing the number of cells in the peripheral circulation. A whole-body dose of 0.25 Gy (25 rad) produces measurable hematologic depression within a few days. This dose by far exceeds normal doses sustained by the working population of the radiation industry. Therefore the use of blood tests for purposes of dosimetry are not valid.

Most blood cells are manufactured in bone marrow. Radiation causes a decrease in the number of immature blood cells (stem, or precursor, blood cells) produced there and hence a reduction, ultimately, of the number of mature blood cells in the bloodstream. The higher the radiation dose received by the bone marrow, the greater the severity of the resulting cell depletion.

If the bone marrow cells have not been destroyed by exposure to ionizing radiation, they can repopulate after a period of recovery. The time necessary for recovery depends on the severity of the radiation dose received. If a relatively low dose (below 1 Gy or 100 rad) of radiation is received, bone marrow repopulation occurs within a few weeks after irradiation. Moderate (1 to 10 Gy or 100 to 1000 rad) to high (10 or more Gy or 1000 or more rad) doses, which severely deplete the number of bone marrow cells, require a longer recovery period. Very high doses of radiation can cause a permanent decrease in the number of stem cells.

Radiation affects primarily the stem cells of the hematopoietic (blood-forming) system. Erythrocytes (precursors of red blood cells) are among the most sensitive of human tissues. As with all cells that transform from an immature, undifferentiated state to a mature functional state, the mature red blood cells are much less radiosensitive. Because the population of circulating red blood cells is high and their life span long, depletion of red cells is not usually the cause of death in high-dose (i.e., several Gy delivered to the whole body) irradiation. Death, if it occurs, is more typically caused by infection that cannot be overcome by the immune system because of the destruction of myeloblasts (precursors of granulocytes, a type of white blood cell) and internal hemorrhage resulting from destruction of megakaryoblasts (precursor of platelets).

Human beings who receive whole-body doses in excess of 5 Gy (500 rad) may die within 30 to 60 days because of effects related to initial depletion of the stem cells of the hematopoietic system. The use of antibiotics or isolation from pathogens in the environment (e.g., placing the patient in a sterile environment, feeding only sterilized food) has been shown to mitigate these effects in animals and human beings. Human beings, however, recover more slowly than do laboratory animals. Thus lethal dose in animals is usually specified as LD 50/30 (dose that produces death in 50% of the subjects within 30 days), and lethal dose in human beings is usually given as LD 50/60. In either case the lethal dose for human beings is generally estimated to be 3 to 4 Gy (300 to 400 rad) without treatment—higher if medical intervention is available.

White blood cells are collectively called *leukocytes*. A subgroup of this group of blood cells are **lymphocytes.** These cells defend the body against foreign antigens by producing antibodies to combat disease. Lymphocytes live only for about 24 hours, having the shortest life span of all the blood cells. Lymphocytes manufactured in bone marrow are the most radiosensitive blood cells in the human body. A radiation dose as low as 0.25 Gy (25 rad) is sufficient to depress the number of these cells present in the circulating blood.

When significant numbers of lymphocytes are damaged by radiation exposure, the body loses its natural ability to combat infection and becomes more susceptible to bacteria and viral antigens.

The normal white blood cell count for an adult ranges from 5000 to 10,000/mm^3 of blood. The number of lymphocytes present in circulating blood decreases when low doses of radiation (0.25 Gy or less or 25 rad or less) are received. At this dose level, complete blood cell recovery occurs shortly after irradiation. However, when a moderate dose of whole-body radiation (0.5 to 1 Gy or 50 to 100 rad) is received, the lymphocyte count decreases to zero within a few days. Full recovery generally requires a period of several months after the exposure.

Neutrophils, another kind of white blood cell, also play an important role in fighting infection. If radiation exposure causes a decrease in the number of these cells, a person's susceptibility to infection increases. A dose of 0.5 Gy (50 rad) of ionizing radiation can cause a reduction in the number of neutrophils present in the circulating blood. When they receive moderate doses of radiation, however, these cells decrease in number to the lowest level possible within a few weeks of irradiation. A few months after the exposure the number of neutrophils present in the blood returns to its original value.

Granulocytes are a scavenger-type of white blood cell that fight bacteria. They remain alive in the circulating blood for only a few days. These cells respond to irradiation by suddenly increasing in number. After this sudden increase the granulocytes decrease in number, rapidly at first and then more slowly. Depending on the dose of radiation received, these cells may fully repopulate within about 2 months after their irradiation.

Thrombocytes, or platelets, initiate blood clotting and prevent hemorrhage. They have a life span of about 30 days. The normal platelet count in the human adult ranges from 150,000 to 350,000/mm^3 of blood. A dose of radiation greater than 0.5 Gy (50 rad) lessens the number of platelets in the circulating blood, but when exposed in the 1 to 10 Gy (100 to 1,000 rad) range, these cells only begin to regain their original numbers approximately 2 months after being irradiated.

Neither the blood nor the blood-forming organs of patients should suffer appreciable damage from radiation exposure received during diagnostic radiologic procedures. However, numerous studies indicate chromosome aberrations in circulating lymphocytes that received radiation doses within the diagnostic radiology range. Prime candidates for such aberrations are those in whom high-level fluoroscopy was employed and those in whom very long fluoro exposure times occurred (e.g., cardiac catheterization).

A therapeutic dose of ionizing radiation causes a decrease in the blood count. Patients who are undergoing radiation therapy treatment are monitored frequently (in the form of weekly or biweekly blood counts) to determine whether the platelet count is adequate.

As previously discussed, a periodic blood count is not recommended as a method for monitoring occupational radiation exposure because biologic damage has already been sustained when an irregularity is seen in the blood count. Because one objective of radiation monitoring is to discover elevated exposure levels before they present a biologic hazard, blood count results are not as useful as other methods. Also, blood count is a relatively insensitive test that is unable to indicate exposures of less than 10 cGy (10 rad). Film badge dosimeters (see Chapter 9) detect exposures in the milliroentgen range and may therefore be used to discover potentially hazardous working conditions before actual hazards appear.

Epithelial tissue

Epithelial tissue lines and covers body tissue. The cells of these tissues lie close together, with little or no substances between them. Epithelial tissue contains no blood vessels, and it regenerates through the process of mitosis. These cells are found in the lining of the intestines, mucous lining of the respiratory tract, pulmonary alveoli, and lining of blood and lymphatic vessels. Because epithelial tissue is constantly being regenerated by the body, the cells that compose this tissue are highly radiosensitive.

Muscle tissue

Muscle tissue contains fibers that affect movement of an organ or part of the body. Because muscle tissue

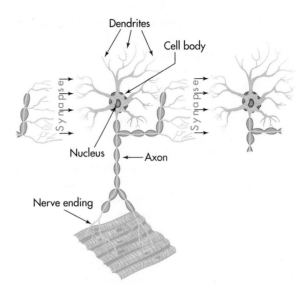

Fig. 6-15 A nerve cell (neuron). Nerve cells relay messages to and from the brain. A message enters a nerve cell through its dendrites, passes through the cell body, and exits the cell through the axon, which transmits the message across a synapse, the communication area leading to the next nerve cell in the chain.

cells are highly specialized and do not divide, they are relatively insensitive to radiation.

Nervous tissue

Nervous tissue (conductive tissue) is found in the brain and spinal cord. A nerve cell (neuron) (Fig. 6-15) consists of a cell body and two kinds of processes (very fine stringlike tissue segments that extend outward), dendrites (processes extending from the cell body that carry impulses toward it), and an axon (a long single process extending from the cell body that carries impulses away from it). Nerve cells relay messages to and from the brain. A message enters the nerve cell through the dendrites. It passes through the cell body and exits the cell through the axon, which transmits the message across a synapse, the communication area leading to the next nerve cell in the chain.

In the adult, nerve cells are highly specialized. They perform specific functions for the body and, similar to muscle cells, do not divide. Nerve cells contain a nucleus. If the nucleus of one of these cells is destroyed, the cell dies and is never restored. If the cell nucleus has been damaged but not destroyed by exposure to radiation, the damaged nerve cell may still be able to function; however, its function may be partially impaired. Radiation also can cause temporary or permanent damage to a nerve's processes (dendrites and axon). When this occurs, communication with and control of some areas of the body may be disrupted. Whole-body exposure to very high doses of radiation causes severe damage to the central nervous system. A single exposure in excess of 50 Gy (5000 rad) of ionizing radiation in humans may lead to death within a few hours or days after irradiation.

Developing nerve cells in the embryo-fetus are more radiosensitive than the mature nerve cells of the adult. Irradiation of the embryo may lead to central nervous system anomalies, microcephaly (small head circumference), and mental retardation. The Japanese atomic bomb survivors provide strong evidence of a "window of maximal sensitivity" extending from 8 to 15 weeks after gestation. This time span covers the end of the period of neuronal organogenesis, a period of development and change of the nerve cells, and extends into the beginning of the fetal period. A lower level of risk remains until week 25, at which time the risk is not found to be significantly different than for young adults. During the window of maximal sensitivity a 0.1 Sv (10 rem) fetal dose is associated with as much as a 4% risk of mental retardation. This level of risk is considered significant compared with the normal risks of pregnancy. Therefore special consideration is given to the irradiation of the abdomen or pelvis of a pregnant patient, particularly during the window of maximal sensitivity. However, the fetal dose associated with routine abdominal fluoroscopy is generally less than 0.05 Sv (5 rem). Thus if the referring physician and radiologist believe that the diagnostic study is vital to the medical management of the mother or offspring, the risk associated with radiation exposure may be justified.

Reproductive cells

Human reproductive cells (germ cells) are relatively radiosensitive, although the exact responses of male and female germ cells to ionizing radiation differ because their processes of development from immature to mature states differ. The male testes contain both mature and immature spermatogonia. Because the mature spermatogonia are specialized and do not divide, they are relatively insensitive to ionizing radiation. The immature spermatogonia, however, are unspecialized and divide rapidly; these germ cells are extremely radiosensitive. A radiation dose of 2 Gy (200 rad) may cause temporary sterility for as long as 12 months, and a dose of 5 or 6 Gy (500 to 600 rad) may cause permanent sterility. Even small doses of ionizing radiation, doses as low as 0.1 Gy (10 rad), may depress the male sperm population. Male reproductive cells that have been exposed to a radiation dose of 0.1 Gy (10 rad) or more may cause genetic mutations in future generations. To prevent mutations from being passed on to offspring, males receiving this level of testicular radiation dose should refrain from unprotected sex for a few months after such an exposure. By that time, cells that were irradiated during their most sensitive stages will have matured and disappeared. It should be noted that germ cells of patients undergoing diagnostic radiologic procedures almost never receive doses of as much as 0.1 Gy (10 rad). Medical radiographers, working under normal occupational conditions, would never receive a gonadal dose of this level.

The ova, the mature female germ cells, do not divide constantly. After puberty, one of the two ovaries expels a mature ovum about every 28 to 36 days (the exact number of days varies among women). During the reproductive life of a woman (from approximately age 12 to 50), 400 to 500 mature ova are produced. Radiosensitivity of ova varies considerably throughout the lifetime of the germ cell. Immature ova are very radiosensitive, whereas more mature ova have little radiosensitivity. After irradiation a mature ovum can still unite with a male germ cell during conception. However, these irradiated cells may contain damaged chromosomes. If fertilization of an ovum with damaged chromosomes occurs, genetic damage may be passed on to the offspring. If the offspring receives damaged chromosomes, the child may be born with congenital abnormalities. In general, whenever chromosomes in male or female germ cells are damaged by exposure to ionizing radiation, mutations may be passed on to succeeding generations. Even low doses received from diagnostic procedures may cause chromosomal damage. For this reason, appropriate shielding of reproductive organs should take place whenever possible.

Exposure to ionizing radiation also may cause female sterility. The dose necessary to produce this consequence depends partly on the age of the subject. Sterility occurs when radiation exposure destroys new and/or mature ova. The ovaries of the female fetus and a young child are very radiosensitive because they contain a large number of stem cells (oogonia) and immature cells (oocytes). As the female child matures from birth to puberty, the number of immature cells (oocytes) decreases. Hence the ovaries become less sensitive. This decrease in sensitivity continues up to the age of 30 years. Actually, women between the ages of 20 and 30 are at the lowest level in sensitivity. After a woman reaches age 30, the sensitivity of the ovaries increases constantly until menopause because the new ova being destroyed are not replenished. Because the ovaries of a younger woman are less sensitive than the ovaries of an older woman, a higher dose of radiation is required to cause sterility in the younger woman.

Temporary sterility usually results from a radiation dose of 2 Gy (200 rad) to the ovaries. A dose of 5 Gy (500 rad) generally causes permanent sterility in mature women. Even small doses of ionizing radiation, doses as low as 0.1 Gy (10 rad), may cause menstrual irregularities such as delay or suppression of menstruation. Although some evidence suggests that immature ova are capable of repairing radiation damage, women who have received 0.1 Gy (10 rad) or more are sometimes advised to postpone conception for 30 days or more to allow the damaged immature ova to be expelled. Because all the ova a woman will ever possess are present from birth until the time they are fertilized or expelled, the best alternative is to avoid substantial exposures in the first place.

Organic Damage from Ionizing Radiation

Radiation-induced damage at the cellular level may lead to measurable somatic and genetic damage in the organism as a whole. Some examples of measurable biologic damage are cataracts, leukemia, and genetic mutations.

Radiation dose–response relationship

The **radiation dose–response relationship** may be demonstrated graphically through a curve with distinct characteristics. Such curves map the effects of radiation observed in relation to the dose of radiation received. As this dose escalates, so do most effects. In a dose-response curve the variables, or numbers, are plotted along both axes of the graph to demonstrate the relationship between the dose received (horizontal axis) and the effects observed (vertical axis). The curve is either linear (straight line) or nonlinear (curved to some degree) and depicts either a threshold dose or nonthreshold dose (Fig. 6-16, *A* and *B*).

In a 1980 report the Committee on the Biological Effects of Ionizing Radiation (BEIR), under the auspices of the National Academy of Sciences, revealed that the majority of stochastic somatic effects (e.g., cancer) and genetic effects at low-dose levels from low-LET radiations, such as those employed in diagnostic radiology, appear to follow a linear-quadratic nonthreshold curve, which is a more conservative approach for establishing radiation protection standards. New risk models and updated dosimetry techniques have provided better follow-up study of Hiroshima and Nagasaki atomic bomb survivors. In 1990 the BEIR Committee's revised risk estimates indicated the risk of radiation to be about three to four times greater than was previously projected. Currently the committee recommends the use of the linear, nonthreshold curve of radiation dose-response for most types of cancer. The linear, nonthreshold curve implies that the biologic response to ionizing radiation is directly proportional to the dose (Fig. 6-17).

The term **threshold** may be defined as the point at which a response or reaction to an increasing stimulation first occurs. If ionizing radiation functions as the stimulus and the biologic effects it produces are the response, and if a linear, **nonthreshold** relationship exists between radiation dose and biologic response (Fig. 6-17), some biologic effects will be caused in living organisms by even the smallest doses of ionizing radiation. Consequently, no radiation exposure level is absolutely safe. Currently, some experts theorize that all radiation exposure levels possess the potential to cause biologic damage and medical radiographers must employ thoughtful radiation safety

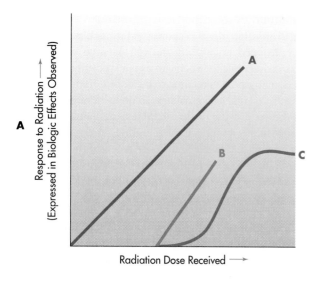

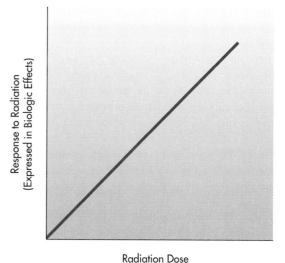

A

B

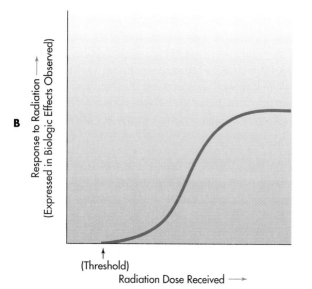

Fig. 6-16 A, *A* represents a hypothetical linear (straight-line), nonthreshold curve of radiation dose-response relationship. *B* represents a hypothetical linear (straight-line), threshold curve of radiation dose-response relationship. *C* represents a hypothetical nonlinear, nonthreshold curve of radiation dose-response relationship. **B,** Hypothetical sigmoid (S-shaped, hence nonlinear) threshold curve of radiation dose-response relationship generally employed in radiation therapy to demonstrate high-dose response.

Fig. 6-17 Hypothetical linear (straight-line), nonthreshold curve of radiation dose-response relationship. The straight-line curve passing through the origin in this graph indicates both that the response to radiation (in terms of biologic effects) is directly proportional to the dose of radiation and no known level of radiation dose exists below which the chance of sustaining biologic damage is zero. In contrast to the case of a cell survival curve, both the vertical and horizontal axes of a dose-response curve are ordinary linear scales.

measures whenever human beings are exposed to radiation during diagnostic radiologic procedures. The linear-quadratic, nonthreshold curve (Fig. 6-18) estimates the risk associated with low-level radiation. As previously stated, the BEIR Committee believes it is a more accurate reflection of stochastic somatic and genetic effects at low-dose levels from low-LET radiations. Leukemia, breast cancer, and heritable damage are presumed to follow this curve. The linear-quadratic, nonthreshold curve is supported by an analysis of the leukemia occurrences in Nagasaki and Hiroshima using a recent reevaluation of the radiation dose distribution in these two cities.[4,5]

The continued use of the linear dose-response model for radiation protection standards has the potential to exaggerate the seriousness of radiation effects at lower-dose levels from low-LET radiations. However, it accurately reflects the effects of high-LET

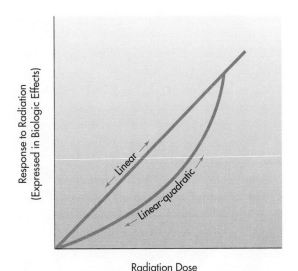

Fig.   6-18 Hypothetical   linear-quadratic,   nonthreshold dose–response relationship. The curve estimates the risk associated with low-dose levels from low-LET radiations.

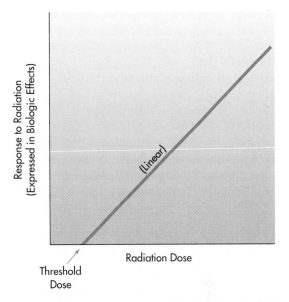

Fig. 6-19 Hypothetical linear, threshold curve of radiation dose-response. This depicts those cases for which a biologic response does not occur below a specific radiation dose.

radiations (neutrons and alpha rays) at higher doses. In establishing radiation protection standards, the regulatory agencies have chosen to be conservative.

Nonstochastic effects of significant radiation exposure such as skin erythema and hematologic depression may be demonstrated graphically through the use of a linear, threshold curve of radiation dose-response (Fig. 6-19). Here, a biologic response does not occur below a specific dose level. Laboratory experiments on animals and data from human populations observed after acute high doses of radiation provided the foundation for this curve. The sigmoid, or "S-shaped," (nonlinear) threshold curve of radiation dose-response relationship (Fig. 6-16, *B*) is generally employed in radiation therapy to demonstrate high-dose response. This curve indicates the existence of a threshold, a minimal dose of ionizing radiation below which observable effects will not occur. Different effects require different minimal doses. The tail of the curve indicates that limited recovery occurs at low radiation doses. At the highest radiation doses the curve gradually levels off and then veers downward because the affected living specimen or tissue dies before the observable effect appears.

Factors on which the amount of somatic and genetic damage depends

The amount of somatic and genetic biologic damage a human being suffers as a result of radiation exposure depends on several factors. The following are most important:

1. The quantity of ionizing radiation to which the subject is exposed
2. The ability of the ionizing radiation to cause ionization of human tissue
3. The amount of body area exposed
4. The specific body parts exposed

Ionizing radiation produces the greatest amount of biologic damage in the human body when a large dose of densely ionizing (high-LET) radiation is delivered to a large or radiosensitive area of the body.

Somatic effects

When living organisms (such as human beings) that have been exposed to radiation suffer biologic damage, the effects of this exposure are classified as **somatic effects.** Depending on the length of time from the moment of irradiation to the first appearance of

symptoms of radiation damage, the effects are classified as either early or late somatic effects.

Early (acute) somatic effects

Early (acute) somatic effects are those that appear
within minutes, hours, days, or weeks of the time of
radiation exposure. A substantial dose of ionizing radiation is required to produce biologic effects so soon
after irradiation. With the exception of certain lengthy
high-dose-rate fluoroscopic procedures, diagnostic
radiologic examinations do not usually impose radiation doses sufficient to cause early effects. The high-
dose effects include nausea, fatigue, **erythema** (diffused redness over an area of skin after irradiation)
(Fig. 6-20), **epilation** (loss of hair), blood disorders,
intestinal disorders, fever, dry and moist **desquamation** (shedding of the outer layer of skin) (Fig. 6-21),
depression of the sperm count in the male, temporary
or permanent sterility in the male and female, and injury to the central nervous system (at extremely high
radiation doses). The various types of organic damage
may be related to the cellular effects discussed previously in this chapter. For example, intestinal disorders
are caused by damage to the sensitive epithelial tissues
lining the intestines. When the whole body is exposed
to a dose of 6 Gy (600 rad) of ionizing radiation, many
of these manifestations of organic damage occur in
succession. These early somatic effects are called
acute radiation syndrome.

Acute radiation syndrome. **Acute radiation syndrome (ARS),** or radiation sickness, occurs in human
beings after whole-body reception of large doses of
ionizing radiation delivered over a short period of
time. Data from epidemiologic studies of human populations exposed to doses of ionizing radiation sufficient to cause this syndrome have been obtained from
atomic bomb survivors at Hiroshima and Nagasaki,
the Marshall Islanders who were inadvertently subjected to high levels of fallout during an atomic bomb
test, nuclear radiation accident victims such as those
injured in the Chernobyl disaster, and radiation therapy patients.

Syndrome is a medical term that means a collection of symptoms. Hence the disorder acute radiation
syndrome is actually a collection of symptoms associated with high-level radiation exposure. Three sepa-

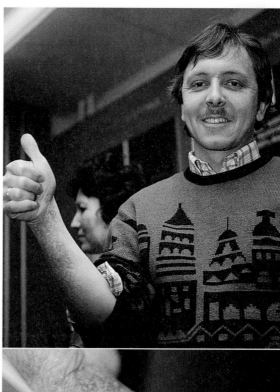

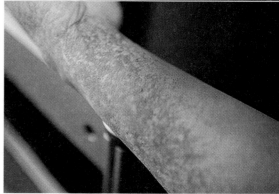

Fig. 6-20 Radiation burn or erythema on the arm of a former worker who was present at the Chernobyl nuclear plant
during the 1986 radiation accident. (From Ken Graham Photography.)

rate dose-related syndromes occur as part of the total-
body syndrome: hematopoietic syndrome, gastrointestinal syndrome, and cerebrovascular system syndrome.

Acute radiation syndrome manifests itself in four
major stages: prodromal, latent period, manifest illness, and recovery or death. The prodromal stage, also

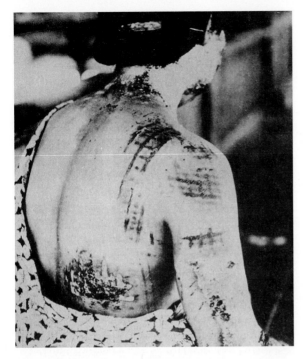

Fig. 6-21 Dry and moist desquamation. The back of this female Japanese atomic bomb survivor demonstrates the pattern of the kimono she was wearing at the time of the bombing. Radiation burns resulting in the shedding of the outer layer of skin are visible. (From PhotoAssist, Inc.)

tion, exhaustion, vomiting, severe diarrhea, fever, headaches, infection, hemorrhage, and cardiovascular collapse. In severe high-dose cases, emaciated human beings eventually die. Hence a primary effect of acute radiation syndrome is shortening of the life span.

If, after a whole-body sublethal dose such as 2 or 3 Gy (200 to 300 rad), exposed persons pass through the first three stages but show less severe symptoms than those seen after super-lethal dosages of 6 to 10 Gy (600 to 1000 rad), recovery may occur in about 3 months. However, those who recover may show some signs of radiation damage and experience late effects.

The massive explosion that blew apart a reactor at the nuclear power station in Chernobyl, Russia, on April 26, 1986, provides a recent example of human beings suffering from acute radiation syndrome. During the explosion, several tons of burning graphite, uranium dioxide fuel, and other contaminants such as cesium 137, iodine 131, and plutonium 239 were ejected vertically into the atmosphere in a 3-mile-high, radioactive plume of intense heat. Of 444 people working at the power plant at the time of the explosion, 2 died instantly and 29 died within 3 months of the accident as a consequence of thermal trauma (burns) and severe injuries from doses of whole-body ionizing radiation of approximately 6 Gy (600 rad) or more.[6-8]

Without effective physical-monitoring devices, biologic criteria such as the occurrence of nausea and vomiting played an important role in the identification of radiation casualties during the first 2 days after the nuclear disaster. Acute radiation syndrome caused the hospitalization of at least 203 people.[8,9] A determination of the lapse of time from the incidental exposure of the victims to the onset of nausea and/or regurgitation completes the biologic criteria. Dose assessment was determined from **biologic dosimetry.** This included serial measurements of levels of lymphocytes and granulocytes in the blood and a quantitative analysis of dicentric chromosomes (chromosomes having two centromeres) in blood and hematopoietic cells coming from bone marrow. The data were compared with doses and effects from earlier radiation mishaps.[7,8]

The Japanese atomic bomb survivors of Hiroshima and Nagasaki are examples of a human population af-

called the *prodromal syndrome,* occurs within hours after a whole-body absorbed dose of 1 Gy (100 rad) or more. Nausea, vomiting, diarrhea, fatigue, and leukopenia (an abnormal decrease of white blood corpuscles usually below 5000/mm^3) characterize this initial stage. The severity of these symptoms is dose related. The higher the dose, the more severe are the symptoms. The length of time involved for this stage to run its course may be hours or a few days. After the prodromal stage comes a latent period of about 1 week during which no visible symptoms occur. Actually, it is during this period that recovery or lethal effects begin. Toward the end of the first week, the next stage commences. This phase is called *manifest illness* because it is the period when symptoms become visible. Some of these symptoms are apathy, confusion, a decrease in the number of red and white blood cells and platelets in the circulating blood, dehydration, epila-

flicted with acute radiation syndrome as a consequence of war. Follow-up studies of the survivors who did not die of acute radiation syndrome, however, have demonstrated late effects of ionizing radiation. The atomic bombing of Japan and the nuclear accident at Chernobyl have made the medical community recognize the need for a thorough understanding of acute radiation syndrome and appropriate medical support of persons afflicted.

Hematopoietic syndrome. The **hematopoietic form** of acute radiation syndrome, or "bone marrow syndrome," occurs when human beings receive whole-body doses of ionizing radiation ranging from 1 to 10 Gy (100 to 1000 rad). The hematopoietic system manufactures the corpuscular elements of the blood and is the most radiosensitive vital organ system in humans. Radiation exposure causes the number of red cells, white cells, and platelets in the circulating blood to decrease. Dose levels that cause this syndrome also may damage cells in other organ systems, causing the affected organ or organ system to fail. For example, radiation doses ranging from 1 to 10 Gy (100 to 1000 rad) may cause a decrease in the number of bone marrow stem cells. When the cells of the lymphatic system are damaged, the body loses some of its ability to combat infection. Because the number of platelets also decreases with a loss of bone marrow function, the body loses a corresponding amount of its blood-clotting ability when exposed to radiation doses in this range. This makes the body more susceptible to hemorrhage.

For persons affected with this syndrome, survival time decreases as the radiation dose increases. Because more bone marrow cells are destroyed as radiation dose increases, the body becomes more susceptible to infection, mostly from its own intestinal flora, and more prone to hemorrhage. When death occurs, it is as a consequence of bone marrow destruction.

Death may occur 6 to 8 weeks after irradiation in some sensitive human subjects who receive a whole-body dose exceeding 2 Gy (200 rad). As the whole-body dose increases from 2 to 10 Gy (200 to 1000 rad), irradiated individuals die sooner. If the radiation exposure is not lethal, perhaps in the 1 to 2 Gy (100 to 200 rad) range, bone marrow cells repopulate to a level adequate to support life in most individuals. Many of these people recover 3 weeks to 6 months after irradiation. The actual dose of radiation received and the irradiated person's general state of health at the time of irradiation determine the possibility of recovery.

Survival of patients with hematopoietic syndrome may be enhanced by intense supportive care and special hematologic procedures. As an illustration, victims who received doses in excess of 5 Gy (500 rad) like those of the nuclear power station accident in Chernobyl, benefited from bone marrow transplants from appropriate histocompatible donors. During the operation, hematopoietic stem cells are transplanted to facilitate bone marrow recovery. This operation, however, is not an absolute cure for patients suffering from hematopoietic syndrome because many individuals undergoing bone marrow transplant die of burns or other damages of radiation they sustained before the transplanted stem cells have had a chance to support the individual.

Gastrointestinal syndrome. In human beings the gastrointestinal form of acute radiation syndrome appears at a threshold dose of approximately 6 Gy (600 rad) and peaks after a dose of 10 Gy (1000 rad). Without medical support to sustain life, exposed persons receiving doses between 6 and 10 Gy (100 to 1000 rad) may die 3 to 10 days after being exposed. Even if medical support is provided, the exposed person will live only a few days longer. Survival time does not change with dose in this syndrome.

A few hours after the dose required to cause the gastrointestinal syndrome has been received, the prodromal stage occurs. Severe nausea, vomiting, and diarrhea persist for as long as 24 hours. This is followed by a latent period, which lasts as long as 5 days. During this time the symptoms disappear. The manifest illness stage follows this period of false calm. Again, the human subject experiences severe nausea, vomiting, and diarrhea. Other symptoms that may occur are fever (as in hematopoietic syndrome), fatigue, loss of appetite, lethargy, anemia, leukopenia (a decrease in the number of white blood cells), hemorrhage (gastrointestinal tract bleeding occurs because the body loses its blood-clotting ability), infection, electrolyte imbalance, and emaciation. Death occurs primarily because of catastrophic damage to the epithelial cells that line the gastrointestinal tract. Such severe damage to these cells results in the exposed person dying from infection, fluid loss, or electrolyte imbalance within 3 to 5 days of irradiation. Death from gastrointestinal syndrome results not only from damage to the bowel but also from damage to the bone marrow. The latter, incidentally, is usually sufficient to cause death in hematopoietic syndrome.

In the gastrointestinal tract the small intestine is the most severely affected part. Because epithelial cells function as an essential biologic barrier, their breakdown leaves the body vulnerable to infection (mostly from its own intestinal flora), dehydration, and severe diarrhea. Some epithelial cells regenerate before death occurs. However, because of the large number of epithelial cells damaged by the radiation, death may occur before cell regeneration is accomplished. The workers and firefighters at Chernobyl are examples of human beings who have died as a result of gastrointestinal syndrome.

Cerebrovascular syndrome. The cerebrovascular form of acute radiation syndrome results from the central nervous system and cardiovascular system receiving doses of 50 Gy (5000 rad) or more of ionizing radiation. A dose of this magnitude can cause death from a few hours to several days (2 or 3) after exposure. After irradiation the prodromal stage begins. Symptoms include excessive nervousness, confusion, severe nausea, vomiting, diarrhea, loss of vision, a burning sensation of the skin, and loss of consciousness. A latent period lasting up to 12 hours follows. During this time, symptoms lessen or disappear. After the latent period the manifest illness stage occurs. During this period the prodromal syndrome recurs with increased severity, and other symptoms appear. These symptoms are disorientation and shock, periods of agitation alternating with stupor, ataxia (confusion and lack of coordination), edema, loss of equilibrium, fatigue, lethargy, convulsive seizures, electrolyte imbalance, meningitis, prostration, respiratory distress, vasculitis, and coma. Damaged blood vessels and permeable capillaries permit fluid to leak into the brain, causing an increase in fluid content. This creates an increase in intracranial pressure, which causes more tissue damage. The final result of this damage is failure of the central nervous and cardiovascular systems, which causes death in a matter of minutes. Because

the gastrointestinal and hematopoietic systems are more radiosensitive than the central nervous system, they also are severely damaged and fail to function after a dose of this magnitude. However, because death occurs quickly, the consequences of the failure of these two systems is not demonstrated.

LD 50/30. The term **LD 50/30** signifies the whole-body dose of radiation that can be lethal to 50% of the exposed population within 30 days. This is a quantitative measurement. For adult human beings the LD 50/30 is about 3.0 Gy (300 rad). For x-rays and gamma rays, this is equal to a dose equivalent of 3.0 Sv (300 rem). Whole-body doses greater than 6 Gy (600 rad) may cause death of the entire population in 30 days without medical support. With medical support, human beings have tolerated doses as high as 8.5 Gy (850 rad).[10]

Other measures of lethality also are quoted, such as LD 10/30, LD 50/60, and LD 100/60. All these measures refer to the percentage of subjects who survive after a certain number of days. The values reported in the literature vary widely because most lethal dose data represent an estimate of the role played by radiation in fatalities in which other factors (e.g., fire at Chernobyl, physical effects of a large explosion at Hiroshima and Nagasaki, chemical contamination in a few nuclear accidents) also were present. Specifications of lethal effects are further complicated by the medical treatment the patient may receive during the prodromal and latent stages, before many of the symptoms of acute radiation syndrome appear. When medical treatment is given promptly, the patient is supported through initial symptoms, but the question of long-term survival may simply be delayed. Thus survival over a 60-day period may be a more relevant indicator of outcome than survival over a 30-day period. Table 6-1 gives estimates of lethal doses, including the treatment that has been given in populations studied. Regardless of treatment, whole-body equivalent doses of greater than 12 Gy (1200 rad) are considered fatal.[11]

Repair and recovery. Because cells contain a repair mechanism inherent in their biochemistry (repair enzymes), repair and recovery may occur when cells are exposed to sublethal doses of ionizing radiation. After irradiation, surviving cells begin to repopulate. This permits an organ that has sustained functional damage

Table 6-1		
Lethal Dose Values for Healthy Adults Who Receive the Specified Medical Treatment after Exposure to Low-LET Radiation at Dose Rates of More Than 100 mGy/min		
Effect	Treatment	Dose in Gy
LD 50/60	Minimal	3.2-4.5
LD 50/60	Optimal supportive	4.8-5.4
LD 50/60	Autologous bone marrow transplantation	11

From Fry RJM: Acute radiation effects. In Wagner LK et al: *Radiation bioeffects and management: test and syllabus,* Reston, Virginia, 1991, American College of Radiology.

as a result of radiation exposure to regain some or most of its functional ability. However, the amount of functional damage sustained determines the organ's potential for recovery. In the repair of sublethal damage, oxygenated cells receiving more nutrients have a better prospect for recovery than do hypoxic (i.e., poorly oxygenated) cells receiving less nutrients. If both oxygenated and hypoxic cells receive a comparable dose of low-LET radiation, the oxygenated cells will be more severely damaged but those that survive will repair themselves and recover from the injury. Even though they are less severely damaged, the hypoxic cells do not repair and recover as effectively.

Research has shown that repeated radiation injuries have a cumulative effect. Hence a percentage (about 10%) of the radiation-induced damage is irreparable, whereas the remaining 90% may be repaired over time. When the processes of repair and repopulation work together, they aid in healing the body from radiation injury and promote recovery.

Late somatic effects

Late somatic effects are effects that appear months or years after exposure to ionizing radiation. These effects may result from previous whole- or partial-body acute, high radiation doses, or they may be the product of individual low doses and chronic low-level doses sustained over several years.

These low-level doses are a consideration for patients and personnel exposed to ionizing radiation as a result of diagnostic radiologic procedures. The risk estimate for human beings of contracting cancer from low-level radiation exposure is still controversial. No conclusive proof exists that low-level ionizing radiation doses below 0.1 Sv (10 rem) cause a significant increase in the risk of malignancy. The risk, in fact, may be negligible. Low-level radiation must be defined in broad terms to encompass the various sources of ionizing radiation, such as x-rays and radioactive materials used for diagnostic purposes in the healing arts, employment-related exposures in medicine and industry, and natural background exposure. Such low-level radiation has been defined as "an absorbed dose of [0.1 Sv] 10 rem or less delivered over a short period of time" and "a larger dose delivered over a long period of time, for instance, [0.5 Sv] 50 rem in 10 years."[12] Numerous laboratory experiments on animals and studies on human populations exposed to high doses of ionizing radiation have been conducted to determine health effects. Using all data available on high radiation exposure, members of the scientific and medical communities have determined that there are three categories of health effects that require study at low-level exposures: cancer induction, damage to the unborn from irradiation in utero, and genetic effects.

Cells that survive the initial irradiation and then retain a "memory" of that event are responsible for producing late effects. As discussed in Chapter 4, such randomly occurring effects are nonthreshold and referred to as stochastic events. For these, it is the probability of their occurrence rather than the severity that is proportional to the dose. This means that the greater the dose received by an individual, the greater is the chance that a specific late effect will be seen. However, the severity of the effect does not increase as a consequence of increased dose. Cancer and genetic disorders are examples of stochastic effects that probably do not have a threshold. When the biologic effects demonstrate the existence of a threshold (a dose below which a person has a negligible chance of sustaining specific biologic damage) and the severity of that biologic damage increases as a consequence of increased absorbed dose, the events are considered nonstochastic effects. Cataract formation and repro-

---

Box 6-1
Major Types of Late Somatic Effects

Stochastic Effects
1. Carcinogenesis
2. Embryologic effects (birth effects)

Nonstochastic Effects
1. Cataractogenesis
2. Nonspecific life span shortening

---

ductive cell damage leading to impaired fertility are examples of late nonstochastic effects. Nonstochastic effects usually occur at much higher doses than those initiating stochastic effects.

The four major types of late somatic effects are carcinogenesis, cataractogenesis, life span shortening, and embryologic effects (birth effects). Of these, carcinogenesis and embryologic effects are considered stochastic events, and cataractogenesis and life span shortening are regarded as nonstochastic effects (Box 6-1).

Risk estimates for causing cancer in humans. Exposure to ionizing radiation may cause cancer as a late somatic effect. At high doses, for groups such as the atomic bomb survivors, the risk is measurable in human populations. At low doses, below 0.1 Sv (less than 10 rem), which includes groups such as occupationally exposed individuals and virtually all patients in diagnostic radiology, this risk is not directly measurable in population studies. Either the risk is overshadowed by the natural incidence of cancer in humans, or else the risk is zero. Current radiation protection philosophy assumes that risk still exists and may be determined by extrapolating (extending the risk versus dose curve) from high-dose data, where risk has been directly observed, down to the low doses, where it has not been observed.

Risk estimates may be given in terms of absolute risk or relative risk caused by a specific exposure to ionizing radiation (over and above background exposure). Both models predict the number of excess cancers, or cancers that would not have occurred in the population in question without the exposure to ioniz-

ing radiation. The **absolute risk** model predicts that a specific number of excess cancers will occur as a result of exposure. The **relative risk** model predicts that the number of excess cancers will increase as the natural incidence of cancer increases in a population with age. It is relative in the sense that it predicts a percentage increase in incidence rather than a specific number of cases. Recent studies of atomic bomb survivors tend to support the relative risk model over the absolute risk model.

Epidemiologic studies suggest that although the radiation doses encountered in diagnostic radiology are a concern, the benefit to the patient of the information gained from a radiologic examination greatly exceeds the minimal theoretic risk to the patient of developing cancer as a late effect. Even at the relatively high doses encountered by the Japanese atomic bomb survivors, the probability of causation of an excess fatal cancer is surprisingly low—approximately 5% per Sv (100 rem).[13]

Researchers commonly use two models for extrapolation of risk from high-dose to low-dose data, the linear and the linear-quadratic models. For the linear model (Fig. 6-22, *A*), both high and low doses are assumed to have the same risk per centigray (rad). This means that the occurrence of cancer follows a straight-line (linear, or proportional) progression throughout the entire dose range. Although this model may fit the high-dose data, it may overestimate the risk at low doses. The linear-quadratic model (Fig. 6-22, *B*) involves extra mathematical terms that produce some curvature at low doses so that the risk per centigray (rad) is actually predicted to be less at low doses than at high doses. The 1989 BEIR V Report supported the linear-quadratic model for leukemia only. For all other cancers the BEIR V Committee recommended adoption of the linear model to fit the available data.[14]

Carcinogenesis. Cancer is the most important late somatic effect caused by exposure to ionizing radiation. As previously discussed, this stochastic effect is a random occurrence that probably does not have a threshold, and the severity of the disease is not dose related. Somatic cells provide an example wherein the probability of the induction of malignancy increases with dose, but the severity of the cancer is not dose dependent.

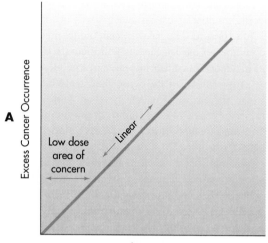

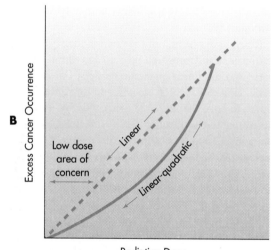

Fig. 6-22 **A,** Hypothetical linear model used to extrapolate the occurrence of cancer from high-dose information to low doses. This model suits current high-dose information satisfactorily but exaggerates the actual risk at low doses and dose rates. **B,** Hypothetical linear-quadratic model used to extrapolate the occurrence of cancer from high-dose information to low doses. This model suits current high-dose information satisfactorily, but risk at low doses may be underestimated.

Laboratory experiments with animals and statistical studies of human populations exposed to ionizing radiation (e.g., the Japanese atomic bomb survivors) prove that radiation induces cancer. In human beings, these radiation-induced cancers may take 5 or more years to develop. Distinguishing radiation-induced cancer by its physical appearance is difficult because it does not appear different from cancers caused by other agents. Cancer from natural causes frequently occurs, and the number of cancers induced by radiation is small when compared with the natural incidence of malignancies. Therefore cancer caused by low-level radiation is difficult to discover. Human evidence for radiation **carcinogenesis** comes from observation of irradiated humans and from **epidemiologic studies** conducted many years after subjects were exposed to high doses of ionizing radiation. Examples of these data follow.

Radium watch-dial painters. During the early years of this century (1920s and 1930s), a radium watch-dial painting industry flourished in some factories in New Jersey. Young girls employed in these factories hand-painted the luminous numerals on watches and clocks with a radium-containing paint. The girls used sable brushes to apply the paint. To do the fine work required, some would place the paint-saturated brush tip to their lips to draw the bristles to a fine point. The girls who followed this procedure ingested large quantities of radium. Because it is chemically similar to calcium, the radium localized in the bone. The accumulation of this toxic substance eventually caused development of osteoporosis (decalcification of the bone), osteogenic sarcoma (bone cancer), and other malignancies, such as carcinomas of the epithelial cells lining the nasopharynx and paranasal sinuses. The bones most frequently affected included the pelvis, femur, and mandible. Doses of 5 Gy (500 rad) or more are assumed to have induced the aforementioned malignancies. The number of head carcinomas attributed to the radium watch-dial painting industry is significant. Of 1474 women in the industry, 61 were diagnosed with cancers of the paranasal sinuses and 21 with cancers of the mastoid air cells. Studies attribute the death of at least 18 of the radium watch-dial painters to radium poisoning.

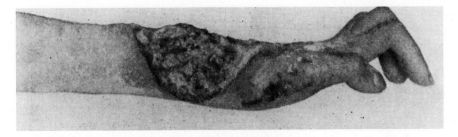

Fig. 6-23 Carcinoma of the distal arm and hand developing after an x-ray burn (1904). (From Eisenberg RL: *Radiology: An illustrated history,* St Louis, 1992, Mosby.)

Uranium miners. During the early years of this century, people worked in European mines to extract pitchblende, a uranium ore. Uranium is a radioactive element with a very long half-life (for U 238 the half-life is 4.5 billion years); it decays through a series of radioactive nuclides by emitting alpha, beta, and gamma radiation.

One of the most important members of its decay family is radium (atomic number = 88). Radium, itself radioactive, decays with a half-life of 1622 years to the radioactive element radon (atomic number = 86). Radon, unfortunately, is a gas that decays with a half-life of 3.8 days by way of alpha particle emission. This gas emanates through tiny gaps in the rocks, creating an insidious airborne hazard to miners. Throughout many years of employment, some miners inhaled significant amounts of radon. Possessing high LET, alpha particles passing through a person's lungs have a high probability of producing a great deal of cellular damage. About 50% of the miners eventually succumbed to lung cancer.

During the 1950s and 1960s, at the height of the Cold War between the United States and Russia, the U.S. government needed fuel for nuclear weapons and plants. The Navajo people of Arizona and New Mexico mined uranium to meet this need. Because the government did not regulate working conditions in the mines to ensure safety from exposure—despite an awareness of risk—some 15,000 Navajos and Caucasians who worked in the uranium mines sustained lethal doses of ionizing radiation by breathing radioactive dust and drinking radioactive water. Experts estimate each miner unknowingly received an approx-

imate dose equivalent of 10 Sv (1000 rem) or more.[15] This resulted in an alarmingly high number of miners dying from cancer and other respiratory diseases. Compounding this tragedy, the families of the miners also were affected. Because the miners had no knowledge of the adverse effects of ionizing radiation, they did not promptly change their work clothing on returning home. Because the clothing was contaminated by radioactive material, the miners' immediate families were made extremely vulnerable to radiation-induced cancers.

Early medical radiation workers. A number of the first generation of radiation workers (radiologists, dentists, and technologists) were exposed to large amounts of ionizing radiation. This resulted in some severe radiation injuries. Many radiologists and dentists developed cancerous skin lesions on their hands as a result of occupational exposure (Fig. 6-23). When compared with their nonradiologist counterparts, many early radiologists showed a higher incidence of blood disorders such as aplastic anemia and leukemia. Because all worked without the benefit of protective devices and some received doses estimated at more than 1 Gy/yr (100 rad/yr), the occurrence of these radiation-induced injuries is understandable. As a result of programs stressing radiation safety education and the development and use of acceptable, effective protective devices, radiation workers employed in medical imaging today need not experience any adverse health effects as a consequence of their work. Studies of radiographers and physicians who began their careers in radiology after the 1940s reveal that these radiation workers have shown no increase in

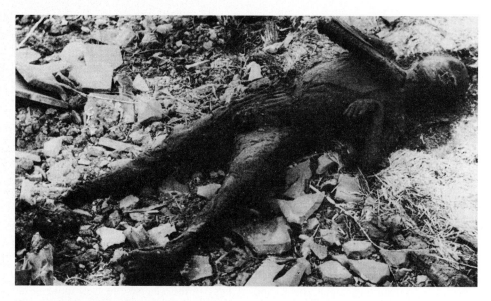

Fig. 6-24 Charred human remains found in the epicenter of Nagasaki after the detonation of the atomic bomb on August 9, 1945. (From Magnum Photos, Inc/Photographer: Yosuke Yamahata.)

adverse health effects as a result of their occupational exposure. This may be attributed to increased knowledge and use of proper protective measures and devices.

Infants treated with x-radiation to reduce an enlarged thymus gland. During the 1940s and early 1950s, physicians diagnosed thymus gland enlargement in many infants suffering from respiratory distress. The thymus is located adjacent to the thyroid in the mediastinal cavity, which extends into the neck as far as the lower edge of the thyroid gland. Functioning as a vital part of the immune mechanism, this gland plays a crucial role in the body's defense against infection. Shortly after birth the thymus glands in these infants responded to infection by enlarging. To reduce the size of the gland, physicians treated the infants with therapeutic doses (1.2 to 60 Gy, or 120 to 6000 rad) of x-radiation. Because the thyroid gland is adjacent to the thymus, the thyroid also received a substantial radiation dose. This resulted in the development, some 20 years later, of thyroid nodules and carcinomas in many of the children whose thymuses had been irradiated.

Children of the Marshall Islanders. Thyroid cancer also occurred in the children of the Marshall Is-

landers who were inadvertently subjected to high levels of fallout during an atomic bomb test (code name BRAVO) on March 1, 1954. During the detonation of a 15-megaton thermonuclear device on Bikini Atoll, the wind shifted and carried the fallout over the neighboring islands. As a consequence of this exposure, the children received substantial absorbed doses to the thyroid from both external exposure and internal ingestion of radioiodine. Estimates indicate that inhabitants of Rongelap Atoll received a mean dose of radiation to the thyroid gland of 21 Gy (2100 rad), and the inhabitants of Utrik Atoll received 2.80 Gy (280 rad).[16,17]

Japanese atomic bomb survivors. On August 6, 1945, the United States dropped the first atomic bomb on the Japanese city of Hiroshima, marking the pivotal moment in World War II. Three days later, on August 9, 1945, a second bomb was dropped on the city of Nagasaki. These bombings killed approximately 88,000 people and injured at least 70,000 more. Many of those who died were killed by the heat and blast (Fig. 6-24). Many of those who survived became the victims of radiation injuries. These individuals have been observed since that time for signs of stochastic somatic late effects of radiation.

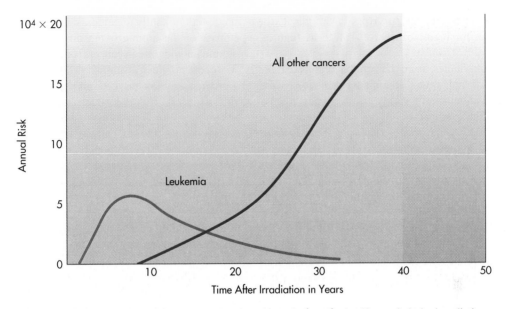

Fig. 6-25 Nominal risk of malignancy from a dose of 0.1 Gy (1 rad) of uniform whole-body radiation. (Modified from Sinclair WK: Radiation protection recommendations on dose limits: the role of the NCRP and the ICRP and future developments, *J Radiat Oncol Biol Phys* 2(31)387, 1995.)

Epidemiologic studies of approximately 100,000 Japanese survivors of the atomic bombings at Hiroshima and Nagasaki indicate that ionizing radiation causes leukemia (proliferation of the white blood cells). According to estimates, atomic bomb survivors *(hibakusha)* exposed to radiation doses of about 1 Gy (100 rad) or more showed a significant increase in the incidence of leukemia. When compared with the spontaneous incidence of leukemia in the Japanese population at the time of the bomb, the incidence of leukemia in the irradiated population increased about 100-fold after the high dose of radiation was received. "Studies of the atomic bomb survivors in both Hiroshima and Nagasaki show a statistically significant increase in leukemia incidence in the exposed population compared with the nonexposed population. In the period 1950 to 1956, 117 new cases of leukemia were reported in the Japanese survivors; approximately 64 of these can be attributed to radiation exposure."[1]

The incidence of leukemia has slowly declined since the late 1940s and early 1950s. However, the occurrence rates of other radiation-induced malignancies have continued to escalate since the late 1950s and early 1960s. Among these are a variety of solid tumors such as thyroid, breast, lung, and bone cancers. As identified by Warren K. Sinclair,[18] Fig. 6-25 demonstrates the nominal risk of malignancy from a dose of .01 Gy (1 rad) of uniform whole-body radiation. The graph indicates that leukemia occurs approximately 2 years after the initial exposure, rises to its highest level between 7 and 10 years, and then declines to almost zero at about 30 years. Unlike leukemia, solid tumors take approximately 10 years to develop and generally increase in occurrence at the same rate that cancer increases as people age. Whether the risk for solid tumors continues to rise beyond 40 years or declines as with leukemia is still unknown. Follow-up studies of the atomic bomb survivors may eventually provide the answer.

In general, Japanese women have a lower natural incidence of breast cancer compared with American and Canadian women.[3] The female Japanese atomic bomb survivors provide strong evidence that ionizing radiation can induce breast cancer. The incidence of breast cancer in these women rises with radiation dose. It follows a linear, nonthreshold curve. Numerous studies of the female survivors have indicated a relative risk for breast cancer of 4:1 to as high as 10:1.

Although studies from Hiroshima and Nagasaki confirm that high doses of ionizing radiation cause cancer, radiation is not a highly effective cancer-causing agent. For example, follow-up studies of approximately 82,000 atomic bomb survivors from 1950 to 1978 reveal an excess of only 250 cancer death attributed to radiation exposure. Instead of the expected 4500 cancer deaths, 4750 actually occurred. This means that of about every 300 atomic bomb survivors, one died of a malignancy attributed to an average whole-body radiation dose of approximately 0.14 Sv (14 rem).

Epidemiologic data on the Hiroshima atomic bomb survivors also indicate that a linear relationship exists between radiation dose and radiation-induced leukemia. In other words, the chance of contracting leukemia as a result of exposure to radiation is directly proportional to the magnitude of the radiation exposure. Available information of the kind necessary to establish the existence of a threshold dose-response relationship (i.e., whether a harmless dose exists) is inconclusive. Hence radiation-induced leukemia follows a linear-nonthreshold dose-response relationship compared with a population that has not been exposed to ionizing radiation.[10] Recent reevaluation of the quantity and type of radiation that was released in the cities of Hiroshima and Nagasaki provides a better foundation for radiation dose and damage assessment. Originally, neutrons were credited with the damage in Hiroshima. However, when recent studies revealed that the uranium-fueled bomb dropped on Hiroshima provided more gamma radiation exposure and less neutron exposure than previously believed, data on the survivors were updated to reflect this more accurate information. Researchers have established that gamma radiation and neutrons each provided about 50% of the radiation dose inflicted on the population of Hiroshima. On the other hand, the inhabitants of Nagasaki, who were exposed to a plutonium bomb, received only 10% of their exposure from neutrons and 90% from gamma radiation. Based on the revised atomic bomb data, radiation-induced leukemias and solid tumors occurring in the survivors may be attrib-

uted predominantly to gamma radiation exposure. The impact of the atomic bomb dosimetry revision is a significant increase in cancer risk estimates. The BEIR V Report provides a summary of the new estimates.

Evacuees from the Chernobyl nuclear power station disaster. The 1986 nuclear power station accident at Chernobyl requires long-term follow-up studies to assess the magnitude and severity of late effects on the exposed population. Detailed observations investigating potential increases in the incidence of leukemia, thyroid problems, and other possible radiation-induced malignancies must continue.

Within 36 hours of the nuclear catastrophe, 49,360 people residing in Pripyat, a city 2 miles from the plant, were evacuated. An additional 85,640 people, most of whom were living in a 10-mile (30-km) radial zone of Chernobyl, also were evacuated over a period of 14 days after the disaster. In general the 135,000 evacuees received an average dose equivalent of 0.12 Sv (12 rem) per person. Of the 135,000, approximately 24,000 people received a dose equivalent of about 0.45 Sv (45 rem). The remaining 111,000 people received from 0.03 to 0.06 Sv (3 to 6 rem).[7, 8] If the evacuees are monitored for at least the next 30 years, important estimates of radiation-induced leukemias, thyroid cancers, and other malignancies may be obtained.

The possibility of late effects occurring from the Chernobyl power station disaster is still a source of concern worldwide. Because winds carried the radioactive plume in several different directions during the 10 days after the accident, more than 20 countries received fallout as a consequence of the catastrophe. Approximately 400,000 people received some exposure to fallout. In February 1989, Dr. Richard Wilson, Professor of Physics at Harvard University in Cambridge, Massachusetts, estimated "that about 20,000 people throughout the world"[22] will develop a radiation-induced malignancy from the Chernobyl accident.

Iodine 131 is one of the radioactive materials that became airborne in the radioactive plume. Iodine 131 concentrates in the thyroid gland and may cause cancer many years after the initial exposure. In an attempt to prevent thyroid cancer resulting from accidental overdose to iodine 131, physicians administered

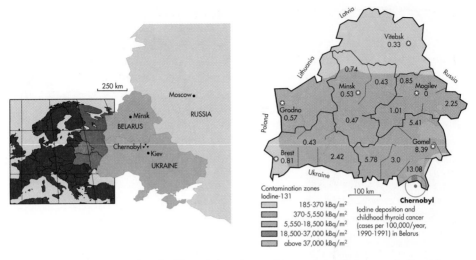

Fig. 6-26 In the 10 years after the Chernobyl nuclear accident a dramatic increase in thyroid cancer was seen among children living in the regions of Belarus, Ukraine, and Russia, where the heaviest contamination occurred. (From *Science*: vol 272, April 19, 1996.)

potassium iodide to children in Poland and some other countries after the Chernobyl accident. By offering a substitute for take-up by the thyroid gland, potassium iodide is intended to block effectively the gland's up-take of iodine 131. The degree of effectiveness of this preventive treatment remains to be determined. In other accidentally exposed populations, thyroid cancer has occurred in some individuals at doses of 1 Gy (100 rad) or less. The approximate time for the appearance of such radiation-induced thyroid malignancies is usually between 10 and 20 years after exposure.

In the 10 years after the Chernobyl disaster the incidence of thyroid cancer increased dramatically among children living in the regions of Belarus, Ukraine, and Russia (Fig. 6-26) where the heaviest radioactive iodine contamination occurred. Thyroid cancer has been identified as the "most pronounced health effect" of the radiation accident.[19] As of April 1996, more than 700 cases of thyroid cancer have been diagnosed in children residing in the areas previously identified. The number of new thyroid cancer cases diagnosed since the Chernobyl incident is significantly higher than anticipated. Radiation scientists from the Western and Eastern hemispheres are collaborating to determine the reason for this increase. Some possible explanations for the higher-than-expected number of

thyroid cancers are (1) chronic iodine deficiency during the years preceding the accident in the children living in the regions contaminated[19] and (2) genetic predisposition to developing thyroid malignancy after radiation exposure in some subgroups of the exposed population.[19] If the first theory is valid, the thyroid gland of these individuals would have assimilated isotopes of the radioactive material inhaled from a cloud or ingested from contaminated milk supplies. If the second theory is valid, some of the exposed individuals may have a disorder that prevents the mechanisms normally used by healthy cells to initiate repair and mend the genetic damage.

From the discussion of the Japanese atomic bomb survivors earlier in this chapter, we have learned that radiation causes leukemia and the disease follows a linear, nonthreshold dose-response curve. However, studies of the Chernobyl victims[20] have not demonstrated a significant increase in the incidence of leukemia, possibly because the radioactive iodine and cesium expelled into the environment during the accident could produce damaging health effects in different ways. For example, ^{131}I has a relatively short half-life (measured in days) and is assimilated by the body and quickly distributed to the thyroid gland, thereby delivering an abrupt, acute dose to that organ. Ra-

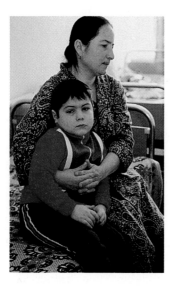

Fig. 6-27 Mother with son, who is suffering from radiation-induced leukemia. The child is a victim of the 1986 nuclear power plant explosion at Chernobyl. (From Ken Graham Photography.)

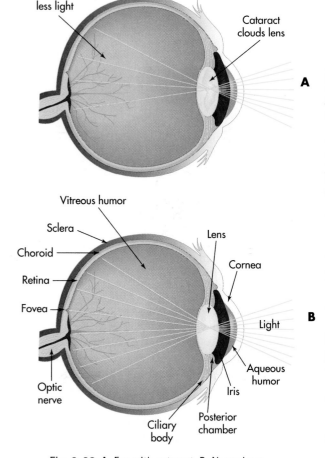

Fig. 6-28 A, Eye with cataract. **B,** Normal eye.

dioactive cesium, on the other hand, has a longer life. It causes whole-body irradiation over time through its presence in the environment and food supply lines. This probably increases the incidence of childhood leukemia (Fig. 6-27). However, this increase is difficult to detect without very sensitive and reliable monitoring procedures. Further investigation is necessary to determine more accurately the actual increase in leukemia induced by radiation.

Continued studies may impart a great deal of information about the link between ionizing radiation and cancer. A more thorough understanding of the effects of low-level ionizing radiation also may be gained. However, because the actual levels of risk from the accident are still unknown because of the limited data provided by the Russians, the risk for development of radiation-induced malignancies is difficult to determine.

Cataractogenesis. The lens of the eye contains transparent fibers that transmit light. The retina receives the light focused by the lens and permits the image formed by the lens to be received (Fig. 6-28,

B). The probability that a single dose of ionizing radiation of approximately 2 Gy (200 rad) will induce the formation of cataracts (opacity of the eye lens) is high (Fig. 6-28, *A*). This results in a partial or complete loss of vision. Laboratory experiments with mice prove that cataracts may be induced with doses as low as 0.1 Gy (10 rad). Highly ionizing neutron radiation is extremely efficient in inducing cataracts. A neutron dose as low as 0.01 Gy (1 rad) has been known to cause cataracts in mice. Radiation-induced cataracts in human beings follow a threshold, nonlinear dose-response relationship. Evidence for human radiation cataractogenesis comes from observation of small groups of people who accidentally received substantial doses to the eyes. These groups include Japanese atomic bomb survivors, nuclear physicists working with cyclotrons (units that produce high-energy particles such as protons) between 1932 and 1960, and patients undergoing radiotherapy who received significantly high exposures to the eyes during treatment.

Life span shortening. Laboratory experiments on small animals indicate that animals exposed to both acute and chronic doses of ionizing radiation die younger than animals that have never been irradiated. Both exposed and unexposed animals die of the same diseases; however, the exposed animals develop diseases at an earlier age and also die at an earlier age. Because no specific diseases associated with radiation-induced life span shortening can be identified, this reduction in the life cycle is termed **nonspecific life span shortening.**

In addition to causing tissue degeneration, radiation apparently accelerates the aging process. Premature aging seems to make animals more susceptible to several diseases. Early demise of the experimental animals results from the induction of cancer.

Studies of physicians practicing radiology during the early years (before 1940) of the profession provide evidence of radiation-induced life span shortening in humans. When compared with the general population and nonradiologist physicians, early radiologists experienced an average life span shortening of about 5 years. At the present time, the life spans for radiologists and nonradiologists appear to be the same. This may be attributed to the implementation of appropriate radiation protection procedures and the use of modern equipment designed with safety features.

Embryologic effects (birth effects). All life forms seem to be most vulnerable to radiation during the embryonic stage of development. The period of gestation during which the embryo-fetus is exposed to radiation governs the effects (death or congenital abnormality) of the radiation on it. Gestation in humans is divided into three stages: (1) preimplantation, which corresponds to 0 to 9 days; (2) organogenesis, which corre-

sponds to 10 days to 6 weeks postconception; and (3) the fetal stage, which corresponds to 6 weeks postconception to term (Fig. 6-29).

Because embryonic cells begin dividing and differentiating after conception, they are extremely radiosensitive and hence may easily be damaged by exposure to ionizing radiation. The first trimester seems to be the most crucial period as far as irradiation of the embryo-fetus is concerned because the embryo-fetus contains a large number of stem cells during this period of gestation. Because the central nervous system and related sense organs contain many of these stem cells, they are extremely radiosensitive and are therefore susceptible to radiation-induced damage. Irradiation of the embryo during the first 8 weeks of development to dose equivalents in excess of 200 mSv (20 rem) frequently results in death or causes congenital abnormalities.

During the preimplantation stage (approximately 0 to 9 days after conception) the fertilized ovum divides and forms a ball-like structure containing undifferentiated cells. If this structure is irradiated with a dose in the range of .05 Gy to 0.15 Gy (5 to 15 rads), embryonic death will occur. Malformations resulting from radiation exposure do not occur at this stage. Because organogenesis (the stage in which the undifferentiated cells are implanted in the uterine wall) occurs between the second and sixth week after conception, the developing fetus is most susceptible to radiation-induced congenital abnormalities during this period. This is actually the time when the undifferentiated cells are beginning to differentiate into organs. The central nervous system in the growing human fetus, however, remains undifferentiated and does not normally complete development until approximately the twelfth year of life. Abnormalities occurring as a consequence of irradiation during the period of organogenesis may include growth inhibition, mental retardation, microcephaly, genital deformities, and sense organ damage. During the late stages of organogenesis the presence of fatal abnormalities in the fetus will cause neonatal death (death at birth). High doses of radiation also will cause this to occur during the fetal stage (a growth period) of development. Skeletal damage from radiation expo-

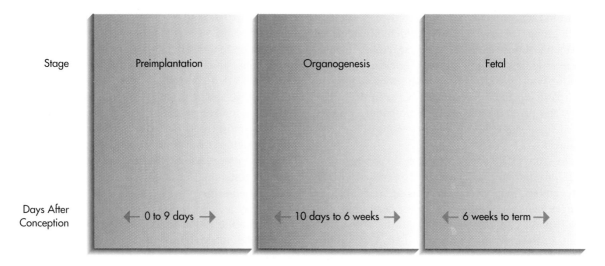

| Stage | Preimplantation | Organogenesis | Fetal |

Fig. 6-29 Division of gestation in humans.

sure occurs most frequently during the period from the third to the twentieth week of development. The development of cancer or functional disorders during childhood are other possible effects of irradiation during the fetal stage.

Fetal radiosensitivity decreases as gestation progresses. Hence during the second and third trimesters, the developing fetus is less sensitive to ionizing radiation exposure. However, even in these later trimesters, congenital abnormalities and functional disorders such as sterility may be caused by radiation exposure. A great deal of the evidence for radiation-induced congenital abnormalities in human beings comes from more than 4 decades of follow-up studies of children exposed in utero during the atomic bomb detonations in Hiroshima and Nagasaki. Although the risk of radiation-induced leukemia is greater when the embryo-fetus is irradiated during the first trimester, leukemia also may be induced by exposure to radiation during the second and third trimesters. Even with some studies of children irradiated in utero[21] indicating an excess of cancer and leukemia deaths, studies of children exposed in utero during the atomic bomb detonations in Hiroshima and Nagasaki have not demonstrated significant rates of cancer and leukemia deaths.

Of the 135,000 evacuees from the 18-mile (30-km) radial zone of the Chernobyl nuclear power plant, approximately 2000 were pregnant women. Each received an average total-body dose equivalent of 0.43 Sv (43 rem). No obvious abnormalities were observed in the 300 live babies born by August of 1987. On the television program *Nova*, Dr. Yelena Lukinova made the following statement: "1950 babies were born after the accident from pregnant women in the zone. All are as healthy as 600 born before the accident."[22]

Fetal effects such as mortality, induction of malformations, mental retardation, and childhood cancer were reviewed by the United Nations Scientific Committee on the Effects of Atomic Radiation (UNSCEAR).[23] This group proposed an upper limit combined radiation risk for the aforementioned fetal effects "of 3 chances per 1000 children for each rem of fetal dose."[24] If each effect was estimated individually, the estimate would be a little lower. Without radiation, these fetal effects have an estimated normal total risk of "60 chances per 1000 children (6%)."[24]

In 1990 the International Chernobyl Project was initiated in response to a request for assistance from the former Soviet Union. The Director of the Radiation Effects Research Foundation in Hiroshima, Japan, led this project. The study compared seven contaminated Russian villages with six uncontaminated villages. By 1990, no significant increases in fetal and genetic abnormalities were seen in this population.[25] However, because of the relatively long latency period for radiogenic cancer, particularly solid tumors, researchers expect that more time will be required before the ultimate impact on the population of Russia is known. Estimates of as many as 500 excess cancers in the former Soviet Union during the next 50 to 60 years have been made.[26]

The effect of low-level ionizing radiation on the embryo-fetus can only be estimated. Documentation on the effects of low-level radiation on the unborn irradiated in utero is still insufficient because some type of abnormality occurs in a small percentage of all live births in the United States. In addition, no birth abnormalities unique to high levels of radiation have appeared. Abnormalities in this context are the same as those that happen naturally; however, if the exposure occurs during a period of major organogenesis, the abnormality may be more pronounced. Assessment of radiation-induced birth abnormalities from low-level exposure also may be more difficult because human genes vary naturally or as a consequence of the environment.

Because the embryo-fetus is relatively sensitive to radiation, radiation workers should exercise caution and employ appropriate safety measures when performing diagnostic radiographic procedures that result in any dose to the unborn. Most diagnostic procedures result in dose equivalents less than 0.01 Sv (1 rem). Such doses are not usually considered dangerous to the unborn.

Genetic effects

Biologic effects of ionizing radiation on future generations are termed **genetic effects.** These effects occur as a result of radiation-induced damage to the DNA molecule in the sperm or ova of an adult. When these germinal mutations occur, faulty genetic information is transmitted to the offspring. This faulty genetic information may manifest itself as various diseases or malformations.

Normally, mutations in genetic material occur spontaneously, without a known cause. Mutations in genes and DNA that occur at random as a natural phenomenon are called *spontaneous mutations.* Because these genetic alterations are permanent and heritable, they can be transmitted from one generation to the next. Spontaneous mutations in human genetic material cause a wide variety of disorders or diseases, some of which include hemophilia, Huntington's chorea, Down syndrome (mongolism), Duchenne's muscular dystrophy, sickle cell anemia, cystic fibrosis, and hydrocephalus. Some genetic disorder is present in approximately 10% of all live births in the United States.

In each generation, some genetic mutations occur as part of the natural order of events. However, certain agents such as elevated temperatures, ionizing radiations, viruses, and chemicals can increase the frequency of mutation. These agents are called **mutagens,** and ionizing radiation is one of the more effective mutagens known. Any nonlethal radiation dose received by the germ cells can cause chromosome mutations, which may be transmitted to successive generations.

When radiation interacts with DNA macromolecules, it can modify the structure of these molecules by causing breaks in the chromosomes or change the amount of DNA belonging to a cell by causing a deletion or an alteration in the sequence of nitrogen bases. Such modifications change the cell's genetic information. A mutation of this type may eventually lead to genetic disease in subsequent generations.

Enzymes attempt to repair cellular damage by mending structural breaks in chromosomes that have been hit by ionizing radiation. If repair is successful, the cell continues to function normally. If repair does not occur, the cell may suffer functional impairment or die.

Mutant genes cannot properly govern the cell's normal chemical reactions or properly control the sequence of amino acids in the formation of specific proteins. These incapacities of mutant genes result in various genetic diseases. For example, sickle cell anemia results from the defective synthesis of the protein hemoglobin. About 300 amino acids combine to form the hemoglobin molecule; sickle cell anemia is caused by the substitution of only one vital amino acid.

Point mutations (genetic mutations at the molecular level) may be either dominant (probably expressed in the offspring) or recessive (probably not expressed for several generations). Radiation is thought to cause primarily recessive mutations, if any. For a recessive mutation to appear in the offspring, both parents must have the same genetic defect. This means that the defect must be located on the same part of a specific DNA base sequence in each parent. Because this rarely occurs, the effects of recessive mutations are not likely to appear in a population. However, an increase in the number of individuals who receive radiation increases the likelihood that two individuals having the same type of mutation will have offspring. Therefore imaging professionals should limit not only the amount of radiation received by an individual but also the radiation exposure of the entire population. Damage from recessive mutations sometimes manifests itself more subtly and may appear as allergies, a slight alteration in metabolism, decreased intelligence, nonspecific life span shortening, and predisposition to certain diseases.

The only concrete evidence showing that ionizing radiation causes genetic effects comes from extensive experimentation with fruit flies and mice at high radiation doses. The data on mice may be extrapolated to low doses and then applied to humans. The information obtained from the experiments indicates that genetic effects do not have a threshold dose—in other words, a dose of ionizing radiation at which genetic effects begin to occur and below which they cannot occur. Because this implies that even the smallest radiation dose may cause some genetic damage, no such thing as a "100% safe" gonadal radiation dose exists.

Existing data on radiation-induced genetic effects in humans are inconclusive. Some of the data accumulated come from observation of test groups of children conceived after one or both parents had been exposed to radiation resulting from the atomic bomb detonation in Hiroshima or Nagasaki. As of the third generation, no radiation-induced genetic effects are known. However, this does not mean that effects will not be seen in subsequent generations. J.F. Crow, a geneticist who spent many years experimenting with fruit flies, stated the following: "The most frequent

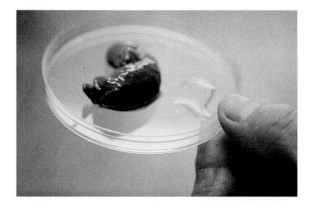

Fig. 6-30 Stillbirth. (From Magnum Photos, Inc.)

mutations in man are not those leading to freaks or obvious hereditary diseases, but those causing minor impairments leading to higher embryonic death rates, lower life expectancy, increase in disease, or decreased fertility."[27]

Animal studies of radiation-induced genetic effects have led to the development of the **doubling dose** concept. This dose measures the effectiveness of ionizing radiation in causing mutations. Doubling dose is the radiation dose that causes the number of spontaneous mutations occurring in a given generation to increase to two times their original number. For example, if 7% of the offspring in each generation are born with mutations, the doubling dose eventually increases the number of mutations to 14%. The radiation doubling dose for humans, as determined from the offspring of the atomic bomb survivors of Hiroshima and Nagasaki, is estimated to have a mean value of 1.56 Sv (156 rem) based on the genetic indicators of untoward pregnancy outcome (e.g., stillbirths [Fig. 6-30], major congenital abnormalities [Fig. 6-31], death during the first postnatal week), childhood mortality, and sex chromosome aneuploidy (possessing an abnormal number of chromosomes). For this reason, the administration of even low doses of radiation to the gonads must be strictly controlled to reduce the risk of genetic damage in future generations. This precaution will help preserve the biologic fitness of the human race.

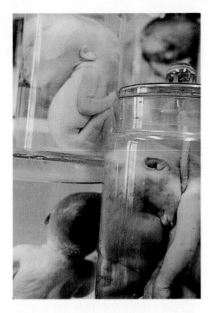

Fig. 6-31 Major congenital abnormalities. (From Magnum Photos, Inc.)

energy neutrons also fall in this category. For radiation protection, these high-LET radiations are of greatest concern when the possibility of internal contamination exists. Damage caused by these radiations may be irreparable because multiple-strand breaks in DNA are possible. Such damage cannot be undone by repair enzymes. As the LET of radiation increases, so does biologic damage. The relative biologic effectiveness (RBE) is the means by which this relative effect is quantitatively described. RBE may be expressed as follows:

$$RBE = \frac{\text{Dose in Gy from 250 k Vp x-rays (reference radiation)}}{\text{Dose in Gy of test radiation}}$$

The amount of cellular injury (e.g., lethality) for a species of ionizing radiation may be obtained by using a comparative measure called *oxygen enhancement ratio (OER)*. This ratio may be expressed as follows:

$$OER = \frac{\text{Radiation dose required to cause biologic response without } O_2}{\text{Radiation dose required to cause biologic response with } O_2}$$

Radiation-induced biologic damage in living systems may be observed on the molecular, cellular, and organic levels. If a sufficient number of somatic cells are damaged by radiation, entire body processes may be disrupted. Radiation damage to the germ (reproductive) cells may be passed on to future generations in the form of genetic mutations. The action of radiation on the cell is classified as either direct or indirect depending on the site of interaction. When biologic damage occurs as a result of the ionization of atoms on DNA molecules causing these molecules to become inactive or functionally altered, the action is termed *direct*. Indirect action involves the effects of reactive free radicals created by the interaction of radiation with water molecules. These agents can cause substantial disruption to DNA molecules, resulting in cell death. The mechanisms of direct and indirect action have been covered in detail in the chapter. High-LET radiations are more likely to cause biologic damage through direct action than are low-LET radiations. Approximately 95% of the effects of x-radiation and

Summary

The principles of radiation biology relevant to radiation protection have been presented in this chapter. The concepts of linear energy transfer (LET), relative biologic effectiveness (RBE), and oxygen enhancement ratio facilitate understanding of the way ionizing radiation causes injury or changes the severity of injury in biologic tissue. As ionizing radiation passes through and interacts with a medium, it deposits energy along its path. The average energy deposited per unit of path length is termed *linear energy transfer* and is generally described in units of kiloelectron volts (keV) per micron (1 micron [μm] = 10^{-6} m). X-rays and gamma rays are external electromagnetic radiations classified as low-LET radiations. When they interact with biologic tissue, they cause damage mainly through an indirect action. Repair enzymes can usually reverse cellular damage caused by sublethal damage to DNA induced by low-LET radiation. Alpha particles, ions of heavier nuclei, and charged particles released from interactions between neutrons and atoms are classified as high-LET radiations. Low-gamma radiation in macromolecules of living systems occur as a result of indirect action. The energy of the radiation may be transferred to the master molecule (DNA) and rupture one of its chemical bonds, thereby potentially severing one of the sugar-phosphate chain siderails (single-strand break), causing a point mutation. Such mutations commonly occur with low-LET radiations. This damage can be reversed by repair enzymes. Additional breaks in the siderails of the DNA structure may occur with further exposure of the affected DNA macromolecule. These double-strand breaks may be repaired but not as easily as the breaks in the single strand. The life of the cell is threatened when double-strand breaks are not repaired because further separation of the DNA chain may occur. Double-strand breaks of DNA are associated with high-LET radiation. Because repair of this type of damage is not likely to occur, the chance of producing a lethal alteration of nitrogenous bases within the genetic sequence is far greater.

Large-scale structural changes in a chromosome brought about by ionizing radiation also may have serious consequences for the cell. Chromosome breaks may occur in both somatic and genetic cells. After chromosomes break, fragments with broken ends are produced. These sticky ends can adhere to other broken fragments. Possible combinations include the rejoining of the broken fragments in their original configuration, failure to rejoin and the creation of an aberration (lesion or anomaly), and the rejoining of other broken ends and the creation of new chromosomes that may or may not look structurally altered compared with the chromosome before irradiation.

DNA is believed to be the master, or key, molecule that maintains normal cell function. If it is by chance directly or indirectly inactivated by exposure to radiation, the cell will die. This concept is known as the target theory. When the cell's nucleus is damaged by exposure to ionizing radiation, damage may manifest itself in one of the following ways: (1) instant death; (2) reproductive death; (3) apoptosis, or programmed cell death (interphase death); (4) mitotic, or genetic, death; (5) mitotic delay; (6) interference of function; and (7) chromosome breakage. A detailed description of each event may be found in the chapter.

The cell survival curve may be used to display the radiosensitivity of a particular type of cell. Information obtained from this curve is valuable in determining the types of cancer cells that will respond to radiation therapy. The degree of radiosensitivity of various types of body cells and tissues varies. Factors that affect the cell's radiosensitivity include cell specialization (differentiation), rate of division, and degree of maturity. According to the law established by Bergonié and Tribondeau in 1906, the most pronounced radiation effects occur in cells having the least maturity and specialization, the greatest reproductive activity, and the longest mitotic phases. This law is true for all types of cells in the human body. In accordance with the Bergonié-Tribondeau law, in diagnostic radiology the embryo-fetus is more susceptible to radiation damage than is the child or the adult. When cells are more mature and specialized in performing specific functions, they are less sensitive to radiation. Blood cells may be adversely affected by exposure to ionizing radiation. The number of cells in the peripheral circulation may become depressed. A measurable hematologic depression may occur within a few days after a whole-body dose of 0.25 Gy (25 rad). A dose of this magnitude is not likely to be sustained by radiation workers today. Lymphocytes that are manufactured in bone marrow are the most radiosensitive blood cells in the human body. When these cells are damaged by radiation exposure, the body loses its natural ability to combat infection and becomes more susceptible to bacterial and viral antigens. Patients receiving radiation exposure from a diagnostic radiologic procedure are not expected to sustain appreciable damage to either the blood or blood-forming organs as a consequence of the examination.

Epithelial tissue lines and covers body tissue. It is highly radiosensitive. Muscle tissue and nervous tissue in the adult are relatively insensitive to radiation and can tolerate higher radiation doses than other body tissues. However, developing nerve cells in the embryo-fetus are relatively radiation sensitive. Irradiation of the embryo may lead to central nervous system anomalies, microcephaly, and mental retardation. During the end of the neuronal organogenesis stage (from the eighth to the fifteenth week of gestation), the fetus is most susceptible to damage from radiation exposure. Therefore special consideration is given to the irradiation of the abdomen or pelvis of a pregnant patient during this period. Human germ cells are relatively radiosensitive. In the male, temporary sterility lasting as long as 12 months can be caused by a radiation dose of 2 Gy (200 rad). Permanent sterility may be induced by a dose of 5 or 6 Gy (500 to 600 rad). Temporary sterility also may be caused in the female from a radiation dose of 2 Gy (200 rad) to the ovaries. In the mature female a dose of 5 Gy (500 rad) generally causes permanent sterility.

When exposure to ionizing radiation causes sufficient damage at the cellular level, measurable somatic and genetic damage (cataracts, leukemia, and genetic mutations) occurs in the organism as a whole. Curves that graphically demonstrate the effects of radiation observed in relation to the dose of radiation received are used to demonstrate the radiation dose–response relationship. The curve is either linear or nonlinear and depicts either a threshold or nonthreshold dose. The linear, nonthreshold curve of radiation dose response for most types of cancers is currently being used because of revised radiation risk estimates. Even the smallest doses of ionizing radiation cause biologic effects in living organisms. An absolutely safe radiation exposure level does not exist. For this reason, thoughtful radiation safety measures must be employed during all diagnostic radiologic procedures. Nonstochastic effects of significant radiation exposure may be graphically demonstrated through the use of a linear, threshold curve of radiation dose response. High dose response such as occurs during radiation therapy treatment may be graphically demonstrated through the use of the sigmoid threshold curve.

The greatest amount of biologic damage (somatic and genetic) in the human body occurs when a large dose of high-LET radiation is delivered to a large or radiosensitive area of the body. Somatic effects are consequences of radiation exposure that affect the exposed living organism. If the effects occur within minutes, hours, days, or weeks after irradiation, they are called *early somatic effects.* Some examples of these effects are nausea, fatigue, erythema, epilation, and blood and intestinal disorders. When the whole body is exposed to a dose of 6 Gy (600 rad) of ionizing radiation, many of these effects occur in succession. This is called *acute radiation syndrome (ARS).* Three separate syndromes occur as part of the total-body syndrome: hematopoietic syndrome, gastrointestinal syndrome, and cerebrovascular syndrome. Each of these syndromes has been described in detail in the chapter. ARS actually manifests in four stages: prodromal, latent period, manifest illness, and recovery or death. Several radiation accident victims from the 1986 nuclear power plant disaster in Chernobyl, Russia, exemplify the effects of ARS. The Japanese atomic bomb survivors of Hiroshima and Nagasaki are earlier examples of a human population afflicted with ARS.

The term *LD 50/30* is used to signify the whole-body dose of ionizing radiation that can be lethal to 50% of the exposed population within 30 days. For adult human beings, LD 50/30 is about 3.0 Gy (300 rad) absorbed dose. Lethal dose in human beings is usually given as LD 50/60 and is estimated to be 3 to 4 Gy (300 to 400 rad) without treatment, higher if medical intervention is available.

When cells are exposed to sublethal doses of ionizing radiation, repair and recovery are possible. Surviving cells begin to repopulate. This permits a functionally damaged organ to regain some or most of its functional ability. Oxygenated cells have a better chance for recovery than do hypoxic cells. Repeated radiation injury causes a cumulative effect. Approximately 90% of the radiation-induced damage may be repaired over time, and about 10% is irreparable.

When effects of ionizing radiation appear after a period of months or years after irradiation, they are called *late somatic effects.* The following four major types are common: carcinogenesis, cataractogenesis, life span shortening, and embryologic effects (birth effects). No conclusive proof exists that low-level ionizing radiation doses below 0.1 Sv (10 rem) cause a significant increase in the risk of malignancy. At low doses, below 0.1 Sv (less than 10 rem), the risk is not directly measurable in human population studies. Risk estimates may be given in terms of absolute risk or relative risk. These models predict the number of excess cancers that would not have occurred in the population in question without the exposure to ionizing radiation. The absolute risk model predicts that a specific number of excess cancers will occur as a result of the exposure. The relative risk model predicts that the number of excess cancers will rise as the natural incidence of cancer increases in a population with age. The linear and the linear-quadratic models are used for extrapolation of risk from high-dose to low-dose data. Cancer is the most important late somatic effect caused by exposure to ionizing radiation. In human beings, radiation-induced cancers may take 5 or more years to develop. Such cancers cannot be distinguished by physical appearance from cancers arising from other causes. The probability that cataracts in human beings may be induced by a single dose of ionizing radiation of about 2 Gy (200 rad) is high. This effect follows a threshold, nonlinear dose-response relationship. The following groups of people experienced cataractogenesis: Japanese atomic bomb survivors, nuclear physicists working with cyclotrons, and patients undergoing radiation therapy who received significant doses to the eyes. When small animals are exposed to both acute and chronic doses of ionizing radiation under laboratory conditions, they die younger than the animals that have never been irradiated. Both groups die of the same diseases, but the animals that have been irradiated develop the disease sooner and die sooner. All life forms seem to be most vulnerable to radiation during the embryonic stage of development. The effects of radiation on the embryo-fetus depend on the gestation period when the exposure was received. The first trimester of pregnancy seems to be the most critical period for radiation exposure of the embryo-fetus. Radiation-induced congenital abnormalities occur most frequently when the embryo-fetus is irradiated during the period of major organogenesis (between the second and sixth week after conception). Radiation exposure during the third to the twentieth week of development usually results in skeletal damage. As gestation progresses, fetal radiosensitivity decreases, but exposure to radiation in the later trimesters can cause congenital abnormalities, functional disorders, and a predisposition for the development of cancer during childhood. The effects of low-level radiation on the embryo-fetus can only be estimated. Documentation is still insufficient. Because radiation workers are aware that the embryo-fetus is relatively sensitive to radiation, they should exercise caution and employ appropriate safety measures when they are performing diagnostic radiographic procedures.

Genetic effects of ionizing radiation are biologic effects on generations yet unborn. Radiation-induced damage to the DNA molecule in the sperm or ova of an adult cause these effects. The offspring of such persons receives faulty genetic information that may eventually manifest in the form of various diseases or malformations. Point mutations may be dominant or recessive. Radiation is thought to cause primarily recessive mutations. Fruit flies and mice still provide the only concrete evidence that ionizing radiation causes genetic effects. Genetic effects do not appear to have a threshold dose. This implies that even the smallest radiation dose can cause some genetic damage. Hence no 100%-safe gonadal radiation dose exists. The doubling dose concept is an outgrowth of animal studies of radiation-induced genetic effects. This dose measures the effectiveness of ionizing radiation in causing mutations. The doubling dose is the radiation dose that causes the number of spontaneous mutations occurring in a given generation to increase to twice their original number. For human beings, it is estimated to have a mean value of 1.56 Sv (156 rem). To reduce the risk of genetic damage in future generations, all medical radiation exposure must be strictly controlled.

Review Questions

1. Radiation damage is observed on which of the following three levels?
   A. Molecular, cellular, and osmotic
   B. Molecular, cellular, and organic
   C. Microscopic, molecular, and organic
   D. Organic, inorganic, and cellular

2. The term *LD 50/30* denotes the radiation dose required to kill which of the following?
   A. 50% of the exposed population in 30 days
   B. 30% of the exposed population in 50 days
   C. 50% of the exposed population in 50 days
   D. 30% of the exposed population in 30 days

3. Which action of ionizing radiation is *most* harmful to the human body?
   A. Direct action
   B. Indirect action
   C. Epidemiologic action
   D. Mitotic action

4. With respect to the law of Bergonié and Tribondeau, which of the following would *best* complete this statement? "The most pronounced radiation effects occur in cells having the _____."
   A. Least reproductive activity, shortest mitotic phases, and most maturity."
   B. Greatest reproductive activity, shortest mitotic phases, and most maturity."
   C. Greatest reproductive activity, longest mitotic phases, and least maturity."
   D. Least reproductive activity, shortest mitotic phases, and least maturity."

5. Which of the following groups of cells are *most* radiosensitive?
   A. Lymphocytes
   B. Adult nerve cells
   C. Erythrocytes
   D. Muscle cells

6. Which molecules in the human body are most commonly directly acted on by ionizing radiation to produce molecular damage through an indirect action?
   A. Protein
   B. Carbohydrate
   C. Fat
   D. Water

7. Which of the following is considered to be low-LET radiation?
   1. X-rays
   2. Alpha particles
   3. Gamma rays
   A. 1 only
   B. 2 only
   C. 1 and 3 only
   D. 2 and 3 only

8. When does ionizing radiation cause complete chromosome breakage?
   A. When a single strand of the sugar-phosphate chain sustains a direct hit
   B. When two direct hits occur in the same rung of the DNA macromolecule
   C. When two direct hits occur in different rungs of the DNA macromolecule
   D. When two direct hits are sustained at opposite ends of the DNA macromolecule

9. Which of the following is *most* radiosensitive?
   A. A mature person
   B. The embryo-fetus during the first trimester of gestation
   C. The fetus during the third trimester of gestation
   D. A 5-year-old child

10. Which of the following are classified as early (acute) somatic effects of ionizing radiation?
    A. Erythema, cataractogenesis, life span shortening
    B. Nausea, epilation, intestinal disorders
    C. Male and female sterility, embryologic effects, carcinogenesis
    D. Blood disorders, fever, nonspecific life span shortening

11. Which of the following is not a form of acute radiation syndrome?
    A. Carcinogenic syndrome
    B. Hematopoietic syndrome
    C. Gastrointestinal syndrome
    D. Cerebrovascular system syndrome

12. Uranium miners in the Colorado plateau who developed lung cancer years after exposure provide an example of which of the following?
    A. Early somatic effects
    B. Late somatic effects
    C. Early genetic effects
    D. Late genetic effects

13. Cancer and genetic defects are examples of _____ effects.
    A. Stochastic
    B. Nonstochastic
    C. Birth
    D. Early somatic

14. Radiation can induce genetic damage by which of the following?
    A. Interacting with somatic cells of only one parent
    B. Interacting with somatic cells of both parents
    C. Altering the essential base coding sequence of DNA
    D. None of the above

15. Most radiation-induced genetic mutations are _____.
    A. Dominant mutations
    B. Expressed in first-generation offspring
    C. Spontaneous mutations that are unique to radiation only
    D. Recessive mutations

16. Based on current data, which of the following would be considered a *safe* radiation dose for the gonads?
    A. 5 Gy
    B. 3 Gy
    C. 1 Gy
    D. 0 Gy

17. Which of the following groups of cells are *least* radiosensitive?
    A. Adult nerve cells
    B. Nerve cells in the embryo-fetus
    C. Lymphocytes
    D. Immature spermatogonia

18. Which of the following gonadal radiation doses will cause permanent sterility in a human male?
    A. 0.01 Gy
    B. 1 Gy
    C. 2.0 Gy
    D. 6 Gy

19. On which of the following factors does somatic or genetic radiation-induced damage depend?
    1. The amount of body area exposed
    2. The quantity of ionizing radiation to which the subject is exposed
    3. The specific parts of the body that are exposed
    A. 1 only
    B. 2 only
    C. 3 only
    D. 1, 2, and 3

20. Revised atomic bomb data for Hiroshima and Nagasaki suggest that radiation-induced leukemias and solid tumors occurring in the survivors may be attributed to exposure to which of the following?
    A. X-rays
    B. Gamma radiation
    C. Neutrons
    D. Various nonionizing radiations

21. For an accurate estimate of the number of radiation-induced leukemias and other malignancies that may occur in some of the 135,000 evacuees from the 1986 nuclear power station accident in Chernobyl, Russia, the exposed population must _____.

    A. Not be permitted to receive any additional medical radiation exposure for the next 20 years
    B. Not be permitted to intermingle with the unexposed population
    C. Be monitored for only the next 10 years
    D. Be monitored for at least the next 30 years

22. Acute radiation syndrome manifests itself in four major stages. In what order do these stages occur?

    A. Latent period, prodromal, manifest illness, recovery or death
    B. Manifest illness, prodromal, latent period, recovery or death
    C. Prodromal, latent period, manifest illness, recovery or death
    D. Manifest illness, latent period, prodromal, recovery or death

23. Which of the following systems is the *most* radiosensitive vital organ system in human beings?

    A. Cerebrovascular
    B. Gastrointestinal
    C. Hematopoietic
    D. Skeletal

24. The number of excess cancers that would not have occurred in a given population without the exposure to ionizing radiation may be predicted by which of the following?

    1. The absolute risk model
    2. The biologic risk model
    3. The relative risk model

    A. 1 and 2 only
    B. 1 and 3 only
    C. 2 and 3 only
    D. 1, 2, and 3

25. Of the following late somatic effects caused by exposure to ionizing radiation, which is considered to be *most* important?

    A. Cataract formation
    B. Embryologic or birth effects
    C. Cancer
    D. Life span shortening

26. Which of the following groups of people exposed to ionizing radiation provide proof that low-level radiation exposure produces late effects?

    A. 135,000 evacuees from the 1986 nuclear power station accident in Chernobyl, Russia
    B. Japanese atomic bomb survivors
    C. Children of the Marshall Islanders who were inadvertently subjected to fallout during the atomic bomb test in 1954
    D. None of the above

27. When a prediction is made that the number of excess cancers in a given population will increase as the natural incidence of cancer increases in that population with age, the risk is described by which of the following terms?

    A. Absolute
    B. Excess
    C. Quadratic
    D. Relative

28. Studies of the Japanese atomic bomb survivors demonstrate that the incidence of leukemia has _____ since the late 1940s and early 1950s and the incidence of solid tumors has continued to _____ since the late 1950s and early 1960s.

    A. Slowly declined, escalate
    B. Increased rapidly, decrease
    C. Increased slowly, decrease
    D. Rapidly declined, decrease

29. Radiation-induced cataracts in human beings follow a _____ dose-response relationship.

    A. Nonlinear, nonthreshold
    B. Linear, nonthreshold
    C. Linear, threshold
    D. Nonlinear, threshold

30. After the 1986 nuclear power station accident in Chernobyl, Russia, an attempt was made to prevent thyroid cancer in children in Poland and some other countries as a consequence of accidental overdose to iodine 131. _____ was administered as a substitute for take-up by the thyroid gland to block its uptake of iodine 131.
    A. Potassium bromide
    B. Sodium chloride
    C. Sodium bicarbonate
    D. Potassium iodide

31. Genetic effects from exposure to ionizing radiation occur as a result of radiation-induced damage to the DNA molecule in which of the following?
    1. Sperm of an adult male
    2. Ova of an adult female
    3. Somatic cells of male and female adults
    A. 1 only
    B. 2 only
    C. 3 only
    D. 1 and 2 only

32. Large doses of ionizing radiation sustained by Japanese children in utero during the atomic bomb detonation at Hiroshima and Nagasaki have resulted in some congenital abnormalities. These abnormalities include which of the following?
    A. Mental retardation
    B. Microcephaly
    C. Growth inhibition
    D. A, B, and C

33. Existing data on radiation-induced genetic effects in humans _____.
    A. Prove conclusively that radiation causes major genetic effects
    B. Prove conclusively that radiation causes only minor genetic effects
    C. Are still inconclusive
    D. Prove conclusively that radiation does not cause any genetic effects

34. $OH^* + OH^* =$
    A. H_2O
    B. HOH^+
    C. HOH^-
    D. H_2O_2

35. What is the mean value of the radiation doubling dose for humans, as determined from the offsprings of the atomic bomb survivors of Hiroshima and Nagasaki?
    A. 1.00 Sv (100 rem)
    B. 1.56 Sv (156 rem)
    C. 3.00 Sv (300 rem)
    D. 5.67 Sv (567 rem)

36. Early (acute) effects of ionizing radiation are *not* caused by which of the following?
    A. Doses greater than 3 Gy (300 rad)
    B. Doses greater than 6 Gy (600 rad)
    C. Doses resulting from atomic bomb detonation
    D. Doses encountered in diagnostic radiology

37. Which of the following defines the ratio of the dose of a reference radiation quality (conventionally, 250 kVp x-rays) necessary to produce the same biologic reaction in a given experiment that is produced by a dose of the test radiation delivered under the same conditions?
    A. Linear energy transfer
    B. Relative biologic effectiveness
    C. Quality factor
    D. Low-level radiation effectiveness

38. While passing through a human cell, an x-ray photon interacts with and inactivates the cell's master molecule. What is the consequence for the cell?
    A. Loss of intracellular fluid
    B. Increased pressure on the cell membrane
    C. Disruption of cell chemistry
    D. Death

39. Radiation dose-response may be demonstrated graphically through the use of curves. Which of the following curves would express a linear-quadratic, nonthreshold dose response?
    A.
    B.
    C.
    D.

40. 1 micron (μm) =
    A. 10^{-6} m
    B. 10^{+6} m
    C. 10^{-3} m
    D. 10^{+3} m

41. In which of the following human populations is the risk for causing a radiation-induced cancer not directly measurable?
    1. All patients in diagnostic radiology subjected to radiation doses below 0.1 Sievert (less than 10 rem)
    2. Chernobyl radiation accident victims living in contaminated villages
    3. Japanese atomic bomb survivors
    A. 1 only
    B. 2 only
    C. 3 only
    D. 2 and 3 only

42. Which of the following illustrates the radiation sensitivity of a particular type of cell?
    A. Epidemiologic data curve
    B. Extrapolation curve
    C. Dose-response curve
    D. Survival curve

43. Which of the following terms describe a nonmitotic or nondivision form of cell death that occurs when cells die without attempting division during the interphase portion of the cell life cycle?
    1. Apoptosis
    2. Programmed cell death
    3. Reproductive death
    A. 1 and 2 only
    B. 1 and 3 only
    C. 2 and 3 only
    D. 1, 2, and 3

44. Which of the following terms describes the ratio of the radiation dose required to cause a particular biologic response of cells or organisms in an oxygen-deprived environment to the radiation dose required to cause an identical response under normally oxygenated conditions?
    A. The oxygen enhancement ratio
    B. The oxygen biologic effectiveness ratio
    C. The oxygen dose–response relationship
    D. The oxygen threshold ratio

45. What do agents such as chemicals, elevated temperatures, ionizing radiation, and viruses have in common?
    A. Nothing
    B. They can increase the frequency of mutations in only those members of the population who are already genetically impaired.
    C. They are all mutagens that may increase the frequency of occurrence of mutations.
    D. They always cause spontaneous abortions during the first trimester of pregnancy.

46. A radiation of 0.05 Gy to 0.15 Gy (5 to 15 rads) delivered to a human embryo during the preimplantation stage of development results in which of the following?
    A. Congenital abnormalities
    B. Delayed bone growth
    C. Embryonic death
    D. Microcephaly

47. Which branch of biology is concerned with the effects of ionizing radiation on living systems?
  A. Apoptotic biology
  B. Cytogenic biology
  C. Molecular biology
  D. Radiation biology

48. During the 10 years immediately after the 1986 Chernobyl nuclear power station accident, which of the following was the *most pronounced* health effect observed?
  1. Dramatic increase in the incidence of childhood leukemia
  2. Dramatic increase in thyroid cancer in children living in the regions where the heaviest radioactive contamination occurred
  3. Major increase in the number of solid tumors in the general population of the former Soviet Union
  A. 1, 2, and 3
  B. 1 only
  C. 2 only
  D. 3 only

49. A biologic reaction is produced by 3 Gy of a test radiation. It takes 12 Gy of 250 kVp x-radiation to produce the same biologic reaction. What is the relative biologic effectiveness (RBE) of the test radiation?
  A. 2.5
  B. 3
  C. 4
  D. 8

50. Which of the following means the loss or change of a nitrogenous base in the DNA chain?
  A. Aneuploidy
  B. Bleb
  C. Free radical
  D. Mutation

References

1. Travis EL: *Primer of medical radiobiology,* ed 2, St Louis, 1989, Mosby.
2. Puck TT, Marcus PI: Action of x-rays on mammalian cells, *J Exp Med* 103:653, 1956.
3. Hall EJ: *Radiobiology for the radiologist,* ed 4, Philadelphia, 1994, JB Lippincott.
4. Straume T, Dobson RL: *Health Phys* 41:666, 1981.
5. Webster EW: In *Proceedings No. 3, Critical issues in setting radiation dose limits,* Washington, D.C., 1982, National Council on Radiation Protection.
6. Finch SC: Acute radiation syndrome, *JAMA* 258(5):666, 1987.
7. Gale RP: Immediate medical consequences of nuclear accidents: lessons from Chernobyl, *JAMA* 258(5):625, 1987.
8. Perry AR, Iglar AF: The accident at Chernobyl: radiation doses and effects, *Radiol Technol* 61(4):290, 1990.
9. Linnemann RE: Soviet medical response to Chernobyl nuclear accident, *JAMA* 258(5):639, 1987.
10. Bushong SC: *Radiologic science for technologists: physics, biology and protection,* ed 6, St Louis, 1997, Mosby.
11. Fry RJM: Acute radiation effects. In Wagner LK et al, editors: *Radiation bioeffects and management: test and syllabus,* Reston, Va, 1991, American College of Radiology.
12. Hendee WR, editor: *Health effects of low-level radiation,* Norwalk, Conn, 1984, Appleton-Century-Crofts.
13. International Commission on Radiological Protection: *Recommendations of the International Commission on Radiological Protection,* ICRP Publication No. 60, Ann ICRP 21 (1-3), 1991.
14. National Research Council, Commission of Life Sciences, Committee on Biological Effects on Ionizing Radiation (BEIR V), Board on Radiation Effects Research: *Health effects of exposure to low levels of ionizing radiations,* Washington, D.C., 1989, National Academy Press.
15. Tilke B: Navajo miners battle long-term effects of radiation, *Adv Radiol Technol* 3(31):3, 1990.
16. Hamilton TE, vanBelle G, LoGerfo J: Thyroid neoplasia in Marshall Islanders exposed to nuclear fallout, *JAMA* 258(5):629, 1987.
17. Lessard E et al: *Thyroid absorbed dose for people at Rongelap, Utrik, and Sifo on March 1, 1954,* U.S. Department of Energy publication (BNL) 51-882, Upton, NY, 1985, Brookhaven National Laboratory.
18. Sinclair WK: Radiation protection recommendations on dose limits: the role of the NCRP and the ICRP and future developments, *J Radiation Oncology Biol Phys* 2(31):387, 1995.
19. Balter M: Children become the first victims of fallout, *Science* 272:357, 1996.
20. Williams N: Leukemia studies continue to draw a blank, *Science* 272:358, 1996.
21. Stewart A et al: A survey of childhood malignancies, *Br Med J* 1(5086):1495, 1958.
22. WGBH Transcripts: Back to Chernobyl, *Nova* No. 1604, Boston, 1989 (television program originally broadcast on PBS on February 14, 1989.)

23. United Nations Scientific Committee on the Effects of Atomic Radiation (UNSCEAR): *Biological effects of pre-natal irradiation,* 35th Session of UNSCEAR, Vienna, April 1986, New York, United Nations.

24. Webster EW et al: *A primer on low-level ionizing radiation and its biological effects,* AAPM Report No. 18, New York, 1986, American Institute of Physics (published for the American Association of Physicists in Medicine).

25. Eijgenraam F: Chernobyl's cloud: a lighter shade of gray, *Science, News and Comment* 252:1245, 1991.

26. Goss LB: International team examines health in zones contaminated by Chernobyl, *Physics Today, Search and Discovery,* p 20, Aug 1991.

27. Crow JF: Genetic effects of radiation, *Bull Atomic Scientists* 14:19, 1958.

Bibliography

Anthony CP, Thibodeau GA: *Textbook of anatomy and physiology,* ed 13, St Louis, 1989, Mosby.

Ballinger PW: *Merrill's atlas of radiographic positions and radiologic procedures,* ed 7, vol 1, St Louis, 1991, Mosby.

Ballinger PW: *Merrill's atlas of radiographic positions and radiologic procedures,* ed 6, vol 1, St Louis, 1986, Mosby.

Barannov A et al: Bone marrow transplantation after the Chernobyl nuclear accident, *N Engl J Med* 321(4):205, 1989.

Baron J et al: *Radiation biology: a survey of the measurement of ionizing radiation and the latent effects of low levels of radiation,* Chicago, American Society of Radiologic Technologists.

BEIR V: *Health effects of exposure to low levels of ionizing radiation,* Washington, D.C., 1990, National Academy Press.

Bond VP, Thiessen JW, editors: *Re-evaluation of dosimetric factors: Hiroshima and Nagasaki,* Springfield, Va, 1982, U.S. Department of Energy/U.S. Department of Commerce.

Bushong SC: *Radiologic science for technologists: physics, biology and protection,* ed 6, St Louis, 1997, Mosby.

Bushong SC: *Radiologic science for technologists: physics, biology and protection,* ed 5, St Louis, 1993, Mosby.

Bushong SC: *Radiologic science for technologists: physics, biology and protection,* ed 2, St Louis, 1980, Mosby.

Casarett AP: *Radiation biology,* Englewood Cliffs, NJ, 1968, Prentice-Hall.

Cobb Jr. CE: Living with radiation, *National Geographic* 175(4):403, 1989.

Commission of Life Sciences, Advisory Committee on Biologic Effects of Ionizing Radiation: *Biological effects of radiation, 1989 (BEIR V Report),* Washington, D.C., 1989, National Academy Press.

Committee on the Biological Effects of Ionizing Radiation: *The effects on populations of exposure to low levels of ionizing radiation,* Washington, D.C., 1980, National Academy of Sciences.

Committee on Biological Effects of Ionizing Radiation: *Health effects of exposure of low levels of ionizing radiations,* Washington, D.C., 1990, National Academy of Sciences/National Research Council.

Committee on the Biological Effects of Ionizing Radiation, National Academy of Sciences, National Research Council: *The effects on populations of exposure to low levels of ionizing radiations, 1980 (BEIR III Report),* Washington, D.C., 1980, National Academy Press.

Committee on Biological Effects of Ionizing Radiation, National Research Council, Commission of Life Sciences, Board on Radiation Research: *Health effects of exposure to low levels of ionizing radiation (BEIR V Report),* Washington, D.C., 1989, National Academy Press.

Crouch JE: *Functional human anatomy,* ed 4, Philadelphia, 1985, Lea & Febiger.

Crow JF: Genetic effects of radiation, *Bull Atomic Scientists* 14:19, 1958.

DeRobertis EDP, DeRobertis EMF: *Cell and molecular biology,* ed 8, Philadelphia, 1987, Lea & Febiger.

Diamond J, producer: *Chernobyl: through a doctor's eyes,* ABC News, Show 634, August 28, 1986 (transcript).

Dowd SB: *Practical radiation protection and applied radiobiology,* Philadelphia, 1994, WB Saunders.

Duke RC, Ojcius DM, Young J: Cell suicide in health and disease, *Scientific American,* p 80, Dec 1996.

Early PJ, Sodee DB: *Principles and practice of nuclear medicine,* ed 2, St Louis, 1995, Mosby.

Edwards M: Chernobyl—one year after, *National Geographic* 171(5):632, 1987.

Fabrikant JI: *Radiobiology,* Chicago, 1972, Year Book Medical.

Finch SC: Acute radiation syndrome, *JAMA* 258(5):664, 1987.

Frankel R: *Radiation protection for radiologic technologists,* New York, 1976, McGraw-Hill.

Fullerton GD et al, editors: *Medical Physics Monograph No. 5,* New York, 1980, American Institute of Physics (published for the American Association of Physicists in Medicine).

Gale RP: Immediate medical consequences of nuclear accidents: lessons from Chernobyl, *JAMA* 258(5):625, 1987.

Gurley LT, Callaway WJ, editors: *Introduction to radiologic technology,* ed 3, St Louis, 1992, Mosby.

Hall EJ: *Radiobiology for the radiologist,* ed 4, Philadelphia, 1994, JB Lippincott.

Hall EJ: *Radiobiology for the radiologist,* ed 3, Philadelphia, 1988, JB Lippincott.

Hamilton TE, vanBelle G, LoGerfo JP: Thyroid neoplasia in Marshall Islanders exposed to nuclear fallout, *JAMA* 258(5):629, 1987.

Hendee WR: Estimation of radiation risks: BEIR V and its significance for medicine, *JAMA* 268:620, 1992.

Hendee WR, editor: *Health effects of low-level radiation,* Norwalk, Conn, 1984, Appleton-Century Crofts.

Hendee WR, Ibbott GS: *Radiation therapy physics,* ed 2, St Louis, 1996, Mosby.

Hendee WR, Ritenour ER: *Medical imaging physics,* ed 3, St Louis, 1992, Mosby.

Howl B: *Simplified radiotherapy for technicians,* Springfield, Ill, 1972, Charles C. Thomas.

Lessard E et al: *Thyroid absorbed dose for people at Rongelap, Utrik, and Sifo on March 1, 1954,* U.S. Department of Energy publication (BNL) 51882, Upton, NY, 1985, Brookhaven National Laboratory.

Levy D: Chernobyl linked to kids' cancer, *USA Today,* p D-1.

Linnemann RE: Soviet medical response to the Chernobyl nuclear accident, *JAMA* 258(5):637, 1987.

London treating victim of Chernobyl disaster, *The Tennessean,* p 2A, Jan 6, 1994.

Mallett M: *A handbook of anatomy and physiology for students of medical radiation technology,* ed 3, Mankato, Minn, 1979, Burnell.

March HC: Leukemia in radiologists, *Radiology* 43:275, 1944.

Meck BJ: The effects of radiation on the eye, *RT Image* 1(11):1, 1988.

Melnykonyck A (The *Louisville Courier-Journal*): Chernobyl disaster: 10 years later, children bear Chernobyl's harshest legacy, *USA Today,* p 8A, April 22, 1996.

Miller PE: Biological effects of diagnostic irradiation, *Radiol Technol* 48:11, 1976.

Miller RW: Delayed radiation effects in atomic bomb survivors, *Science* 166:569, 1969.

Miller RW: Effects of ionizing radiation from the atomic bomb on Japanese children, *Pediatrics* 41:257, 1968.

National Council on Radiation Protection and Measurements (NCRP): *Basic radiation protection criteria,* Report No. 39, Washington, D.C., 1971, NCRP Publications.

National Council on Radiation Protection and Measurements (NCRP): *Review of the current state of radiation protection philosophy,* Report No. 43, Washington, D.C., 1975, NCRP Publications.

National Council on Radiation Protection and Measurements (NCRP): *Medical radiation exposure of pregnant and potentially pregnant women,* Report No. 54, Washington, D.C., 1977, NCRP Publications.

National Council on Radiation Protection and Measurements (NCRP): *Recommendations on limits for exposure to ionizing radiation,* Report No. 91, Bethesda, Md, 1987, NCRP Publications.

National Council on Radiation Protection and Measurements (NCRP): *The relative biological effectiveness of radiations of different quality,* Report No. 104, Bethesda, Md, 1990, NCRP Publications.

National Council on Radiation Protection and Measurements (NCRP): *Risk estimates for radiation protection,* Report No. 115, Bethesda, Md, 1993, NCRP Publications.

Noz ME, Maguire Jr. GQ: *Radiation protection in radiologic and health sciences,* ed 2, Philadelphia, 1985, Lea & Febiger.

Perry AR, Iglar HF: The accident at Chernobyl: radiation doses and effects, *Radiol Technol* 61(4):290, 1990.

Pizzarello DJ, Witcofski RL: *Basic radiation biology,* ed 2, Philadelphia, 1975, Lea & Febiger.

Pizzarello DJ, Witcofski RL: *Medical radiation biology,* ed 2, Philadelphia, 1982, Lea & Febiger.

Polednak AP, Stehney AF, Rowland RE: Mortality among women first employed before 1930 in the US radium dial-painting industry, *Am J Epidemiol* 107:179, 1978.

Rafla S, Rotman M: *Introduction to radiotherapy,* St Louis, 1974, Mosby.

Reimenschneider J: Rethinking radiation protection standards, *RT Image* 3(6):1990.

Ritenour ER: *Radiation protection and biology: a self-instructional multi-media learning series,* Denver, 1985, Multi-Media Publishing.

Rowland RE, Stehney AF, Lucas Jr. HF: Dose-response relationships for female radium dial workers, *Radiat Res* 76:368, 1978.

Russell LB, Russell WL: Radiation hazards to the embryo and fetus, *Radiology* 58:369, 1962.

Saccomanno G et al: Lung cancer of uranium miners on the Colorado plateau, *Health Phys* 10:1195, 1964.

Seeram E: *Radiation Protection,* Philadelphia, 1997, Lippincott.

Selman J: *Elements of radiobiology,* Springfield, Ill, 1983, Charles C. Thomas.

Seltser R, Sartwell PE: The influence of occupational exposure to radiation on the mortality of American radiologists and other medical specialists, *Am J Epidemiol* 81:2, 1965.

Stewart AM: *An epidemiologist takes a look at radiation risk,* DHEW Publication No. (FDA-BRH) 73-8024, 1974, Department of Health, Education and Welfare.

Stewart A et al: A survey of childhood malignancies, *Br Med J* 1(5086):1495, 1958.

Stewart A, Kneale GW: Radiation dose effects in relation to obstetric x-ray and childhood cancers, *Lancet* 1:1185, 1970.

Straume T, Dobson RL: Implication of new Hiroshima and Nagasaki dose estimates: cancer risk and neutron RBE, *Health Phys* 41:666, 1981.

Sullivan CA: Chromosome aberrations as a means to determine occupational exposure: an alternative, *Radiol Technol* 52:185, 1980.

Thomas CL, editor: *Taber's cyclopedic medical dictionary,* ed 13, Philadelphia, 1977, FA Davis.

Thompson MA et al: *Principles of imaging science and protection,* Philadelphia, 1994, WB Saunders.

Tilke B: Navajo miners battle long-term effects of radiation, *ADVANCE for Radiologic Technologists* 3(31):3, 1990.

Travis EL: *Primer of medical radiobiology,* ed 2, Chicago, 1989, Year Book Medical.

Tsuya A et al: Capillary microscopic observation of the superficial minute vessels of atomic bomb survivors, Hiroshima, 1972-73, *Radiat Res* 72:353, 1977.

U.S. Department of Health, Education, and Welfare, Public Health Service, Food and Drug Administration, Bureau of Radiological Health: *The biological effects of ionizing radiation: an overview,* HEW Publication FDA 77-8004, Rockville, Md, 1976, HEW.

Vinocur B: New data rekindle radiation debate, *Diagn Imaging,* p 94, Nov 1983.

Watkins GL: Public health risks from low dose medical radiation, *Radiol Technol* 59(2):160, 1987.

Webster EW: In *Proceedings No. 3, Critical issues in setting radiation dose limits,* Washington, D.C., 1982, National Council in Radiation Protection.

Webster EW et al: *A primer on low-level ionizing radiation and its biological effects,* AAPM Report No. 18, New York, 1986, American Institute of Physics (published for the American Association of Physicists in Medicine).

7

Protection of the Patient During Diagnostic Radiologic Procedures

added filtration

aperture diaphragm

bone marrow dose

calcium tungstate screens

cinefluorography

clear lead gonad and breast shielding

compensating filters

computed tomography (CT)

cones

cumulative timer

deterministic effects

double-emulsion x-ray film

entrance skin exposure (ESE)

entrance skin exposure rates

exposure factors

extension cylinders

fetal dose

film speed

filtration

flat contact shields

fluoroscopic exposure switch (the foot pedal)

fluoroscopic field

genetically significant dose (GSD)

genetic effects

gonadal dose

half-value layer (HVL)

high-level-control (HLC) fluoroscopy

high resolution

high-speed film-screen image receptor systems

image intensification fluoroscopy

inherent filtration

intensifying screens

intermittent fluoroscopy

interventional procedures

involuntary motion

late somatic effects

light-localizing variable-aperture rectangular collimator

luminance

mammography

mean active bone marrow dose

off-focus or stem radiation

patient motion

positive beam limitation (PBL)

primary protective barrier

protective shielding

quantum mottle

radiographic grid

radiographic processing

rare-earth screens

scattered radiation

shadow shields

shaped contact shields

silver halide crystals

skin dose

source-to-image receptor distance (SID)

source-to-tabletop distance

specific area shielding

spiral CT

thermoluminescent dosimeters (TLDs)

trough or bilateral wedge filter

total filtration

useful beam (primary beam or umbra)

voluntary motion

wedge filter

x-ray beam limitation devices

10-day rule

After completing this chapter, the reader will be able to perform the following:

- Explain the meaning of a holistic approach to patient care.
- Explain the need for effective communication between imaging department personnel and the patient.
- Explain the significance of adequate immobilization of the patient during a radiographic exposure.
- Describe the various beam-limiting devices, and identify the device that best confines the radiographic beam.
- Explain the importance of luminance of the collimator light source.
- State the requirement for good coincidence between the radiographic beam and the localizing light beam when using a variable rectangular collimator.
- Explain the function of the radiographic collimator's positive beam limitation (PBL) feature.
- Explain the function of x-ray beam filtration in diagnostic radiology.
- List two types of filtration used to filter the diagnostic x-ray beam adequately.
- Describe half-value layer (HVL), and give examples of HVLs required for selective peak kilovoltages.
- State the reason for using gonadal shielding or other specific area shielding during radiologic examinations, and identify the types of shields used.
- Explain the function of a compensating filter when radiographing a body part that varies in thickness, and list two types of such filters.
- Discuss the need to use appropriate radiographic exposure factors for all radiologic procedures.
- Explain the method whereby radiographic exposure factors may be adjusted to reduce patient dose.
- Explain the way high-speed film-screen combinations reduce radiographic exposure for the patient.
- Discuss the value of good radiographic processing techniques in reducing radiographic exposure for the patient.
- Explain the way radiographic grids increase patient dose.

Continued

During a diagnostic radiologic procedure a holistic approach to patient care is essential. This means treating the whole person rather than just the area of concern. Holistic patient care must begin with real communication between the radiographer and patient. Effective communication alleviates the patient's uneasiness and increases the chance for cooperation and successful completion of the procedure. To deal appropriately with all patients, the reader must develop effective communications skills.

Radiographers must limit the exposure of the patient to ionizing radiation by correctly employing appropriate techniques and devices. Patient exposure may be limited by proper immobilization, use of appropriate beam limitation devices, correct filtration, use of gonadal or other specific area shielding, selection of appropriate exposure factors in conjunction with high-speed film-screen combinations, good radiographic processing techniques, and a minimum of repeat radiographs. This chapter provides an overview of techniques used to protect patients, from unnecessary radiation exposure during diagnostic radiologic procedures.

Effective Communication

When words, or verbal messages, and unconscious actions or body language, or nonverbal messages, are understood as intended, communication between the radiographer and patient is effective. Communication encourages closeness, reduces anxiety and emotional stress, enhances the professional image of the radiographer as a person who cares about the patient's well-being, and increases the chance for successful completion of the radiologic examination. Everyone within the medical imaging department should always behave as compassionate professionals. Words and actions must demonstrate understanding and respect for human dignity and individual uniqueness.

Patient protection during a diagnostic radiologic procedure should begin with clear, concise instructions (Fig. 7-1). When patients understand the procedure and their responsibilities, they can more fully cooperate. When health care professionals do not thoroughly explain procedures, patients fear the unknown and become anxious, especially during lengthy procedures. To alleviate the problem, the radiographer must take adequate time to explain the procedure in simple terms that the patient can understand. The radiographer also should give patients the opportunity to ask questions. The radiographer must listen attentively to these questions and answer them truthfully in an appropriate tone of voice and in accordance with ethical guidelines. This creates a sense of trust between the patient and the radiographer and encourages further communication.

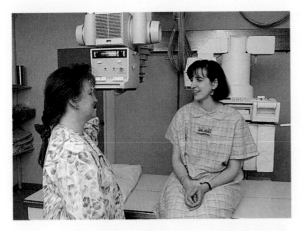

Fig. 7-1 Clear, concise instructions promote effective communication between the radiographer and the patient.

If the radiographic procedure (e.g., angiocatheterization, other contrast media injection) will cause pain, discomfort, or any strange sensations, the patient must be informed before the procedure begins (Fig. 7-2). However, to prevent the patient from imagining more pain or discomfort than the procedure will actually cause, the radiographer should try not to overemphasize this aspect of the examination.

Repeat radiographs may sometimes be attributed to poor communication between the radiographer and patient. Inadequate or misinterpreted communication may cause a communication gap, which may result in the patient's inability to cooperate. For example, during an interventional radiographic examination that creates some thermal discomfort, patients may move because they are surprised or want to inform the technologist or physician that something is wrong. This movement may result in an unnecessary repeat exposure. Effective communication between radiographer and patient can prevent this problem from occurring.

Immobilization

If a patient moves during a radiographic exposure, the radiographic image will be blurred. Because such radiographs have little or no diagnostic value, a re-

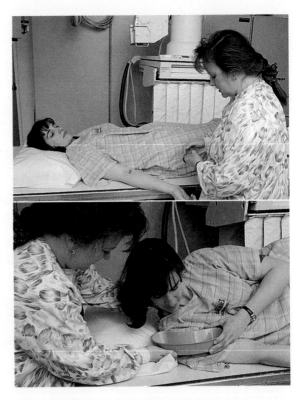

Fig. 7-2 Before the procedure begins, inform the patient of any pain, discomfort, or strange sensations that will be experienced during the procedure.

peat examination is necessary, although it results in additional radiation exposure for the patient and radiographer.

Two types of patient motion exist: voluntary and involuntary. Motion controlled by will is classified as **voluntary motion.** To eliminate the problem of voluntary patient movement during radiography, the radiographer must gain the cooperation of the patient or adequately immobilize the patient during the radiographic exposure (Fig. 7-3). A variety of suitable restraining devices is available to immobilize either the whole body or individual body part to be radiographed. These radiographic aids should be used whenever necessary.

Involuntary motion, caused by muscle groups such as those associated with the digestive organs or

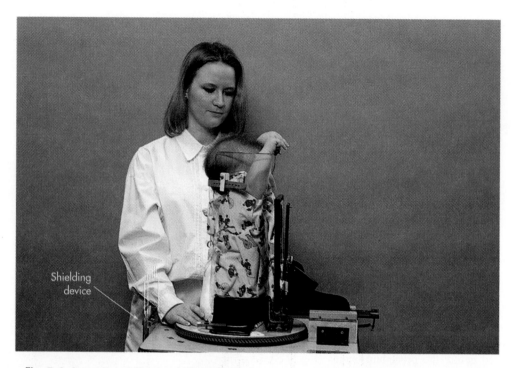

Shielding
device

Fig. 7-3 Proper immobilization during radiographic examinations eliminates voluntary motion. This restraint has a shield *(left)* that may be raised or lowered to shield the infant's reproductive organs.

the heart, cannot be willfully controlled. This type of motion may be reduced by shortening exposure time and using very-high-speed image receptors.

X-Ray Beam Limitation Devices

Basic **x-ray beam limitation devices** include aperture diaphragms, cones and cylinders, and collimators. These devices confine the **useful beam (primary beam or umbra)** *before* it enters the area of clinical interest, thereby limiting the quantity of body tissue irradiated. This also reduces the amount of **scattered radiation** in the tissue, preventing unnecessary exposure to tissues not under examination.

Aperture diaphragm

An **aperture diaphragm** is the simplest of all beam limitation devices. It consists of a flat piece of lead with a hole of a designated size and shape cut in its center. The dimensions of the hole determine the size

and shape of the radiographic beam. Different film sizes and different source-to-image receptor distances require aperture diaphragms of various sizes to accommodate them. Diaphragm openings are rectangular, square, or round, with the rectangular shape being most common.

Placed directly below the window of the x-ray tube, the aperture diaphragm confines the primary radiographic beam dimensions suitable to cover a given size of film at a specified **source-to-image receptor distance (SID)** (Fig. 7-4). Use of an aperture diaphragm reduces scattered radiation because the diaphragm limits field size (the area of the body irradiated); the amount of scattered radiation produced is a function of the volume of tissue irradiated.

Cones

Cones are circular metal tubes that attach to the x-ray tube housing or variable rectangular collimator to limit the x-ray beam to a predetermined size and

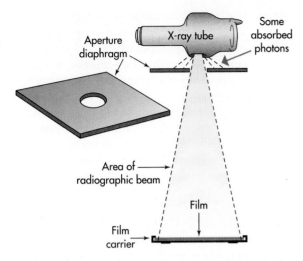

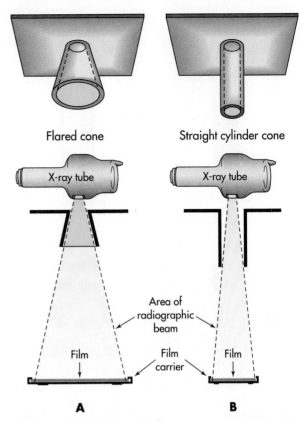

Fig. 7-4 An aperture diaphragm, a flat piece of lead with a hole of a designated size and shape cut in its center, is placed directly below the window of the x-ray tube to confine the primary radiographic beam dimensions suitable to cover a given size of film at a specified source-to-image receptor distance (SID).

Fig. 7-5 Cones are circular metal tubes that attach to the x-ray tube housing or variable rectangular collimator to limit the radiographic beam to a predetermined size and shape. **A,** Cone fashioned in the form of a flared metal tube. **B,** Cone fashioned in the form of a straight cylinder.

shape. The design of this collimating device is simple, consisting of either a flared metal tube with the diameter of the upper end smaller than the diameter of the lower end, or a straight cylinder with the diameter the same at both the upper and lower ends (Fig. 7-5, *A* and *B*). Although the length and diameter of cones vary, it is primarily the lower rim of the cone that governs beam limitation. Sharper size restriction is achieved when the cone or cylinder is longer. Field size at selected SIDs should be indicated on the cone.

Spot, or very small field, radiography is best accomplished through the use of **extension cylinders,** which are cylindric metal tubes with a 10- to 20-inch metal extension at the far end of the barrel (Fig. 7-6). The use of this extension piece further limits the size of the useful beam.

Light-localizing variable-aperture rectangular collimators have replaced cones for most radiographic examinations. However, cones are still frequently used for radiographic examinations of the head (e.g., cone-down view of the sella turcica or views of the paranasal sinuses), vertebral column, and chest.

Beam-defining cones are widely used in dental radiography. Because dental x-ray equipment is usually less bulky than general purpose equipment, a one-piece beam limitation device, such as a cone made of plastic, is convenient. Some dental cones are lined with lead. When dentists use lead-lined cones instead of the conventional plastic cones, patient exposure is reduced because the source of secondary radiation (the plastic cone itself) is eliminated.[1]

Collimators

The collimator is the most versatile device for defining the size and shape of the radiographic beam. The **light-localizing variable-aperture rectangular**

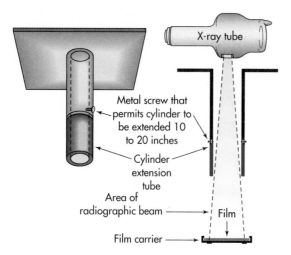

X-ray tube

Metal screw that permits cylinder to be extended 10 to 20 inches

Cylinder extension tube

Area of radiographic beam

Film

Film carrier

Fig. 7-6 Extension cylinder used for spot or very small field radiography.

collimator (Fig. 7-7, *A*) is the type of collimator most often used with multipurpose x-ray units. It is box shaped and contains the radiographic beam-defining system (Fig. 7-7, *B*), which consists of two sets of adjustable lead shutters mounted within the device at different levels, a light source to illuminate the x-ray field and permit it to be centered over the area of clinical interest, and a mirror to deflect the light beam toward the object to be radiographed.

The first set of shutters, the upper shutters, are mounted as close as possible to the tube window to reduce the amount of **off-focus or stem radiation** (x-rays emitted from parts of the tube other than the focal spot) coming from the primary beam and exiting at various angles from the x-ray tube window. This radiation can never be completely eliminated because the metal shutters cannot be placed immediately beneath the actual focal spot of the x-ray tube, but placing the first set or upper shutters as close as possible to the tube window can reduce it significantly. This practice reduces patient exposure resulting from off-focus radiation.

The second set of collimator shutters, the lower shutters, are mounted below the level of the light source and mirror and function to confine further the radiographic beam to the area of clinical interest (Fig. 7-7, *B* and *C*). This set of shutters consists of two

pairs of lead plates oriented at right angles to each other. Each set may be adjusted independently so that a variety of rectangular shapes can be selected. In this way the field is not limited to the circular or square shapes that sometimes irradiate areas of the patient not requiring imaging.

To minimize skin exposure to electrons produced by photon interaction with the collimator, the patient's skin surface should be at least 15 cm below the collimator. Some collimator housings contain "spacer bars," which project down from the housing to prevent the collimators from being closer than 15 cm to the patient.

Luminance is a scientific term referring to the brightness of a surface. Specifically, luminance quantifies the intensity of a light source (i.e., the amount of light per unit area coming from its surface). Luminance is determined by measuring the concentration of light over a particular field of view. This may be understood by examining the units used to describe luminance. The primary unit is the candela per square meter, known more simply as the nit. One candela corresponds to 3.8 million billion photons per second being emitted from a light source through a conelike field of view. A good analogy for this is the sound intensity emerging from a drill sergeant with a megaphone held to his lips. With appropriate dimensions the megaphone's larger opening corresponds to the conelike field of view associated with the candela. Luminance of the collimator light source must be adequate to permit the localizing light beam to outline the margins of the radiographic beam adequately on the patient's anatomy. If the light field were not sufficiently bright, a radiographer might improperly position the x-ray field on a patient or at the very least have great difficulty in accurately centering the x-ray beam, especially in the case of a dark-skinned patient. Another potential problem with insufficient brightness is that the x-ray unit may fail a state inspection because the luminance is so low that it cannot sufficiently illuminate a calibrated light meter. The light meter reading must not be below 15 "foot-candles." A foot-candle is approximately equivalent to 10.76 nit (the unit of luminance). Therefore 15 foot-candles corresponds to a collimator light source with a luminance of about 161 nit or candela per square meter. If

A

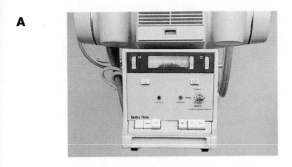

B

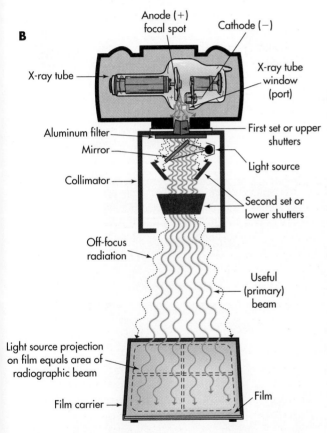

C

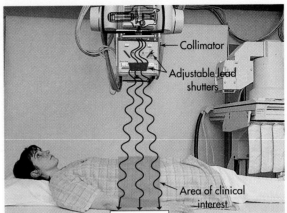

Fig. 7-7 A, Light-localizing variable-aperture rectangular collimator. **B,** Diagram of a typical collimator demonstrating radiographic beam-defining system: *1,* anode focal spot; *2,* x-ray tube window; *3,* mirror; *4,* light source; *5,* first set or upper shutters; *6,* second set or lower shutters; and, *7,* aluminum filter. The metal shutters collimate the radiographic beam so that it is no larger than the image receptor (the film). **C,** Collimator containing the radiographic beam-defining system, which establishes the parameters (margins) of the beam. Adjustable lead shutters limit the crosssectional area of the beam and confine it to the area of clinical interest.

the luminance of the collimator light source is adequate, the localizing light beam should adequately outline the margins of the radiographic beam on the area of interest on all patients.

When using a light-localizing variable-aperture rectangular collimator, good coincidence (i.e., both physical size and alignment) between the radio-

graphic beam and the localizing light beam is essential. Both alignment and length and width dimensions of the radiographic and light beams must correspond to within 2% of the SID. As an example, 40 inches, which is equal to 101.6 cm, is the most commonly used SID in radiography. At this SID the maximal allowable difference in either length or width dimensions of the projected light field in relation to the radiographic beam at the level of the image receptor must be no more than 2% of 40 inches (0.8 inches) or 2% of 101.6 cm, or approximately 100 cm (2 cm).

In the collimation system described so far, the radiographer could inadvertently use a film size much smaller than the size of the radiation field. Thus areas of the patient would be irradiated that would not be recorded on film. Either the radiation field size should be smaller (if the anatomy is not of diagnostic interest) or the film should be larger (if the anatomy is indeed of diagnostic interest). To prevent such a mismatch,

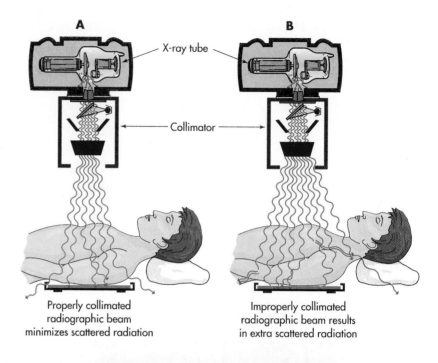

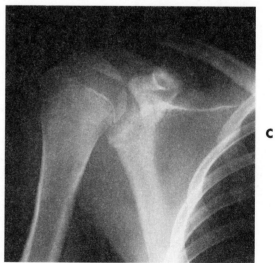

Fig. 7-8 Collimate the radiographic beam so that it is no larger than the image receptor (the film). Limiting the beam to the area of clinical interest decreases the amount of tissue irradiated and minimizes patient exposure by reducing the amount of scattered and absorbed radiation. **A,** Good collimation. **B,** Poor collimation. **C,** AP radiograph of the shoulder demonstrating good collimation.

radiographic collimators now include a feature called **positive beam limitation (PBL).** The PBL feature consists of electronic sensors in the film cassette holder that send signals to the collimator housing. When PBL is activated, the collimators are automatically adjusted so that the radiation field size matches the film size. The PBL feature may be deactivated by turning a key if some special conditions require that the radiographer have complete control of the system. However, in such a circumstance a warning light is automatically lit to indicate that the PBL system has been deactivated.

The PBL system illustrates an important principle of patient protection during radiographic procedures. The radiographer must ensure that collimation is adequate by applying the following principle: *Collimate the radiographic beam so that it is no larger than the image receptor (the film)* (Fig. 7-8, *A* to *C*). The regulatory standard is that an accuracy by 2% of the SID is required with PBL.

Filtration

Filtration of the radiographic beam reduces exposure to the patient's skin and superficial tissue by absorbing most of the lower-energy photons (long-wavelength or soft x-rays) from the heterogeneous beam (Fig. 7-9). This increases mean energy, or "quality," of the x-ray beam. This change in beam quality also is referred to as "hardening" of the beam.

Because filtration absorbs some of the photons in a radiographic beam, it decreases the overall intensity (quantity or amount) of radiation. The remaining photons, however, are as a whole more penetrating and therefore less likely to be absorbed in body tissue. Hence the absorbed dose to the patient decreases when proper filtration is placed in the path of the radiographic beam. If adequate filtration were not present, very-low-energy photons (20 keV or lower) would always be absorbed in the body, increasing the patient's radiation dose but contributing nothing to the image process. They should be removed from the radiographic beam through the process of filtration.

Two types of filtration are available:
1. Inherent filtration
2. Added filtration

Inherent filtration includes the glass envelope encasing the x-ray tube, the insulating oil surrounding the tube, and the glass window in the tube housing. This inherent material amounts to approximately 0.5-mm aluminum equivalent. An additional 1-mm aluminum equivalent is provided by the light-localizing variable-aperture rectangular collimator. The reflective surface of the collimator mirror provides most of this aluminum equivalent.

Added filtration usually consists of sheets of aluminum (or its equivalent) of appropriate thickness. This additional filtration is located outside the glass

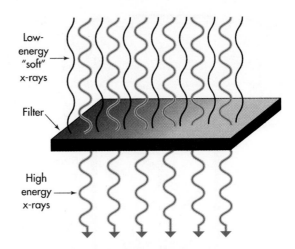

Fig. 7-9 Filtration removes low-energy photons (long-wavelength or "soft" x-rays) from the beam by absorbing them and permits higher-energy photons to pass through. This reduces patient dose.

window of the tube housing above the collimator shutters. It is readily accessible to service personnel and may be changed as the x-ray tube ages. The inherent and added filtration combine to equal the required amount of total filtration necessary to filter the useful beam adequately.

The peak kilovoltage of a given x-ray unit determines the total amount of filtration required. **Total filtration** of 2.5-mm aluminum equivalent for fixed x-ray units operating above 70 kVp is the regulatory standard (Fig. 7-10). Because such fixed x-ray equipment comes from the manufacturer with inherent filtration of 0.5-mm aluminum equivalent and 1-mm aluminum equivalent is attributed to the collimator components, the manufacturer needs to place only an additional 1-mm aluminum equivalent filter between the tube housing and collimator to meet the total filtration requirement. Mobile diagnostic units and fluoroscopic equipment also require 2.5-mm aluminum equivalent total permanent filtration.

Fixed radiographic equipment requires total filtration of 1.5-mm aluminum equivalent for x-ray units operating from 50 to 70 kVp.[2] Proper filtration also is necessary for mammographic equipment. Metallic elements such as molybdenum and rhodium are frequently employed as filters. These materials facilitate

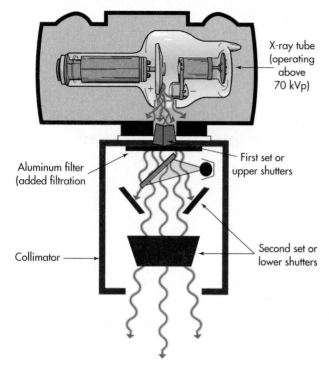

X-ray tube
(operating
above
70 kVp)

Aluminum filter
(added filtration

First set or
upper shutters

Collimator

Second set or
lower shutters

Fig. 7-10 A minimum of 2.5-mm aluminum equivalent total filtration is required for fixed radiographic units operating above 70 kVp.

image contrast over the clinical extent of compressed breast thicknesses by preferentially selecting a particular range or window of energies from the x-ray spectrum emerging from the x-ray tube target. Molybdenum filters allow a lower-energy window than rhodium filters. Molybdenum filters are therefore suitable for small and average breast thickness, and rhodium filters are better for larger breasts (i.e., compression thickness of 6 cm and greater). The intelligent use of such materials has the effect of reducing the mean glandular dose in firm breast tissue. Maintaining and enhancing subject contrast is important in mammography. Beryllium takes the place of glass in the window of the mammographic x-ray tube to accommodate this need. This light, strong metal permits the relatively soft characteristic radiation produced by the tube to pass through and improve subject contrast.

In general diagnostic radiology, aluminum (atomic number 13) is the metal most widely selected as filter material because, without severely decreasing the x-ray beam intensity, it effectively removes low-energy (soft) x-rays from a polyenergetic (heterogeneous) x-ray beam. Also, aluminum is lightweight, sturdy, relatively inexpensive, and readily available. In compliance with the Radiation Control for Health and Safety Act of 1968 a diagnostic x-ray beam must always be adequately filtered. This means that a sufficient quantity of low-energy photons have been removed from a beam produced at a given peak kilovoltage. The **half-value layer (HVL)** of the beam must be measured to verify this. *HVL* may be defined as the thickness of a designated absorber (customarily a metal such as aluminum) required to decrease the intensity (quantity or amount) of the primary beam by 50% of its initial value. This measurement should be obtained by a radiologic physicist at least once a year and also after an x-ray tube is replaced or repairs have been made on the diagnostic x-ray tube housing or collimation system. For diagnostic x-ray beams the HVL measurement is expressed in millimeters of aluminum. Because HVL is a measure of beam quality, a certain minimal HVL is required at a given peak kilovoltage. Examples of required HVLs for selective peak kilovoltages are listed in Table 7-1.

Protective Shielding

Radiation exposure to radiosensitive body organs or tissues requires the use of **protective shielding** to reduce or eliminate radiation dose that would otherwise result in biologic damage. Some organs or tissues that should be shielded from the useful beam whenever possible include the lens of the eye, the breast, and the reproductive organs. Selective shielding of these areas may be accomplished through the use of specific area shielding.

Gonadal shielding devices

Gonadal shielding devices are used during radiologic procedures to protect the reproductive organs from exposure to the useful beam when they are in or within approximately 5 cm of a properly collimated beam. Gonadal shielding is used unless it will compromise the diagnostic value of the examination. Gonadal shielding should be a secondary protective measure, not a substitute for a properly collimated beam. Proper

Table 7-1	
HVL Required by the Radiation Control for Health and Safety Act of 1968 and Detailed by the Bureau of Radiological Health* in 1980	

Peak kilovoltage	Required HVL in millimeters of aluminum
30	0.3
40	0.4
50	1.2
60	1.3
70	1.5
80	2.3
90	2.5
100	2.7
110	3.0
120	3.2

*The Bureau of Radiological Health changed its name to the Center for Devices and Radiological Health in 1982.

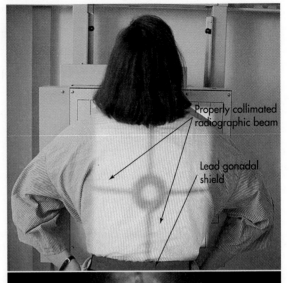

A

Properly collimated radiographic beam

Lead gonadal shield

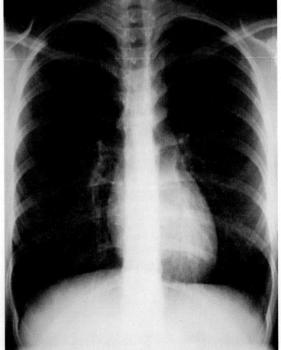

B

collimation of the radiographic beam (Fig. 7-11, *A* and *B*) must always be the first step in gonadal protection.

As a consequence of their anatomic location, the female reproductive organs receive about three times more exposure during a given radiographic procedure involving the pelvic region than do the male reproductive organs. However, gonadal exposure for both men and women may be greatly reduced through the application of appropriate gonadal shielding. For female patients the use of a flat contact shield (containing 1 mm of lead) placed over the reproductive organs reduces exposure by about 50%. Primary beam exposure for male patients may be reduced by 90% to 95% through the use of a shaped contact shield (also containing 1 mm of lead). Gonadal shielding should always be used whenever it will not obscure necessary clinical information. Every imaging department should establish a written shielding protocol for each of its radiologic procedures. This contributes to a reduction in the cumulative population gonad dose.

Four basic types of gonadal shielding devices are used:

1. Flat contact shields
2. Shadow shields

Fig. 7-11 A, Proper collimation of the radiographic beam must always be the first step in gonadal protection. **B,** When the gonads are not in the area of clinical interest, proper collimation of the radiographic beam reduces gonadal exposure.

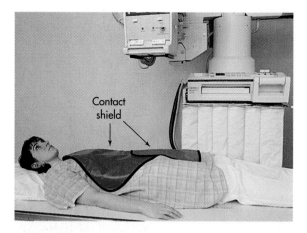

Fig. 7-12 An uncontoured, flat contact shield of lead-impregnated material may be placed over the patient's gonads to provide protection from x-radiation.

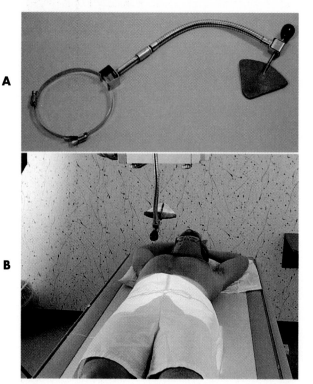

Fig. 7-13 A, Shadow shield components. **B,** A shadow shield suspended above the radiographic beam-defining system casts a shadow over the protected body area, the gonads. (Courtesy Nuclear Associates, Inc.) **C,** The radiograph demonstrates effective gonadal shielding resulting from the use of a shadow shield.

3. Shaped contact shields
4. Clear lead

Flat contact shields

Flat contact shields are made of lead strips or lead-impregnated materials. These shields may be placed directly over the patient's reproductive organs (Fig. 7-12) or secured to the patient with tape. These shields are most effective when used as protective devices for patients having anteroposterior (AP) or posteroanterior (PA) radiographs while in a recumbent position. Flat contact shields are not suited for nonrecumbent positions or projections other than AP or PA. If the flat contact shield is used during a fluoroscopic examination, it must be placed under the patient to be effective because the x-ray tube is located under the radiographic table.

Shadow shields

Shadow shields (Fig. 7-13, *A*) are made of a radiopaque material. Suspended from above the radiographic beam-defining system, these shields hang over the area of clinical interest to cast a shadow in the primary beam over the patient's reproductive organs (Fig. 7-13, *B* and *C*). The clear lead filter illustrated in Fig. 7-14 functions as a shadow shield and is used to shield breasts and gonads. The beam-defining light casts the shadow of the shield over the anatomy. The beam-defining light must be accurately positioned to ensure proper placement of the shadow shield. When the shield is properly positioned, it provides protec-

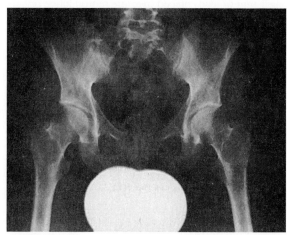

C

tion from the radiographic beam as efficiently as the contact shield. If the shield is not properly positioned, it may necessitate a repeat exposure, thus increasing patient dose. The shadow shield is not suitable for use during fluoroscopy because no localizing light field exists and the field of view is usually moved about during a study. However, the shadow shield may be used effectively to provide gonadal protection in a sterile field or when examining incapacitated patients. Shadow shields have the advantage of reducing patient embarrassment by generally eliminating the need for the radiographer to palpate the patient's anatomy in the area of the reproductive organs before placing the shield in the appropriate position.

Shaped contact shields

Shaped contact shields are made of radiopaque material contoured to enclose the male reproductive organs. Disposable or washable athletic supporters or jockey-style briefs function as carriers for these shields. The carriers each contain a pouch into which the shield is placed (Fig. 7-15). The cuplike shape of the shield permits comfortable placement over the scrotum and penis whether the patient is in a recumbent or a nonrecumbent position. To ensure privacy and reduce embarrassment, the patient can don the garment containing the shield in the confines of the dressing room.

Because the shaped contact shield is securely held in place by the carrier, AP, oblique, and lateral radiographs may be obtained with maximal gonadal protection. This shield also is suitable for use during fluoroscopic examinations. Shaped contact shields are not recommended for PA projections because the shield covers the anterior surface of the reproductive organs and the x-ray beam enters from the posterior surface; therefore the shield does not protect the gonads.

Clear lead

Some of the basic gonadal shielding devices such as the shaped contact shield and first-generation shadow shield previously described are being replaced by **clear lead gonad and breast shielding** (Fig. 7-14). These shields are made of transparent lead-plastic material impregnated with approximately 30% lead by weight. Examples of gonad and breast shielding are provided in Fig. 7-16, which demonstrates a full-spinal scoliosis examination. Along with the clear lead gonad and breast shields, a lightweight, fully transparent clear lead filter is incorporated to provide uniform density throughout the spinal canal (Fig. 7-16, *A*)

Specific area shielding

Radiosensitive organs and tissues other than the reproductive organs may be selectively shielded from the primary beam during a diagnostic radiographic examination. Contact lens shields for the lens of the eye can reduce or eliminate exposure to that highly sensi-

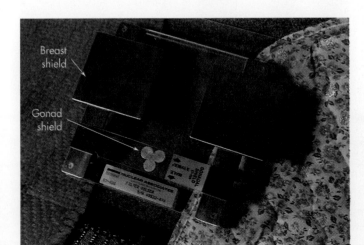

Fig. 7-14 Lead filter with breast and gonad shielding device. This shield functions as a shadow shield. (Courtesy Nuclear Associates, Inc.)

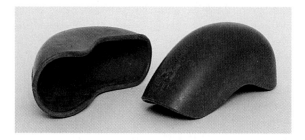

Fig. 7-15 Shaped contact shields (cuplike in shape) may be held in place with a suitable carrier.

tive area. Shielding of particularly sensitive breast tissue may be accomplished using a clear lead shadow shield (Fig. 7-14). This shielding is of vital importance in providing protection during juvenile scoliosis examinations. Radiation dose to the breast of a young patient may be further reduced by performing the scoliosis examination with the radiographic beam entering the posterior surface of the patient's body instead of the anterior surface. The use of the PA projection results in a lower entrance exposure dose to the anterior body surface, thereby significantly reducing the dose to the breast.

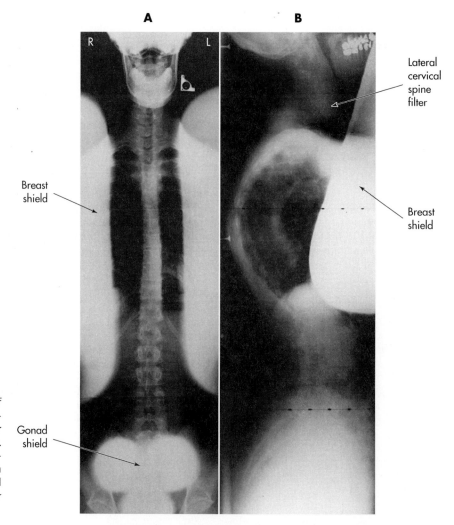

Fig. 7-16 A, AP radiograph of a full-spine scoliosis examination demonstrating lead filter with breast and gonad shields. **B,** Lateral radiograph of full-spine scoliosis examination with lateral cervical filter and breast shield. (Courtesy Nuclear Associates, Inc.)

In summary, effective shielding programs may be established in any facility by providing the appropriate shields. Because substantial gonadal dose reduction can be achieved through effective shielding, patients with the potential to reproduce should be shielded during radiologic procedures whenever the diagnostic value of the examination is not compromised. This protective measure minimizes the number of potentially deleterious x-ray–induced mutations expressed in future generations. **Specific area shielding** for selective body areas other than the gonads significantly reduces radiation exposure to those areas and should be used whenever possible.

Compensating Filters

Dose reduction and uniform radiographic imaging of body parts that vary considerably in thickness or tissue composition may be accomplished by use of **compensating filters** constructed of aluminum, lead-acrylic, or other suitable materials. These devices partially attenuate x-rays that are directed toward the thinner, or less dense, area while permitting more x-radiation to strike the thicker, or more dense, area. For example, the **wedge filter** (Fig. 7-17, *A* and *B*) may be used to provide uniform density when radiographing the foot in the dorsoplantar projection. For this examination the wedge is attached to the lower rim of the collimator and positioned with its thickest part toward the toes and its thinnest part toward the heel. The **trough, or bilateral wedge, filter,** which is used in some dedicated chest radiographic units, provides another example of a compensating filter. This filter is thin in the center to permit adequate x-ray penetration of the mediastinum and thick laterally to reduce exposure to the aerated lungs. With this device a radiographic image with uniform average density is obtained.

Exposure Factors

Selection of appropriate **exposure factors** for each radiographic examination is essential to ensure a diagnostic radiograph with minimal patient dose. The technique chosen must ensure sufficient penetration of the area of clinical interest, appropriate radiographic

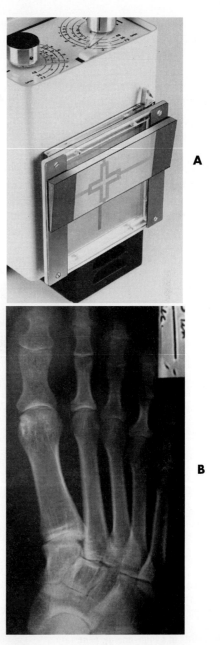

A

B

Fig. 7-17 A, Wedge-shaped lead compensating filter used to provide uniform density for **(B),** a dorsoplantar projection of the foot.

film density (exposure), and an adequate amount of radiographic contrast between adjacent tissue densities. The appropriate factors are determined by factors such as (1) the mass per unit volume of tissue of the area of clinical interest, (2) the effective atomic numbers and electron densities of the tissues involved, (3) the film-screen combination, (4) the SID, (5) the type and quantity of filtration employed, (6) the type of x-ray generator used (single phase, three phase, or high frequency), and (7) the balance of radiographic density and contrast required.

To ensure uniform selection of radiographic exposure factors, efficient imaging departments use standardized technique charts for each x-ray unit. The ra-

diographer is responsible for consulting this chart before making each radiographic exposure to ensure a diagnostic radiograph with minimal patient dose. Neglecting to use standardized technique charts necessitates estimating the exposure factor, which may result in poor-quality radiographs, repeat examinations, and additional, unnecessary exposure for the patient.

Exposure factors that minimize the radiation dose to the patient should be selected whenever possible. The use of higher kilovoltage (kVp) and lower milliamperage and exposure time in seconds (mAs)* re-

---

*mAs (milliampere seconds) are the product of x-ray electron tube current and the amount of time in seconds that the x-ray beam is on.

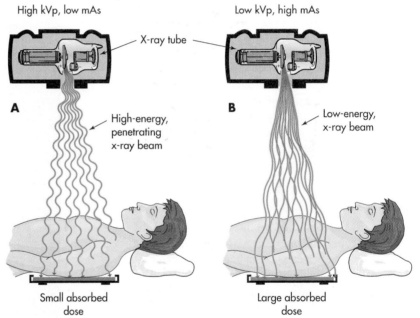

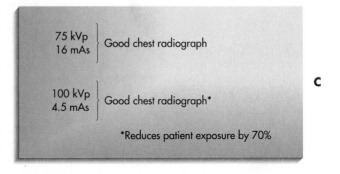

Fig. 7-18 The use of higher kilovoltage (kVp) and lower milliamperage and exposure time in seconds (mAs) reduces patient dose. **A,** The use of high kVp and low mAs results in a high-energy, penetrating x-ray beam and a small patient absorbed dose. **B,** The use of low kVp and high mAs results in a low-energy x-ray beam, most of which is easily absorbed by the patient. **C,** Example of a higher-kVp, lower-mAs technique resulting in a 70% reduction in patient exposure without significantly compromising radiographic quality.

duces patient dose (Fig. 7-18, *A* and *B*). However, this exposure factor combination produces a poorer quality radiograph. As kVp increases and mAs decreases, radiographic contrast is reduced. Consequently, the amount of diagnostically useful information in the image is reduced. A balance in radiographic exposure factors must be achieved to ensure the presence of adequate information in the image and minimize patient dose. To achieve this balance, the radiographer must select the highest kVp and the lowest mAs that will yield sufficient information for each examination (Fig. 7-18, *C*).

Radiographic Processing

Proper **radiographic processing** enhances image quality by making diagnostic information visible on the finished radiograph. Poorly processed radiographs offer inadequate diagnostic information, leading to repeat examinations and unnecessary patient exposure.

To ensure standardization in processing techniques, imaging departments should establish a quality assurance program that includes monitoring and maintenance of all processors in the facility. Such a program ensures the production of high-quality radiographs. A number of excellent reviews have been written on this subject. These reviews include step-by-step procedures for performance, monitoring, and quality control.[3-6]

Film–Screen Combinations

X-ray film, most of which is **double-emulsion x-ray film** (i.e., emulsion coated on both sides of the film), responds strongly to the light emitted by the intensifying screens. **Intensifying screens** enhance the action of x-rays on film by converting x-ray energy into visible light. About 95% of the radiographic density of the recorded image results from the visible light photons emitted by the intensifying screens. Because a single x-ray photon can produce 80 to 95 light photons, this conversion drastically speeds the film exposure process and permits radiographic exposure time to be substantially reduced. This leads to a sizeable reduction in patient dose. At the time of this writing, intensifying screens are predominantly **rare-earth screens.** Because they absorb a higher portion of the incident x-ray beam and can convert the x-ray energy

to light more efficiently, rare-earth screens are noticeably faster than the **calcium tungstate screens** that were used until the 1970s. Rare-earth screens also place less thermal stress on the x-ray tube, increasing its life span. In addition, when rare-earth screens are used, radiation shielding requirements for the x-ray room are decreased because a general reduction of x-radiation in the environment occurs.

To reiterate, **film speed** and the use of intensifying screens significantly influence radiographic exposure time. In general, 200- to 400-speed systems are considered standard at the time of this writing. Changing from a 200-speed system to a 400-speed system reduces patient radiation exposure by approximately 50%. When the amount of **silver halide crystals** (approximately 95% of which are silver bromide) contained in the film emulsion is increased, the speed of the film is increased. This means that less radiation is required to obtain an image. As radiographic exposure decreases, patient dose decreases.

Kilovoltage also affects screen speed. As kilovoltage increases, screen speed increases. This results in a reduction in patient dose.

Although the use of **high-speed film-screen image receptor systems** with calcium tungstate intensifying screens significantly reduced patient dose, a loss of radiographic quality was possible because the recorded image may have had poorer resolution. As a result, the use of these image receptor systems was not practical for all radiography. To be able to select the appropriate image receptor system for a given radiographic examination, the radiographer had to be aware of the capabilities and limitations of the different systems available. Product information of this type was supplied by the manufacturers or distributors.

As mentioned previously, rare-earth intensifying screens are more efficient than calcium tungstate intensifying screens in converting x-ray energy into light photons. Made of rare-earth phosphors such as gadolinium, lanthanum, or yttrium, these screens absorb approximately five times more x-ray energy than the previously used calcium tungstate screens; hence they emit considerably more light. This results in a significant reduction in the radiographic exposure required to obtain an image of acceptable quality. An additional benefit of rare-earth screens is that **high resolution** (the ability of a system to make two adjacent objects visually distinguishable) of the recorded image remains constant. This ensures radiographic quality. Higher-speed rare-earth systems do, however, produce **quantum mottle** (faint blotches) in the recorded image, causing some degradation of the image.

Radiographic Grids

Even though patient dose increases with the use of the **radiographic grid,** the benefit obtained (improved radiographic contrast, making available a greater quantity of diagnostic information) makes the use of the grid a fair compromise. However, care must be taken to ensure that the proper type of grid is being used for a particular examination, or else a repeat may be necessary, which would negate the benefit of increased image quality.

When x-rays pass through an object, photons are scattered away from their original path as a result of coherent and Compton scattering processes. Radiographic quality is highest when scattered photons are not recorded on the radiograph. If scattered photons are recorded, a general darkening of the film occurs, which detracts from the viewer's ability to distinguish between the different structures of the object being radiographed. Thus only those photons that have passed through matter with no deviation from their original path should be recorded. To minimize the influence of scattered photons, a grid is inserted between the patient and the image receptor. The grid acts as a sieve to block the passage of photons that have been scattered at some angle from their original path (Fig. 7-19).

Grids are made of parallel radiopaque lead strips alternated with low-attenuation strips of aluminum, plastic, or wood. Because some fraction of the film is covered with lead, mAs must be increased to compensate for the use of the grid. Hence patient dose increases whenever a grid is used. Because more lead is contained in higher-ratio grids (e.g., 16 : 1), patient dose increases as grid ratio increases.

Repeat Radiographs

The term *repeat radiograph* refers to any radiograph that must be performed more than once because of human or mechanical error during the production of the initial radiograph. This additional exposure increases patient dose. The skin and gonads of the patient receive a "double dose" whenever a repeat examination occurs. For this reason, repeat radiographs must be minimized. An occasional repeat radiograph is permissible when recommended by the radiologist for the purpose of obtaining additional diagnostic information. However, repeat examinations resulting from carelessness or poor judgment on the part of the radiographer must be eliminated. The radiographer must select the radiographic techniques and exposure factors that will ensure the production of high-quality radiographs for each examination the first time.

Institutions can benefit significantly by implementing and maintaining a repeat analysis program. By determining the number of repeats and the reasons for producing unacceptable radiographs, existing problems and conditions in an imaging department may be identified. Repeat analysis studies determine the number of radiographs in a given period that must be done

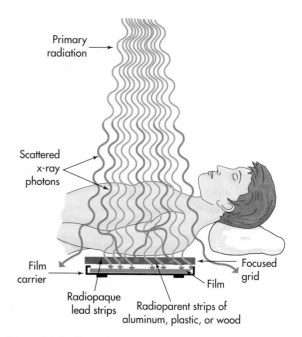

Fig. 7-19 Radiographic grids remove scattered x-ray photons that emerge from the object being radiographed before this scattered radiation reaches the film and decreases radiographic quality.

more than once because of human or mechanical error. Many categories may be established for discarded radiographs. These categories include the following: radiographs too dark or too light because of inappropriate selection of technique, incorrect patient positioning, improper centering of the radiographic beam, improper collimation, patient motion, and processing artifacts.

The presence of a repeat analysis program in an imaging department offers many benefits. First, the program increases awareness among staff and student radiographers of the need to produce optimal-quality images. Second, radiographers generally become more careful in producing their radiographs because they are aware that the radiographs are being reviewed. Third, when the repeat analysis program identifies problems or concerns, in-service education programs covering these specific topics may be designed for radiography personnel.

A repeat analysis program for radiographers also may help reduce an imaging department's repeat volume. A quality-control radiographer or other designated person reviews discarded radiographs with coworkers to point out the causes of various repeats. At the very least, this practice should lead to an improvement in technical skills.

Unnecessary Radiologic Procedures

The responsibility for ordering a radiologic examination lies only with the physician. The physician is therefore responsible for determining the need for any radiologic procedure. To make this decision, the physician must determine whether the benefit to the patient in terms of medical information gained provides sufficient justification to subject the patient to the minimal risk of the absorbed radiation resulting from the examination.

In the past, some radiographic examinations were performed routinely even in the absence of definite medical indications. Some nonessential radiologic examinations include the following:
1. A chest x-ray examination on scheduled admission to the hospital: This examination should not be performed without clinical indications of chest disease or another important concern that justifies exposing the patient to ionizing radiation. This includes presurgical patients. A panel of physicians appointed by the Food and Drug Administration (FDA)[7] concluded that a chest x-ray examination is not necessary for every presurgical patient. Patients admitted for treatment of pulmonary problems or diseases, however, may benefit from a preadmission chest x-ray examination.
2. A chest x-ray examination as part of a preemployment physical: Very little information about previous illness or injury can be gained through this examination, and it is unlikely to be useful to the employer.
3. Lumbar spine examinations as part of a preemployment physical: As with the preemployment chest x-ray examination, this examination provides very little information about previous illness or injury that would be useful to an employer.
4. Chest x-rays or other unjustified x-ray examinations as part of a routine health check-up: Radiologic procedures should not be performed unless a patient exhibits symptoms that merit radiologic investigation.
5. Chest x-ray examination for mass screening for tuberculosis (TB): Such examinations are of little value for most people. Testing for TB may be done with more efficient procedures. However, Bushong[3] indicates that some x-ray screening is still acceptable. This applies to high-risk groups such as members of the medical and paramedical community, people working in fields such as education and food preparation, and selective groups of workers such as miners and workers dealing with materials such as asbestos, beryllium, glass, and silica.

Minimal Source-Skin Distance for Mobile Radiography

Mobile radiographic units require special precautions to ensure patient safety. When operating the unit, the radiographer must use a source-skin distance of *at least* 12 inches (30 cm) (Fig. 7-20). The 12-inch distance limits the effects of the inverse square falloff of radiation intensity with distance. This falloff is more pronounced the shorter the source-skin distance.

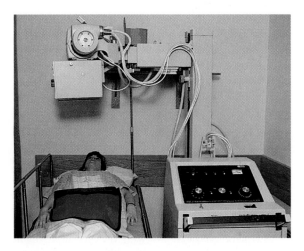

Fig. 7-20 Mobile radiographic examinations require a minimal source-skin distance of 12 inches (30 cm) to limit the effects of the inverse square falloff of radiation intensity with distance.

When the source-skin distance is small, patient entrance exposure is significantly greater than exit exposure. Thus when reasonable techniques are used to obtain an image of midline structures, the entrance surface of the patient receives an unnecessarily high exposure. By increasing source-skin distance, the radiographer maintains a more uniform distribution of exposure throughout the patient.

Mobile (portable) units should be used to perform radiographic procedures only on patients who cannot be transported to a fixed radiographic installation (an x-ray room). Mobile units are not designed to replace specially designed rooms.

Fluoroscopic Procedures

Fluoroscopic procedures (Fig. 7-21) produce the greatest patient radiation exposure rate in diagnostic radiology. In view of this fact the physician should carefully evaluate the need for a fluoroscopic examination to ascertain whether the potential benefit to the patient in terms of information gained outweighs the potentially adverse somatic and/or genetic effects of the examination. If the fluoroscopic procedure is necessary, every precaution must be taken to minimize patient exposure time.

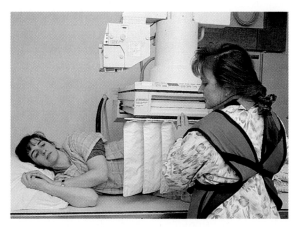

Fig. 7-21 Fluoroscopic procedures produce the greatest patient radiation exposure rate in diagnostic radiology.

Image intensification fluoroscopy

Image intensification fluoroscopy has three significant benefits:

1. Increased image brightness
2. Saving of time for the radiologist
3. Patient dose reduction

The x-ray image intensification system converts the x-ray image pattern into a corresponding amplified visible light pattern. Overall brightness of the fluoroscopic image increases to 7000 times the brightness of the image on a conventional fluoroscopic system operating under the same conditions. This increase in image brightness improves the radiologist's perception of the fluoroscopic image.

Because an image intensification system permits viewing of the fluoroscopic image at ordinary brightness level (regular white light), the radiologist uses photopic, or cone, vision when viewing the image through this system. Because cone vision can be used, the radiologist does not need to go through the process of darkness adaptation; this saves time. Cone vision also considerably improves visual acuity, permitting the radiologist to discriminate better between small fluoroscopic images.

Because an image intensification system significantly increases brightness, image intensification fluoroscopy requires less milliamperage than does conventional fluoroscopy (about 1.5 to 2 mA is required for image intensification systems, whereas 3 to 5 mA is required for conventional fluoroscopy). The consequent decrease in exposure rate results in a reduction in dose for the patient.

Intermittent fluoroscopy

The practice of **intermittent fluoroscopy** (periodic activation of the fluoroscopic tube by the fluoroscopist rather than lengthy, continuous activation) significantly decreases patient dose, especially in long procedures, and helps extend the life of the tube. Many systems include a last-image-hold feature that allows the fluoroscopist to see the most recent image without exposing the patient to another pulse of radiation.

Limitation of the size of the fluoroscopic field

The radiologist must limit the size of the **fluoroscopic field** to include only the area of clinical interest by properly collimating the x-ray beam. Proper collimation involves adjusting the lead shutters placed between the fluoroscopic tube and the patient. When fluoroscopic field size is limited, patient dose decreases substantially.

Primary beam length and width both must be confined within the image receptor boundary. Irrespective of the distance from the x-ray source to the image receptor, the useful beam should not extend outside the image receptor.

Exposure factors

Proper exposure factors must be selected in fluoroscopic procedures to minimize patient dose. Increases in peak kilovoltage and filtration reduce patient radiation exposure rate. Most fluoroscopic examinations performed with image intensification systems employ a range of from 85 to 120 kVp for adult patients, depending on the area of the body being examined. This optimal peak kilovoltage range produces the proper level of fluoroscopic image brightness. Lower peak kilovoltage results in increased patient dose and reduced brightness of the fluoroscopic image. If lower peak kilovoltage (a less energetic and penetrating x-ray beam) is employed for an adult patient, a higher milliamperage (a larger quantity of x-ray photons in the beam) must be used to provide an adequate exposure. This causes an increase in radiation exposure rate, leading to an increase in patient dose. In addition,

to prevent excessive entrance exposure of the patient and reduce the total exposure of both patient and radiographer, the **source-to-tabletop distance** must not be less than 15 inches (38 cm) for fixed fluoroscopes and must not be less than 12 inches (30 cm) for mobile fluoroscopes. A 12-inch (30-cm) minimal distance is required, but a 15-inch (38-cm) minimal distance is preferred for all image-intensification systems.

Exposure factors for fluoroscopic procedures for children necessitate a decrease in peak kilovoltage by as much as 25%. The peak kilovoltage chosen should depend on part thickness just as it does in radiography.

Filtration

The function of a filter in fluoroscopy, as in radiographic procedures, is to reduce the patient's skin dose. Adequate layers of aluminum equivalent material placed in the path of the useful beam remove the more harmful lower-energy photons from the beam by absorbing them. A minimum of 2.5-mm total aluminum equivalent **filtration** must be permanently installed in the path of the useful beam of the fluoroscopic unit. With image intensification systems a total aluminum equivalent filtration of 3.0 mm may be preferred. Patient dose decreases by one fourth during fluoroscopic procedures when aluminum filtration increases from 1-mm aluminum to 3-mm aluminum. Although this increase in filtration causes a slight loss of fluoroscopic image brightness, compensation may be made by increasing peak kilovoltage somewhat.

As in radiography, when filtration of the x-ray beam is questionable, the half-value layer (HVL) of the beam must be measured. In image intensification fluoroscopy an x-ray beam HVL of 3- to 3.5-mm aluminum is considered acceptable when peak kilovoltage ranges from 90 to 100.

Source-to-tabletop distance

The source-to-tabletop distance must be no less than 15 inches (38 cm) for fixed fluoroscopes and no less than 12 inches (30 cm) for mobile fluoroscopes. This standard ensures, as discussed earlier in the chapter, that the entrance surface of the patient does not receive excessive exposure. Maintaining an appropriate source-to-tabletop distance reduces the exposure of the patient and radiographer.

Cumulative timing device

A **cumulative timer** must be provided and used with each fluoroscopic unit. This device times the x-ray exposure and sounds an audible alarm or temporarily interrupts the exposure after the fluoroscope has been activated for 5 minutes. It makes the radiologist aware of the length of time the patient receives exposure for each fluoroscopic examination. When the fluoroscope is activated for shorter periods, the patient, radiologist, and radiographer receive less exposure.

Fluoroscopic unit exposure rate limitation

Current federal standards limit **entrance skin exposure rates** of general-purpose intensified fluoroscopic units to a maximum of 10 roentgen (R) per minute $(10 \times 2.58 \times 10^{-4}$ coulomb [C]/kg/min), whereas nonintensified units may not exceed 5 R per minute $(5 \times 2.58 \times 10^{-4}$ C/kg/min). Measured at tabletop, these standards have been imposed to give consideration to the cumulative small doses of radiation the patient receives over a lifetime. Fluoroscopic equipment equipped with high-level control (HLC) may permit a skin entrance exposure rate of as much as 20 R per minute $(20 \times 2.58 \times 10^{-4}$ C/kg/min). Because fluoroscopic procedures result in some of the largest patient doses in diagnostic radiology, fluoroscopic unit exposure rates must be kept within established limits.

Primary protective barrier

A **primary protective barrier** of 2-mm lead equivalent is required for an image intensifier unit. This barrier is provided by the image intensifier assembly itself. The assembly must be joined with the x-ray tube, which is located underneath the tabletop and interlocked so that the fluoroscopic x-ray tube cannot be activated when the unit is in the parked position.

Fluoroscopic exposure switch

The **fluoroscopic exposure switch (the foot pedal)** must be of the dead-man type (i.e., only continuous pressure applied by the operator [usually a radiologist] can keep the switch activated and the fluoroscopic tube emitting x-radiation). This means that the exposure automatically terminates if the person operating the switch becomes incapacitated (e.g., suffers a heart attack).

C–Arm Fluoroscopy

C-Arm fluoroscopes are frequently used in the operating room for orthopedic procedures (e.g., pinning of a fractured hip). This piece of equipment may be manipulated in almost any position and remain in an energized state for long periods to accommodate the surgeon during the procedure. Personnel routinely operating a C-Arm fluoroscope or those who are in the immediate area of the unit should wear protective aprons. This garment should be 0.5-mm lead equivalent to ensure adequate protection. Appropriate monitoring of personnel (see Chapter 9) normally involved in C-Arm fluoroscopic procedures should be a routine procedure.

Mobile fluoroscopic units are required to have a minimal source-to-skin distance of 12 inches (30 cm). Some type of spacer or collimator extension is usually installed to prevent any part of the patient from violating this minimal distance standard. During C-Arm fluoroscopic procedures, the patient–image intensifier distance should be as short as possible. This reduces patient dose.

Cinefluorography

The techniques to reduce patient dose during fluoroscopy also apply to dose reduction during **cinefluorography.** In cinefluorography, or cine, a movie camera is used to record the image of the output phosphor of the image intensifier. Dose-reduction techniques are especially important in cine, however, because cine procedures tend to result in the highest patient doses of all diagnostic procedures. The high dose resulting from cine is caused by a relatively high inherent dose rate and the length of the procedure, particularly in cardiology and neuroradiology. Thus a percentage decrease in cine dose yields greater actual dose reduction than the same percentage decrease in lower dose procedures.

Patient dose may be inferred from tabletop exposure levels. The amount of exposure varies with a number of operator-adjustable parameters. Typical cine tabletop exposure is approximately 25 mR per frame for 6- to

7-inch mode. This translates to 45 R per min if a frame rate of 30 frames per second is used. Thus any limitation of beam-on time is important as long as the efficacy of the procedure is not compromised. Patient exposure increases when a smaller viewing mode (6 inches, compared with 9 inches) or a lower-speed cine film is used. Exposure increases if the frame rate is increased. For example, switching from a 9-inch to a 6-inch field of view approximately doubles the tabletop exposure rate. If the frame rate is increased from 30 frames per second to 60 frames per second, the exposure rate is doubled. If both adjustments are made at the same time, the exposure rate increases by a factor of four. Other factors such as image intensifier input phosphor exposure level set by the vendor, grid factor, and source-to-skin distance play a role in determining typical dose levels for a system.

Collimating to the area of interest has the same effect in cine as in fluoroscopy. Collimation decreases the integral dose (product of dose and volume of tissue irradiated) while increasing image quality by reducing scatter.

The radiologist or cardiologist can reduce exposure during cine procedures by limiting the time of the cine run, using fluoroscopy when possible to locate the catheter. When fluoroscopy is used, intermittent exposures to verify location and movement of the catheter between exposures can limit total fluoroscopy time as well. Some optional equipment features such as the last-frame-hold feature, in which the most recent fluoroscopic image remains in view as a guide to the radiologist when the x-ray beam is off, also promote lower patient dose.

The typical dose delivered to the patient depends on the procedure. In selective coronary arteriography, most radiation exposure is from the cine. Although the dose rate is lower, the total dose from fluoroscopy may exceed the total dose from cine if the total fluoroscopy time is longer, as is often the case in percutaneous transluminal angioplasty.

High-Dose (High–Level–Control) Interventional Procedures

Interventional procedures are medical procedures performed by a physician during an imaging procedure such as fluoroscopy. The interventional physi-
cian, usually a radiologist or cardiologist, inserts catheters into vessels or directly into patient tissues for the purpose of drainage, biopsy, or alteration of vascular occlusions or malformations. For these procedures, **high-level–control (HLC) fluoroscopy** is the fluoroscopy of choice. HLC fluoroscopy is an operating mode for fluoroscopic equipment in which exposure rates are higher than those normally allowed in routine fluoroscopic procedures. The higher exposure rate allows visualization of smaller and lower-contrast objects that do not usually appear during fluoroscopy. HLC fluroscopy is used for interventional procedures in which visualization of fine catheters or other structures is crucial. An audible signal constantly reminds personnel that the HLC mode is being used.

Some fluoroscopically guided therapeutic interventional procedures have the potential for substantial patient exposure. On September 30, 1994, the FDA issued a public health advisory to alert health care workers to the dangers of overexposure of patients through the use of HLC fluoroscopy. The FDA X-Ray Equipment Standards, enacted in 1974[8], limited the tabletop exposure rate of fluoroscopic equipment for routine procedures to 10 R per min unless an HLC mode was present, in which case routine fluoroscopy was limited to 5 R/min when the system was not in HLC mode and unlimited when it was in HLC mode. The authors of the standards felt that the high-level capability was necessary for certain vital situations involving therapeutic interventional procedures in which the potential risks to the patient of radiation exposure would be subordinate to a successful medical outcome of an intervention. The HLC mode, although allowing unlimited exposure, required continuous, positive-pressure manual operation (e.g., continuously depressing a foot switch) and a continuous audible signal to remind personnel that the high-level fluoroscopic mode was in use. During this mode, patient exposure rates have been estimated to be in the range of 20 to 120 R per min. When the rule was enacted, total patient exposure was limited by the heat-loading capabilities of the x-ray tube. The heat limit of the tube would be reached before any detectable non-stochastic radiation injury could occur. By the early 1990s, advances in x-ray tube technology and the development of vascular interventional procedures that require long fluoroscopy times (Box 7-1) had created a situation in which skin reactions had been reported in some patients. Radiogenic skin injuries such as erythema (diffused reddening) or desquamation (sloughing off of skin cells) are **deterministic effects,** effects in which the severity of the disorder increases with radiation dose. As the data in Table 7-2 show, a half hour of total beam-on time at one location on the skin of a patient is sufficient to produce erythema. The effect does not appear for approximately 10 days. Because manifestation of skin injury is delayed, a radiologist would not usually be the first person to observe the onset of symptoms. Therefore patient monitoring, radiation dosimetry, and record keeping are important for future medical management of adverse reactions. The FDA has recommended that a notation be placed in the patient's record if skin dose is received in the range of 1 to 2 gray (Gy) (100 to 200 rad). The location of the area of the patient's skin that received the absorbed dose should be noted using a diagram, annotated photograph, or narrative description.

Box 7-1

Procedures Involving Extended Fluoroscopic Time

Percutaneous transluminal angioplasty
Radiofrequency cardiac catheter ablation
Vascular embolization
Stent and filter placement
Thrombolytic and fibrinolytic procedures
Percutaneous transhepatic cholangiography
Endoscopic retrograde cholangiopancreatography
Transjugular intrahepatic portosystemic shunt
Percutaneous nephrostomy
Biliary drainage
Urinary or biliary stone removal

From the U.S. Food and Drug Administration: *Public health advisory: avoidance of serious x-ray-induced skin injuries to patients during fluoroscopically guided procedures,* Rockville, Md, FDA, September 30, 1994.

Patient Dose

Because increasing numbers of people in the United States are undergoing diagnostic radiologic procedures each year, concern about the risk of such procedures is growing. Medical imaging personnel must reduce the risk to patients whenever possible by employing radiation control practices that en-

Table 7-2

Radiation-Induced Skin Injuries

| Effect | Typical threshold absorbed dose (Gy)* | Hours of fluoroscopic "on time" to reach threshold† | | Time to onset of effect‡ |
		Usual fluoroscopic dose rate of 0.02 Gy/min (2 rad/min)	High-level dose rate of 0.2 Gy/min (20 rad/min)	
Early transient erythema	2	1.7	0.17	Hours
Temporary epilation	3	2.5	0.25	3 wk
Main erythema	6	5.0	0.50	10 d
Permanent epilation	7	5.8	0.58	3 wk
Dry desquamation	10	8.3	0.83	4 wk
Dermal atrophy	11	9.2	0.92	>14 wk
Telangiectasis	12	10.0	1.00	>52 wk
Moist desquamation	15	12.5	1.25	4 wk
Late erythema	15	12.5	1.25	6-10 wk
Dermal necrosis	18	15.0	1.50	>10 wk
Secondary ulceration	20	16.7	1.67	>6 wk

Modified from Wagner LK, Eifel PJ, Geise RA: Potential biological effects following high x-ray dose interventional procedures, *J Vasc Interv Radiol* 5:71, 1994.
*The unit for absorbed dose is the gray (Gy) in the International System of units. One Gy is equivalent to 100 rad in the traditional system of radiation units.
†Time required to deliver the typical threshold dose at the specified dose rate.
‡Time after single irradiation to observation of effect.

sure safety by minimizing dose.

In general, patient dose from diagnostic radiologic procedures may be specified in four ways: entrance skin exposure (ESE), skin dose, gonadal dose, and bone marrow dose. Although each type of specification has significance in estimating the risk to the patient, ESE is the most frequently reported because it is the simplest to determine.

Entrance skin exposure (ESE)

Entrance skin exposure (ESE) may be converted to patient **skin dose** by using well-documented multiplicative factors. As discussed below, ESE measurements are relatively easy to obtain. When actual patient measurements are not available, reasonably accurate ESE estimates can still be made. This is the reason that ESE is so widely used in the assessment of patient dose.

Thermoluminescent dosimeters (TLDs) are the sensing devices most frequently used to measure skin doses directly. (The characteristics, components, and function of the TLD are described in Chapter 9.) A small, relatively thin pack of TLDs is secured to the patient's skin in the middle of the clinical area of interest and exposed during a radiographic procedure. Because the sensing material in the TLD responds in a manner similar to human tissue when exposed to ionizing radiation, an accurate determination of surface dose can be made (Table 1-3 provides a list of permissible skin entrance exposures for various radiographic examinations.) In fluoroscopy, patient dose may be estimated by measuring the radiation exposure rate at the tabletop.

When direct patient measurements are not available, ESE may be estimated through the use of graphical data, which enable an individual to estimate the output intensity of a specific type of radiographic unit if exposure factors are known or ascertained with a reasonable degree of accuracy.

Another way in which ESE may be determined when patient measurements are unavailable is to have a medical physicist measure the output intensity of a specific radiographic unit in units of mR per mAs for a range of selected kVps. With this data and the patient's thickness at the site of exposure, the entrance exposure to the patient may be simply calculated. The following example illustrates the technique.

Example: AP projection of the pelvis
Collimator size: 14×17 inches
Exposure factors: 100 kVp, 30 mAs, 40-inch SID
Patient AP thickness at pelvis: 10 inches
Medical physicist output measurement of radiographic unit at 40 inches at 100 kVp: 10 mR/mAs

Solution: Entrance exposure to the patient is at a distance of 27 inches from the x-ray tube target (distance from table top to Bucky = 3 inches)
Using the inverse square law (see Chapter 8), the mR per mAs at 27 inches is given by the following equation:

$$10 \times (40/27)^2 = 21.9 \text{ mR per mAs}$$

Therefore the entrance skin exposure to the patient is equal to

$$21.9 \ \frac{mR}{mAs} = 30 \text{ mAs } = 657 \text{ milliroentgens or in SI units:}$$

$$0.657 \text{ R} \times 2.58 \times \frac{10^{-4} \text{ C/kg}}{\text{R}} = 170 \times 10^{-6} \text{ C/kg}$$

Skin dose

Skin dose in general represents the absorbed dose to the most superficial layers of the skin. This region is called the epidermis. It is composed of five layers: the horny or outer layer, translucent or clear layer, granular layer, prickle cell layer and germinal, or basal, cell layer. The thickness of the epidermis varies from one anatomic area to another. It is greater in areas such as the palms of the hands and soles of the feet. The primary function of the epidermis is to provide protection for underlying tissues and structures.

Gonadal dose

Because genetic effects may result from exposure to ionizing radiation, protection of the reproductive organs is of particular concern in diagnostic radiology. (Table 1-6 lists some typical gonadal doses from various radiographic examinations.) For several examinations identified in the table, differences exist between the dosages received by human males and females. Protection of the ovaries by overlying tissue accounts for these differences. In diagnostic radiology, the relatively low **gonadal dose** for a single human is considered insignificant. However, when the low gonadal dose is applied to the entire population, the dose becomes far more significant. The concept of **genetically significant dose (GSD)** is used to assess the impact of this dose. GSD is the dose equivalent to the reproductive organs that, if received by every human, would be expected to bring about an identical gross genetic injury to the total population, as does the sum of the actual doses received by exposed individual population members. In other words, if a maximum of 500 people were inhabiting the earth and each person received a dose equivalent of 0.005 sievert (Sv) (0.5 rem) gonadal radiation, the gross genetic effect would be identical to the effect occurring when 50 individual inhabitants each receive 0.05 Sv (5 rem) of gonadal radiation and no dose equivalent is received by the other inhabitants. In simple terms the GSD concept suggests that the consequences of substantial absorbed doses of gonadal radiation become significantly less when averaged over an entire population rather than applied to just a few of its members.

The GSD takes into consideration the fact that some people receive radiation to their reproductive organs during a given year, whereas others do not. Also, it accounts for the fact that radiation exposure in members of the population who cannot bear children (e.g., those who are beyond reproductive years) has no genetic impact. Hence the GSD is the average annual gonadal dose equivalent to members of the population who are of childbearing age. It includes the number of children who may be expected to be conceived by members of the exposed population in a given year. According to the U.S. Public Health Service, the estimated GSD for the population of the United States is about 0.20 mSv (20 mrem).

Bone marrow dose

In human beings, bone marrow is of great importance because it contains large numbers of stem, or precursor, blood cells that may be depleted or destroyed by substantial exposure to ionizing radiation. The **bone marrow dose** is a dose of radiation delivered to that organ. More precisely, this dose should be referred to as the **mean active bone marrow dose.** This dose may be defined as "the average radiation dose to the entire active bone marrow."[3] For example, if in the course of performing a specific radiographic proce-

dure, 25% of the active bone marrow were in the useful beam and received an average absorbed dose of 0.8 mGy (80 mrad), the mean active bone marrow dose is 0.2 mGy (20 mrad). Radiation dose absorbed by an organ such as bone marrow cannot be measured accurately by a direct method. It can only be estimated. In diagnostic radiology the bone marrow dose provides a measurement of patient absorbed dose even though hematologic effects are generally negligible for doses associated with this discipline.

Table 1-5 provides typical bone marrow doses for various radiographic examinations performed on human adults. The levels indicated in Table 1-5 are usually less for children because the active bone marrow is more evenly spread out and significantly lower radiographic exposure factors are used. Although each dose listed in Table 1-5 results from fragmentary exposure of the human body, it is averaged over the whole body.

Fetal Dose

Only an estimate of **fetal dose** is possible. It is customarily obtained from phantom measurements or computer-generated calculations. Table 1-7 lists typical fetal dose factors as a function of skin entrance exposure. To determine fetal dose according to this table, the reader must first determine the skin entrance exposure for the selected radiologic procedure. The fetal dose is given in millirads per roentgen of entrance exposure.[9]

When the primary x-ray beam passes through the uterus, as it does during radiography of the abdomen or pelvis, fetal dose is highest. However, it is significantly lower when the diagnostic x-ray beam is directed toward a part of the body away from the lower trunk (e.g., head, feet).

Other Important Diagnostic Examinations and Imaging Modalities

Patient dose in mammography

Mammography is used to detect breast cancer that is not palpable in physical examinations (Fig. 7-22). Experts agree that yearly mammographic screening of women 50 years of age and older leads to earlier de-

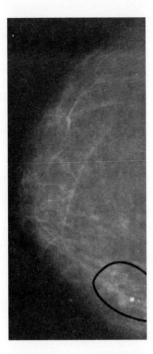

Fig. 7-22 Mammography can be used to detect breast cancer.

tection of breast cancer. Earlier treatment saves lives and reduces suffering. The value of mammography in younger women is somewhat controversial. The controversy has very little to do with radiation risk. Although it is still mentioned occasionally in the popular press, cancer researchers generally agree that radiation risk resulting from the relatively small doses associated with mammography is negligible in all women[10-12]. Federal regulations for FDA certification of screening mammography facilities state that the maximal dose to the glandular tissue of a 4.5-cm compressed breast using a screen-film mammography system should not exceed 3 mGy (300 mrad) per view.[13] Studies have shown that well-calibrated mammographic systems are capable of providing optimal imaging performance with an average glandular dose of less than 2 mGy (200 mrad).[14] The age recommendation for screening is controversial because mammography is less accurate in the detection of breast cancer in younger women and likely to result in many false positive readings, leading to unnecessary biopsies in that population. The increased density of the

breasts of younger women tends to reduce radiographic contrast, and therefore mammography may be less sensitive in the average younger woman than in the average older woman. Nevertheless, earlier detection of more aggressive cancers is assumed to save lives in general. Consequently, the efficacy of screening mammography in women under 50 is a subject that has generated a great deal of interest.

As of this writing, the authors support the recommendations of the American College of Radiology, the American Cancer Society, and the American Medical Association. These groups advocate annual mammography screening for women between the ages of 40 and 49. A baseline mammogram for comparison with mammograms taken at a later age also is recommended between the ages of 35 and 39. The interested reader should contact these organizations for their latest policy statements on this subject.

Patient dose in computed tomography (CT)

As defined by Johnson and Rowberg in *Merrill's Atlas of Radiographic Positions and Radiologic Procedures,* "**computed tomography (CT)** is the process of creating a crosssectional tomographic plane (slice) of any part of the body. The image then is reconstructed by a computer using x-ray absorption measurements collected at multiple points about the periphery of the part being scanned." Although a discussion of CT equipment, function, and procedure is not within the scope of this text, patient dose resulting from exposure to ionizing radiation is relevant because CT is a frequently employed diagnostic x-ray imaging modality.

Two concerns relate to patient dose in CT scanning. One concern is the skin dose, and the other is the dose distribution during the scanning procedure. When compared with any routine radiographic projection of the adult cranium or a single AP projection of the abdomen, the entrance exposure received by the patient after a succession of adjacent scans is greater than the entrance exposure from an individual x-ray projection. However, when a patient undergoes an ordinary but complicated x-ray examination, many radiographs involving different projections are obtained. If the doses from this extensive radiographic series are added together, the sum is comparable to the dose from a CT examination. Still another consideration exists. CT examinations generally expose a smaller mass of tissue than that exposed during an ordinary x-ray series. The reason for this is that the CT x-ray beam is more tightly collimated than the conventional radiographic beam. The entrance exposure from a CT examination also may be compared with the entrance exposure received during a routine fluoroscopic examination. In this instance the entrance exposure received during a CT examination is considerably less than that received during a routine fluoroscopic procedure.

The dose distribution resulting from a CT scan is not the same as the dose distribution occurring in routine radiologic procedures (Fig. 7-23). Because CT scanners use an x-ray beam that is tightly collimated, the amount of scatter radiation generated is lower than the scatter produced by the less tightly collimated radiographic beam. Because CT scanners collimate the x-ray beam so well, the mass of human tissue exposed to radiation falls off rapidly outside the plane of concern during the production of any given scan. Although only one slice is exposed and imaged at a time, some overlap of the margins of the x-ray beam occurs when each single tomographic section is made. Also, when adjacent slices are obtained, some radiation scatters from the slice being made into the adjacent slices (interslice scatter). Both of these contribute to dose increase and are the reason that a succession of adjacent tomographic sections (slices) imparts a higher absorbed dose than would a single tomographic section.

Bushong[3] identifies average skin dose ranges from scans of the cranial region to be from 1 to 3 cGy (1 to

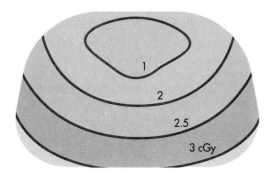

Fig. 7-23 Typical distribution of the doses deposited in a single-slice CT examination. For multiple contiguous slices, the doses may be twice these values.

3 rad) and dose ranges for scans of the body to be from 2 to 6 cGy (2 to 6 rad).[3] Actual doses delivered during any CT scanning procedure depend on the type of scanner being used and the radiation technique selected. The tight collimation of the CT beam makes possible its very accurate placement relative to the area of anatomy to be studied. This permits CT technologists to avoid exposing selected radiosensitive organs (e.g., the eyes).

Direct patient shielding is not typically used in CT. Because of the rotational nature of the exposure, a shield is no more effective than the collimators that already exist on the device. Because the beam is so tightly collimated to the slice thickness, exposure to anatomy outside the field of view is caused only by internal scatter. Basically, in CT, anatomy does not appear in the primary x-ray beam unless it is part of the intended field of view.

Spiral CT presents a greater challenge for assessing patient dose than does conventional CT. When spiral scan pitch ratio (pitch), which is the relationship between the movements of the patient couch and the x-ray beam collimator, is about 1 : 1, spiral CT patient dose is comparable with that produced by conventional CT. However, when the pitch is higher (e.g., 2 : 1), patient dose is reduced in comparison with conventional CT. The reverse also is true; patient dose increases at a lower pitch.

Patient dose also may be influenced by other factors. Changes in noise level (the random variation in pixel brightness seen when an image is made of too few photons—i.e., if the mA is too low in a CT scan), pixel (individual picture element) size, and slice thickness all affect patient dose. The use of smaller pixel sizes for better resolution, the selection of thinner slices, and the increase of tube mA because of higher noise level each increase the patient's absorbed dose. These relationships are summarized in the following equation:

$$D = K\left[\frac{SNR^2}{e^3h}\right]$$

where *SNR* is the "signal-to-noise" ratio (i.e., the comparison of the average CT number in a region with the statistical variation of CT number in that region), *e* is the size of the smallest resolvable object, and *h* is the slice thickness. *K* is simply a constant of proportionality that depends on the special properties or characteristics of each scanner. The value of this constant is determined by measurement. The signal-to-noise ratio is an indicator of the "smoothness" of the image and is related to the ability to detect low-contrast objects (e.g., a liver tumor within liver tissues). The equation shows that increasing the signal-to-noise ratio (e.g., by increasing the mA) results in a higher dose because dose is proportional to the square of the SNR. Dose also increases if CT technologists insist on being able to resolve smaller objects or set thinner slice widths without sacrificing any SNR.

From a radiation protection point of view, the goal of CT imaging should be to obtain the best possible image while delivering a reasonable dose of ionizing radiation to the patient. The fulfillment of this responsibility lies with the technologist performing the examination.

Pediatric Considerations

With regard to the potential for biologic damage from exposure to ionizing radiation, children are more vulnerable to both the **late somatic effects** and genetic effects of radiation than adults. Hence children require special consideration when undergoing diagnostic radiologic studies. Appropriate radiation protection methods must be used for each procedure. Some of these methods are described in the following sections. Because children have a greater life expectancy, they may easily survive long enough to develop a leukemia induced by radiation or develop a radiogenic malignancy such as lung or thyroid cancer. In fact, according to studies published by Beebe and others in 1978,[15] the risk of a radiation-induced leukemia in children after a substantial dose of ionizing radiation is about two times that of adults. For low doses such as those encountered in diagnostic radiology, data are still inconclusive (see Chapter 6). With this consideration in mind, radiographers must take every precaution to minimize exposure to all pediatric patients.

In general, smaller doses of ionizing radiation suffice to obtain useful images in pediatric radiologic procedures than are necessary for adult radiologic procedures. For example, an entrance exposure below 5 mR[16] will result from an AP projection of an infant's chest, whereas the same projection or a PA projection

of an adult's chest will yield an entrance exposure ranging from 12 to 26 mR (see Table 1-3).

Patient motion is frequently a problem in diagnostic pediatric radiography. Because of the limited ability of children to understand the radiologic procedure and, in most cases, their limited ability to cooperate, children are less likely to remain still during a radiographic or fluoroscopic exposure. To solve or at least minimize this problem, the radiographer must employ very short exposure times by selecting a high mA station and effective immobilization techniques. For some examinations, such as chest radiography, special pediatric immobilization devices are available to hold the pediatric patient securely and safely in the required position, thus providing adequate immobilization (see Fig. 7-3). The use of such techniques along with the use of appropriate radiographic or fluoroscopic exposure factors and proper processing techniques greatly reduces or eliminates the need for repeat examinations that increase patient dose.

The presence of technologists who are experienced in dealing with children is helpful. Rooms specially earmarked for pediatric studies also are beneficial. Such rooms contain not only the appropriate restraint devices but also suitable entertainment and distracting devices such as cartoon posters and puppets. The examination progresses most efficiently with the best hope for patient cooperation when the child feels less intimidated.

The radiographer should be familiar with particular difficulties related to gonadal shielding in pediatric studies. First, if the gonadal tissue is more than 2 cm from the edge of the field of view (assuming proper collimation), the use of a gonadal shield does not significantly affect the gonadal dose because in that case the dose is caused solely by internal scatter. In small girls the variation in anatomic location of the ovaries requires shielding of the iliac wings as well as the sacral area when shielding is needed.[16] Effective shielding may not be possible for some studies because it obscures the anatomy of interest.

Collimation is especially important in pediatric studies. The automatic collimation system reduces the radiation field size to the dimensions of the image receptor, but because many pediatric patients are significantly smaller than the image receptor, further manual adjustment of collimation is sometimes necessary.

As in any other radiographic study, reducing the field size to the anatomy of interest not only reduces patient exposure but also increases image quality by reducing scatter. Projection orientation also is important. Female pediatric patients who may be imaged in either PA or AP projection will receive significantly lower doses to the breast tissues in a PA projection.[17]

Essentially, the same patient protection methods used to reduce the radiation exposure for adults may be employed to reduce the radiation exposure for pediatric patients. In general the techniques discussed in this chapter may be applied to meet the needs of infants or children.

Special Precautions Employed in Medical Radiography to Protect the Pregnant or Potentially Pregnant Patient

Because some evidence suggests that the developing embryo-fetus is especially radiation sensitive, special care is taken in medical radiography to prevent unnecessary exposure of the abdominal area of pregnant females. Unfortunately, most women are not aware that they are pregnant during the earliest stage of pregnancy, which means that exposure of the abdominal area of potentially pregnant (i.e., fertile) women is a concern. In 1970[18] the International Commission on Radiation Protection (ICRP) proposed a **10-day rule.** Based on the low degree of probability that a woman would be pregnant during the first 10 days after the onset of menstruation, this rule suggests that abdominal x-ray examinations of fertile women be postponed until sometime during the first 10 days after the onset of the next menstrual cycle if the results of the examination are not important in connection with an immediate illness. However, such scheduling is difficult in many imaging departments, where sustained contact among the radiologist, the referring physician, and the patient is unlikely. Because most fertile women are not pregnant at any given time, the 10-day rule may result in unnecessary postponement of examinations for the majority of female patients. For these reasons, the 10-day rule is now obsolete. The official position of the American College of Radiology (ACR), the major professional organization of radiologists in the United States, is as follows: "Abdominal radiological exams that have been requested after full consideration of the clinical status of the patient, including the possibility of pregnancy, need not be postponed or selectively scheduled."[19]

When radiologic procedures are not considered urgent by the referring physician, they may be regarded as elective examinations and can be booked at an appropriate time to meet patient needs and safety. In NCRP Report No. 102[20] the following recommendation has been made to facilitate scheduling of elective examinations:

> Ideally, an elective abdominal examination of a woman of childbearing age should be performed during the first few days following the onset of menses to minimize the possibility of irradiation of an embryo. In practice, the timeliness of medical needs should be the primary consideration in deciding the timing of the examination.

In the event that a pregnant patient is inadvertently irradiated, a radiologic physicist should perform the calculations necessary to determine fetal exposure. This may include the taking of measurements using phantoms to simulate the patient and the use of ion chambers to record exposure. The following question sometimes arises: Should a therapeutic abortion be performed to prevent the birth of an infant because of radiation exposure during pregnancy? Studies of groups such as the atom bomb survivors of Hiroshima have shown that damage to the newborn is unlikely for doses below 20 rad. Because most medical procedures result in fetal exposures of less than 1 rad, the risk of abnormality is small. The National Council on Radiation Protection and Measurements states the following[20]:

> This risk is considered to be negligible at 5 rad or less when compared to the other risks of pregnancy, and the risk of malformations is significantly increased above control levels only at doses above 15 rad. Therefore, the exposure of the fetus to radiation arising from diagnostic procedures would very rarely be cause, by itself, for terminating a pregnancy. If there are reasons, other than the possible radiation effects, to consider a therapeutic abortion, such reasons should be discussed with the patient by the attending physician, so that it is clear that the radiation exposure is not being used as an excuse for terminating the pregnancy.

If the physician feels it is in the best interests of a pregnant or potentially pregnant patient to undergo a radiologic examination, the examination should be performed without delay. Under such circumstances, special efforts should be made to minimize the dose of radiation received by the patient's lower abdomen and pelvic region. This can be accomplished by selecting technical exposure factors that are appropriate for the examination (i.e., by using the smallest exposure that will generate a diagnostically useful radiograph) and by adequately and precisely collimating the radiographic beam to include only the anatomic area of interest. When the patient's lower abdomen and pelvic region does not have to be included in the area to be irradiated, it should be protected with a lead apron or other suitable protective contact shield (Fig. 7-24) so that a developing embryo-fetus does not receive unnecessary radiation exposure.

Summary

In this chapter the need for protecting the patient during diagnostic radiologic procedures and the various tools and techniques used therein have been described. Effective communication with the patient is essential. Verbal and nonverbal messages should be congruent so that they are understood as intended. Procedures should be explained in simple terms. Patients must have an opportunity to ask questions and should receive truthful answers within ethical limits.

Adequate immobilization of the patient is necessary to eliminate voluntary motion. Suitable restraining devices are available for this purpose. Involuntary motion can be reduced by shortening exposure time and using very-high-speed image receptors.

X-ray beam limitation devices must be used to confine the useful beam before it enters the area of clinical interest. Aperture diaphragms, cones and extension cylinders, and the light-localizing variable-aperture rectangular collimator are the beam limitation devices used. Of these the collimator is the most versatile. The patient's skin surface should always be at least 15 cm below the collimator to minimize exposure to the epidermis. Good coincidence between the x-ray beam and the light-localizing beam of the collimator is necessary. Both alignment and width dimensions of the two beams must correspond to within 2% of the source-to-image distance (SID). To ensure that the radiographic beam matches the size of the image receptor, radiographic collimators include positive beam limitation (PBL) devices to collimate the beam automatically. According to the regulatory standard presently in effect, 2% of the SID is required with PBL.

Exposure to the patient's skin may be reduced through proper filtration of the radiographic beam. This aluminum equivalent filtration material absorbs the majority of lower-energy photons from the x-ray beam. Inherent filtration amounting to 0.5-mm aluminum equivalent is required. In general, 2 mm more are added outside the glass window of the x-ray tube housing above the collimator shutters. Together the inherent and added filtration compose the total filtration. For fixed x-ray equipment operating above 70 kVp, this filtration equals 2.5-mm aluminum equivalent. This regulation also applies to mobile diagnostic units and fluoroscopic equipment. From 50 to 70 kVp, fixed radiographic units require total filtration of only 1.5-mm aluminum equivalent. The half-value layer (HVL) of the beam is measured to determine whether an x-ray beam is adequately filtered. A radiologic physicist should obtain this measurement annually.

Protective shielding may be used to reduce or eliminate radiation exposure to radiosensitive body organs or tissues. Organs and tissues such as the lens of the eye, the breast, and the reproductive organs may be selectively shielded from the useful beam through the use of specific area shielding. The reproductive organs should be protected from exposure to the useful beam when they are in or within approximately 5 cm of a properly collimated beam unless this would compromise the

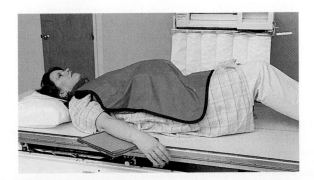

Fig. 7-24 To protect a developing embryo-fetus from unnecessary radiation exposure, place a lead apron over the female patient's lower abdomen and pelvic region when it does not have to be included in the area to be irradiated.

diagnostic value of the study. Because of their location in the pelvic region, the female reproductive organs receive approximately three times more exposure than the male reproductive organs. Appropriate gonadal shielding can greatly reduce the exposure received by both sexes (50% reduction for females, 90% to 95% reduction for males).

The clear lead shadow shield can significantly reduce the dose to the breast of a young patient undergoing a scoliosis examination. The use of the PA projection also may reduce dose to the breast.

Compensating filters such as the wedge filter and trough or bilateral wedge filter are used in radiography to provide uniform imaging of body parts when considerable variation in thickness or tissue composition exists. These devices partially attenuate x-rays that are directed toward the thinner or less dense area while permitting more x-radiation to strike the thicker or more dense area.

Appropriate exposure factors for each examination must be selected. Techniques chosen should ensure a diagnostic radiograph with minimal patient dose. The availability of standardized technique charts for each x-ray unit help provide uniform selection of exposure factors. In the selection of exposure factors the use of high kVp and lower mAs should be chosen whenever possible, as long as acceptable contrast is obtained, to reduce patient dose. Good processing is essential to make the information on the exposed radiographic film visible. Double-emulsion x-ray film used with high-speed rare-earth intensifying screems in system speeds of 200 to 400 are suitable for most examinations because they afford high resolution of recorded detail with a reduction in patient dose. Although the use of radiographic grids increases patient dose in radiography, their use for examination of thicker body parts is a fair compromise because they remove scattered radiation emanating from the patient that would otherwise degrade the recorded image. Grids yield a sharper image. Higher-ratio grids (e.g., 16 : 1) contain more lead and therefore increase patient dose.

Repeat radiographs resulting from human or mechanical error must be minimized to prevent the patient's skin and gonads from receiving a double dose of radiation. Care must be exercised to position the patient properly and select the correct exposure factors to ensure the production of a high-quality radiograph for each examination the first time. Imaging departments can benefit greatly from the implementation and maintenance of a repeat analysis program. When problems or concerns are identified, in-service education programs can be initiated to address them.

To limit the effects of inverse square falloff of radiation intensity with distance during a mobile radiographic examination, a source-skin distance of at least 12 inches (30 cm) must be used. A more uniform distribution of exposure throughout the patient is maintained when source-skin distance is increased.

Fluoroscopic procedures produce the greatest patient radiation exposure rate in diagnostic radiology. Patient exposure times should therefore be minimized whenever possible. To decrease patient exposure further, the fluoroscopist can limit the size of the fluoroscopic field to include only the area of clinical interest and also employ the practice of intermittent fluoroscopy to reduce the overall length of exposure. The selection of proper exposure factors also may help minimize patient dose. An additional method of reducing patient exposure is to ensure that the source-to-tabletop distance is no less than 15 inches (38 cm) for fixed fluoroscopes and no less than 12 inches (30 cm) for mobile fluoroscopes. The fluoroscopic beam itself must be adequately filtered (i.e., a minimum of 2.5-mm total aluminum equivalent filtration must be permanently installed in the path of the useful beam) to reduce the dose to the patient's skin. In image-intensification fluoroscopy an x-ray beam half-value layer of 3- to 3.5-mm aluminum is considered acceptable when peak kilovoltage ranges from 90 to 100. A cumulative timer that sounds an audible alarm or temporarily interrupts the x-ray exposure after the fluoroscope has been activated for 5 minutes must be provided to alert personnel to the length of time the fluoroscope is in use. A maximum of 10 R per minute ($10 \times 2.58 \times 10^{-4}$ C/kg/min) for general purpose intensified fluoroscopic units is the federal regulatory standard limit for entrance skin exposure rates. This rate can be as great as 20 R per minute ($20 \times 2.58 \times 10^{-4}$ C/kg/min) for high-level–control (HLC) fluoroscopic equipment. The image-intensifier assembly functions as a primary protective barrier with a 2-mm lead-equivalent attenuation. The assembly joins with the x-ray tube and interlocks so that the fluoroscopic tube cannot be activated when the unit is in the parked position.

Cinefluorography can result in the highest patient doses of all diagnostic procedures. Patient exposure increases when a smaller viewing mode or a lower-speed cine film is used. Exposure also increases if the frame rate is increased. Using intermittent activation of the fluoroscope to locate the catheter and limiting the time of the cine run reduces patient dose, as does the use of the last-frame-hold feature to view the most recent fluoroscopic image.

HLC fluoroscopy is used for interventional procedures. This operating mode uses exposure rates that may be substantially higher than those allowed for routine fluoroscopic procedures. This equipment emits an audible signal to remind personnel that it is in use. Before new regulatory standards, patient exposure rates were estimated to range as high as 120 R per minute. If skin dose is received in the range of 1 to 2 Gy (100 to 200 rad), the FDA requires that a notation be placed in the patient's record. The area of the patient's skin receiving such a dose also must be noted using a diagram, annotated photograph, or narrative description.

Patient dose from diagnostic radiologic procedures may be specified as entrance skin exposure dose (ESE), skin dose, gonadal dose, or bone marrow dose (mean active bone marrow dose). Of these, ESE is the easiest to obtain and the most widely used. The relatively low gonadal dose in diagnostic radiology is insignificant for a single individual. It becomes far more important when applied to an entire population. The concept of genetically significant dose (GSD) is used to assess the impact of this dose. GSD is the dose equivalent to the reproductive organs that, if received by every human being, would be expected to bring about an identical gross genetic injury to the total population as does the sum of the actual doses received by exposed individual population members. According to the U.S. Public Health Service the estimated GSD for the population of the United States is about 0.20 mSv (20 mrem). The bone marrow dose or mean active bone marrow dose is a dose of radiation delivered to that organ. This dose can only be estimated. In diagnostic radiology, it can provide a measurement of patient absorbed dose even though hematologic effects

are generally negligible for doses associated with this discipline. Fetal dose is another dose that can only be estimated. It is usually obtained from phantom measurements or computer-generated calculations. It is given in millirads per roentgen of entrance exposure.

Nonpalpable breast cancer may be detected through mammography. Annual screening of women 50 years of age and older leads to early detection of breast cancer. Federal regulations in the United States for FDA certification of screening mammography facilities state that the maximal dose to the glandular tissue of a 4.5-cm compressed breast using a screen-film mammography system should not exceed 3 mGy (300 mrad) per view. Annual mammographic screening for women 40 to 49 years of age and a baseline mammogram between the ages of 35 and 39 are presently advocated by the Americal College of Radiology, the American Cancer Society, and the American Medical Association.

Skin dose and dose distribution during the actual scanning procedure are two concerns in the performance of computed tomography (CT) scanning. Actual doses delivered during any CT procedure depend on the type of scanner being used and the radiation technique selected. In spiral CT, patient dose is comparable with that of conventional CT when the pitch ratio is about equal to 1. Patient dose is reduced when the pitch is higher. When the pitch is lower, the patient dose increases. Patient dose also is influenced by other factors such as changes in noise level, pixel size, and slice thickness.

Children are more vulnerable than adults to both the late somatic and genetic effects of ionizing radiation. Hence radiation protection methods and techniques to reduce exposure must be employed whenever possible during radiologic procedures. Effective immobilization techniques are essential to prevent patient motion. The breast tissue exposure in female pediatric patients may be significantly decreased by using a PA projection instead of an AP projection.

A developing embryo-fetus is especially sensitive to exposure from ionizing radiation. Therefore radiation protection methods and techniques should be employed to minimize or eliminate exposure to the unborn whenever an examination of a pregnant patient must be performed. The dose received by the patient's lower abdomen and pelvic region may be minimized by using the smallest exposure factors that will generate a diagnostically useful radiograph and by adequate and precise collimation of the beam to include only the anatomic area of interest. A protective lead apron or other suitable protective contact shield should be placed over the patient's lower abdomen and pelvic region to prevent unnecessary irradiation of that area if it does not need to be included in the examination.

The 10-day rule proposed by the International Commission on Radiation Protection in 1970 is now obsolete. The American College of Radiology presently advocates that "abdominal radiological exams that have been requested after full consideration of the clinical status of the patient, including the possibility of pregnancy, need not be postponed or selectively scheduled." Radiologic procedures that are not considered urgent by the referring physician may be regarded as elective examinations and scheduled at an appropriate time to meet the patient's needs and safety. If a pregnant patient is inadvertently irradiated, a radiologic physicist should perform the calculations necessary to determine fetal dose.

Review Questions

1. The number of repeat radiographs in an imaging department may be reduced by which of the following?
   A. Effective communication between the radiographer and patient
   B. Elimination of voluntary patient motion through adequate immobilization
   C. Careful and appropriate selection of radiation exposure factors by the radiographer
   D. All of the above

2. Which of the following is not an x-ray beam limitation device?
   A. Filter
   B. Aperture diaphragm
   C. Cone
   D. Collimator

3. Which of the following may reduce patient exposure resulting from off-focus radiation?
   A. Placing the second pair of shutters in the collimator below the level of the light source and mirror
   B. Placing the first pair of shutters in the collimator as close as possible to the tube window
   C. Transmitting an electric signal through the collimators first and second pair of shutters
   D. Off-focus radiation in a collimator cannot be reduced.

4. The radiographic beam should be collimated so that it is which of the following?
   A. Slightly larger than the image receptor
   B. No larger than the image receptor
   C. Twice as large as the image receptor
   D. Four times as large as the image receptor

5. What is the function of filtration in diagnostic radiologic procedures?
   A. To decrease beam hardness, thereby reducing patient skin dose
   B. To increase beam hardness, thereby reducing patient skin dose
   C. To eliminate short-wavelength radiation to reduce patient dose
   D. To increase beam hardness, thereby increasing patient skin dose

6. A fixed radiographic unit operating at 90 kVp requires which of the following?
   A. 1.0-mm aluminum equivalent total filtration
   B. 1.5-mm aluminum equivalent total filtration
   C. 2.0-mm aluminum equivalent total filtration
   D. 2.5-mm aluminum equivalent total filtration

7. Which of the following is the first step in providing gonadal protection for a patient during a radiographic exposure of the chest?
   A. Placing a lead shield over the reproductive organs
   B. Increasing total aluminum filtration to 5.0 mm
   C. Properly collimating the radiographic beam to include only the area of clinical interest
   D. Using a grid cassette with a 16 : 1 ratio

8. Which of the following types of gonadal shielding provide the *best* protection for a male patient during most radiologic procedures?
   A. Flat contact shield containing 1 mm of lead
   B. Shadow shield
   C. Shaped contact shield containing 1 mm of lead
   D. None of the above

9. Which of the following combinations of exposure factors reduce patient radiation dose during a radiographic examination?
   A. Lower kVp, higher mAs, decreased filtration
   B. Higher kVp, lower mAs, increased filtration
   C. Higher kVp, higher mAs, decreased filtration
   D. Lower kVp, lower mAs, increased filtration

10. Patient dose *decreases* in which of the following situations?
    A. Lower milliamperage and lower exposure time in seconds (mAs) are used
    B. Rare-earth intensifying screens and appropriate radiographic film are used
    C. Higher kVp techniques are used
    D. All of the above

11. Which of the following result(s) in an *increase* in patient dose?
    A. Using a radiographic grid
    B. Using proper radiographic processing techniques
    C. Using a rare-earth intensifying screen with appropriate radiographic film rather than using a high-speed calcium tungstate intensifying screen with appropriate film
    D. Using the highest practicable kVp with the lowest possible mAs for each examination

12. To reduce the radiation exposure rate and thereby reduce patient dose when operating a mobile radiographic unit, the radiographer must use a minimal source-skin distance of
    A. 6 inches (15 cm)
    B. 12 inches (30 cm)
    C. 15 inches (38 cm)
    D. 18 inches (45 cm)

13. Which of the following examinations yields the highest patient dose?
    A. Multiple radiographs of the hand done with a properly collimated x-ray beam
    B. PA and lateral chest radiographs on an adult patient
    C. Skull radiographs
    D. Fluoroscopy of an adult patient's chest

14. When a fluoroscopic image is electronically amplified by an image-intensification system, which of the following benefits result(s)?
    A. Increased image brightness
    B. Saving of time for the radiologist
    C. Patient dose reduction
    D. All of the above

15. Patient dose decreases and the life of the fluoroscopic tube increases when the radiologist uses which of the following practices?
    A. Restriction of the size of the fluoroscopic field to include only the area of clinical interest
    B. Conventional fluoroscopy rather than image intensification
    C. Intermittent fluoroscopy
    D. Darkness adaptation

16. What is the function of a filter in diagnostic radiology?
    A. To permit only alpha rays to reach the patient's skin
    B. To remove alpha particles from the x-ray beam
    C. To decrease the radiation dose to the patient's skin
    D. To permit only beta particles to interact with the atoms of the patient's body

17. Federal government specifications recommend a minimal total filtration of _____ for fluoroscopic units.
    A. 1.0-mm aluminum equivalent
    B. 1.5-mm aluminum equivalent
    C. 2.0-mm aluminum equivalent
    D. 2.5-mm aluminum equivalent

18. Image-intensifier fluoroscopic systems require a source-to-tabletop distance of at least _____ but preferably a distance of not less than _____.
   A. 6 inches (15 cm), 12 inches (30 cm)
   B. 12 inches (30 cm), 15 inches (38 cm)
   C. 15 inches (38 cm), 18 inches (45 cm)
   D. 9 inches (23 cm), 12 inches (30 cm)

19. Current federal standards limit entrance skin exposure rates of general-purpose intensified fluoroscopic units to a maximum of
   A. 5 R/min ($5 \times 2.58 \times 10^{-4}$ C/kg/min)
   B. 10 R/min ($10 \times 2.58 \times 10^{-4}$ C/kg/min)
   C. 15 R/min ($15 \times 2.58 \times 10^{-4}$ C/kg/min)
   D. 20 R/min ($20 \times 2.58 \times 10^{-4}$ C/kg/min)

20. During fluoroscopy, patient dose may be decreased by one fourth by which of the following?
   A. Increasing filtration from 1-mm aluminum to 3-mm aluminum
   B. Increasing filtration from 1-mm aluminum to 5-mm aluminum
   C. Decreasing filtration from 1-mm aluminum to ½-mm aluminum
   D. Completely removing all aluminum filtration from the path of the x-ray beam

21. Which of the following is true when the radiologist limits fluoroscopic field size to include only the area of clinical interest?
   A. Exposure factors must be increased significantly to provide adequate compensation.
   B. Patient dose decreases significantly.
   C. Patient dose increases somewhat.
   D. Patient dose remains the same.

22. Repeat radiographs result in which of the following?
   A. A double dose of radiation to the patient's skin and gonads
   B. No additional exposure for the patient
   C. Ten times more exposure for the patient
   D. None of the above

23. For protection of the patient's skin from exposure to electrons produced by photon interaction with the collimator, the skin surface should be at least _____ below the collimator.
   A. 6 cm
   B. 12 cm
   C. 15 cm
   D. 20 cm

24. Sharper size restriction of the radiographic beam is achieved when the cone or cylinder is
   A. Made of aluminum
   B. Made of plastic
   C. Shorter
   D. Longer

25. Which of the following is the most versatile type of x-ray beam limitation device?
   A. Cylinder
   B. Light-localizing variable-aperture rectangular collimator
   C. Cone
   D. Aperture diaphragm

26. Both alignment and length and width dimensions of the radiographic and light beams must correspond to within
   A. 1% of the SID
   B. 2% of the SID
   C. 5% of the SID
   D. 10% of the SID

27. HVL may be defined as the thickness of a designated absorber required to do which of the following?
   A. Increase the intensity of the primary beam by 50% of its initial value
   B. Increase the intensity of the primary beam by 25% of its initial value
   C. Decrease the intensity of the primary beam by 50% of its initial value
   D. Decrease the intensity of the primary beam by 25% of its initial value

28. What is the term for any radiograph that must be done more than once because of human or mechanical error in the process of producing the initial radiograph?
A. Blooper
B. Double exposure
C. Practice exposure
D. Repeat

29. The source-to-tabletop distance must not be less than _____ for fixed fluoroscopes and not less than _____ for mobile fluoroscopes to ensure that the entrance surface of the patient does not receive excessive exposure.
A. 15 inches (38 cm), 12 inches (30 cm)
B. 12 inches (30 cm), 6 inches (15 cm)
C. 15 inches (38 cm), 9 inches (23 cm)
D. 18 inches (45 cm), 15 inches (38 cm)

30. Which of the following are considered to be benefits of a repeat analysis program?
1. Increased awareness among staff and student radiographers of the need to produce optimal quality images
2. Radiographers become more careful in producing the radiographs because they are aware that the radiographs are being reviewed
3. When problems or concerns are identified, inservice education programs can be designed for radiography personnel to cover the topic of concern
A. 1 only
B. 2 only
C. 3 only
D. 1, 2, and 3

31. A cumulative timing device times the x-ray exposure and sounds an audible alarm or temporarily interrupts the exposure after the fluoroscope has been activated for what amount of time?
A. 1 minute
B. 3 minutes
C. 5 minutes
D. 10 minutes

32. Skin doses are most frequently assessed by using which of the following?
A. Thermoluminescent dosimeters
B. Filtration equivalent to 4.0-mm aluminum in the path of the beam
C. No filtration in the path of the beam
D. Extension cylinders

33. The genetically significant dose (GSD) for the population of the United States is about
A. 1.00 mSv (100 mrem)
B. 0.80 mSv (80 mrem)
C. 0.40 mSv (40 mrem)
D. 0.20 mSv (20 mrem)

34. Three of the radiographic procedures listed below may be considered unnecessary. Which procedure does *not* fall into this category?
A. Lumbar spine x-ray examinations as part of a preemployment physical
B. Cervical spine x-ray examinations after neck trauma from a motor vehicle accident
C. Chest x-ray examination as part of a routine health check-up
D. Chest x-ray examination on scheduled admission to the hospital for a patient who has no clinical indication of chest disease or other problems associated with the chest

35. Federal regulations in the United States for Food and Drug Administration certification of screening mammography facilities state that the maximal dose to the glandular tissue of a 4.5-cm compressed breast using a screen-film mammography system should *not* exceed which of the following?
A. 1 mGy (100 rad) per view
B. 3 mGy (300 rad) per view
C. 5 mGy (500 rad) per view
D. 7 mGy (700 rad) per view

36. Interslice scatter during a CT scanning procedure results in which of the following?
A. A uniform distribution of dose into all adjacent areas
B. A poorly defined crosssectional image of the anatomy
C. An increase in patient dose
D. A decrease in patient dose

37. Pediatric patients require special consideration and appropriate radiation protection procedures because they are more vulnerable to which of the following?
    A. Both the late somatic effects and genetic effects of radiation
    B. Only the late somatic effects of radiation
    C. Only the genetic effects of radiation
    D. Only the early somatic effects of radiation

38. In image-intensification fluoroscopy an x-ray beam half-value layer of 3- to 3.5-mm aluminum is considered acceptable when peak kilovoltage ranges from
    A. 50 to 70
    B. 70 to 80
    C. 80 to 90
    D. 90 to 100

39. If possible, the radiologic examination of the lower abdomen or pelvis of a fertile woman should be limited to the _____.
    A. Earliest part of the menstrual cycle
    B. Middle of the menstrual cycle
    C. End of the menstrual cycle
    D. Time of the menstrual cycle when ovulation occurs

40. When a pregnant patient must undergo a radiographic examination, radiation exposure may be minimized by which of the following practices?
    A. Selecting technical exposure factors that are appropriate for the part of the body to be radiographed
    B. Opening the x-ray beam collimator as wide as possible to ensure adequate coverage of the image receptor
    C. Adequately collimating the x-ray beam to include only the anatomic area of interest and shielding the lower abdomen and pelvis when this area does not need to be included in the area to be irradiated
    D. A and C

41. Luminance of the collimator light source must be
    A. Adequate to outline the margins of the radiographic beam on the patient's anatomy
    B. Visible on the patient's anatomy only when all white light is turned off in the radiographic room
    C. Below 5 foot-candles
    D. At least 10 foot-candles

42. The use of the PA projection during a juvenile scoliosis radiographic examination results in which of the following?
    A. Poor quality radiographs that necessitate a repeat examination
    B. Higher entrance exposure dose to the anterior body surface, thereby significantly increasing the dose to the breast
    C. Lower entrance exposure dose to the anterior body surface, thereby significantly reducing the dose to the breast
    D. Radiographs that do not adequately demonstrate spinal curvature

43. Which of the following types of filters should be used to provide uniform density when radiographing the foot in the dorsoplantar projection?
    A. Bilateral wedge filter
    B. Trough filter
    C. Thoraeus filter
    D. Wedge filter

44. Making a change from a 200-speed to a 400-speed system will result in which of the following?
    A. An increase in patient radiation exposure by approximately 25%
    B. A decrease in patient radiation exposure by approximately 25%
    C. An increase in patient radiation exposure by approximately 50%
    D. A decrease in patient radiation exposure by approximately 50%

45. A primary protective barrier is provided by the image intensifier of a general-purpose fluoroscopic unit. This barrier must be
A. 1-mm lead equivalent
B. 2-mm lead equivalent
C. 3-mm lead equivalent
D. 4-mm lead equivalent

46. Fluoroscopic equipment equipped with HLC may permit a skin entrance exposure rate as great as which of the following?
A. 5 R per minute ($5 \times 2.58 \times 10^{-4}$ C/kg/min)
B. 10 R per minute ($10 \times 2.58 \times 10^{-4}$ C/kg/min)
C. 20 R per minute ($20 \times 2.58 \times 10^{-4}$ C/kg/min)
D. 50 R per minute ($50 \times 2.58 \times 10^{-4}$ C/kg/min)

47. If in the course of performing a specific radiographic procedure, 75% of the active bone marrow were in the useful beam and received an average absorbed dose of 0.4 mGy (40 mrad), the mean active bone marrow dose would be which of the following?
A. 0.3 mGy (30 mrad)
B. 0.6 mGy (60 mrad)
C. 0.9 mGy (90 mrad)
D. 1.0 mGy (100 mrad)

48. A radiographer uses a 10×12 radiographic film in a cassette equipped with rare-earth intensifying screens to radiograph the chest of a 2-year-old child. The image receptor is larger than the actual size of the child's chest. To reduce patient dose as much as possible and assuming optimal exposure factors are used, the radiographer should do which of the following?
A. Shield the reproductive organs and collimate the radiographic beam so that it is slightly larger than the margins of the image receptor
B. Shield the reproductive organs and collimate the radiographic beam so that it is no larger than the margins of the image receptor
C. Shield the reproductive organs and collimate the radiographic beam so that it is smaller than the margins of the image receptor
D. Not shield the reproductive organs and collimate the radiographic beam so that it is smaller than the margins of the image receptor

49. The 10-day rule is considered obsolete because it can result in which of the following?
A. The irradiation of a large number of embryo-fetuses in a high percent of the pregnant female population
B. Excessive irradiation of the embryo-fetus, resulting in spontaneous abortion
C. Menstrual irregularities
D. Unnecessary postponement of radiologic examinations for the majority of female patients

50. A woman who is 3 months pregnant has been in a motor vehicle accident. Injury to her cervical spine is suspected by the emergency room physician. The physician orders x-rays to aid in determining the extent of the injury. Because the patient is pregnant, the radiographer should
1. Select the smallest technical exposure factors that will generate a diagnostically useful radiograph
2. Adequately and precisely collimate the radiographic beam to include only the anatomic area of interest
3. Shield the patient's lower abdomen and pelvic region with a suitable protective contact shield
A. 1 only
B. 2 only
C. 3 only
D. 1, 2, and 3

References

1. Edwards C, Statkiewicz-Sherer MA, Ritenour ER: *Radiation protection for dental radiographers*, Denver, Colo, 1984, Multi-Media Publishing.
2. National Council on Radiation Protection and Measurements (NCRP): *Medical x-ray, electron beam and gamma ray protection for energies up to 50 MeV: equipment design, performance, and use*, Report No. 102, Bethesda, Md, 1989, NCRP.
3. Bushong SC: *Radiologic science for technologists: physics, biology and protection*, ed 6, St Louis, 1997, Mosby.
4. Gray J et al: *Quality control in diagnostic imaging*, Baltimore, 1983, University Park Press.
5. Hendee WR, Chaney EL, Rossi RP: *Radiologic physics equipment and quality control*, Chicago, 1977, Year Book.
6. McKinney W: *Radiographic processing and quality control*, Philadelphia, 1988, J.B. Lippincott.
7. FDA Publication No. 86-8265, *Pre-surgical chest x-ray screening examinations*, Washington, DC, Superintendent of Documents, U.S. Government Printing Office.
8. Federal Register, August 15, 1972 (37 FR 16461).

9. Ballinger PW, editor: *Merrill's atlas of radiographic positions and radiologic procedures,* ed 8, vol 1, St Louis, 1995, Mosby.

10. Huda W et al: Radiation doses due to breast imaging in Manitoba: 1978-1988, *Radiology* 177:812, 1990.

11. Ritenour ER, Hendee, WR: Screening mammography: a risk vs risk decision, *Invest Radiol* 24:17, Jan 1989.

12. Taubes G: The breast-screening brawl, *Science* 275:1056, Feb 21, 1997.

13. Federal Register, 42CFR494 (d) . 251, 53525.

14. Yaffe M, Mawdslwy GE: Equipment requirements and quality control for mammography, in specification, acceptance testing and quality control of diagnostic x-ray imaging equipment. In Siebert JA, Barnes GT, Gould RG, editors: *American association of physicists in medicine, medical physics monograph No. 20,* College Park, Md, 1994, American Association of Physicists in Medicine.

15. Beebe, GW, Kato H, Land DE: Studies of the mortality of A-bomb survivors. 6. Mortality and radiation dose, 1950-1974, *Radiat Res* 75:138, 1978.

16. National Council on Radiation Protection and Measurements (NCRP): *Radiation protection in pediatric radiology,* Report No. 68, Washington, DC, 1981, NCRP Publications.

17. Bontrager KL: *Textbook of positioning and related anatomy,* ed 4, St Louis, 1997, Mosby.

18. International Commission on Radiation Protection: *Protection of the patient in x-ray diagnosis,* Publication No. 16, Oxford, England, 1970, Pergamon Press.

19. Reynold FB: Prepared remarks for the October 20, 1976, American College of Radiology press conference.

20. National Council on Radiation Protection and Measurements (NCRP): *Medical exposure of pregnant and potentially pregnant women,* Report No. 54, Washington, D.C., 1977, NCRP Publications.

Bibliography

Ballinger PW: *Merrill's atlas of radiographic positions and radiologic procedures,* ed 8, vol 1, St Louis, 1995, Mosby.

Ballinger PW: *Merrill's atlas of radiographic positions and radiologic procedures,* ed 5, vol 1, St Louis, 1982, Mosby.

Beebe GW et al: Studies of the mortality of A-bomb survivors. 6. Mortality and radiation dose, 1950-1974, *Radiat Res* 75:138, 1978.

Boone JM, Levin DC: Radiation exposure to angiographers under different fluoroscopic conditions, *Radiology* 180(3):861, Sept 1991.

Brown RF: Prepared remarks for the October 20, 1976, American College of Radiology press conference.

Bushong S: *Radiologic science for technologists: physics, biology, and protection,* ed 2, St Louis, 1980, Mosby.

Bushong SC. In Ballinger PW, editor: *Merrill's atlas of radiographic positions and radiologic procedures,* ed 7, vol 1, St Louis, 1991, Mosby.

Bushong SC: *Radiologic science for technologists: physics, biology, and protection,* ed 6, St Louis, 1997, Mosby.

Carlton RR, Adler AM: *Principles of radiographic imaging an art and a science,* Albany, NY, 1992, Delmar.

Christensen EE, Curry II TS, Dowdey JE: *An introduction to the physics of diagnostic radiology,* ed 2, Philadelphia, 1978, Lea & Febiger.

Cullinan JE, Cullinan AM: *Illustrated guide to x-ray technics,* ed 2, Philadelphia, 1980, J.B. Lippincott.

Curry II, TS, Dowdey JE, Murry Jr RC: *Christensen's introduction to the physics of diagnostic radiology,* ed 3, Philadelphia, 1984, Lea & Febiger.

Donohue DP: *An analysis of radiographic quality: lab manual and workbook,* Baltimore, 1980, University Park Press.

Donohue DP: *An analysis of radiographic quality: lab manual and workbook,* ed 2, Rockville, Md, 1984, Aspen.

Dorst JP et al. In Ballinger PW, editor: *Merrill's atlas of radiographic positions and radiologic procedures,* ed 7, vol 3, St Louis, 1991, Mosby.

Dowd SB: *Practical radiation protection and applied radiobiology,* Philadelphia, 1994, W.B. Saunders.

Eddy DM et al: The value of mammography screening in women under age 50 years, *JAMA* 259(10):1512, 1988.

Frankel R: *Radiation protection for radiologic technologists,* New York, 1976, McGraw-Hill.

Goss CM, editor: *Gray's anatomy,* ed 29, Philadelphia, 1973, Lea & Febiger.

Hendee WR, editor: *Health effects of low-level radiation,* Norwalk, Conn, 1984, Appleton-Century-Crofts.

International Commission on Radiation Protection: *Protection of the patient in x-ray diagnosis,* Publication No. 16, Oxford, England, 1970, Pergamon Press.

Jayaraman S et al: Analysis of radiation risk versus benefit in mammography, *Appl Radiol,* p45, Mar/Apr, 1986.

Johnson KC, Rowberg AH. In Ballinger PW, editor: *Merrill's atlas of radiographic positions and radiologic procedures,* ed 7, vol 3, St Louis, 1991, Mosby.

Mallett M, editor: *Handbook of anatomy and physiology for students of medical radiation technology,* ed 3, Mankato, Minn, 1979, The Burnell Company/Publishers.

Malott JC, Fodor III, J: *The art and science of medical radiography,* ed 7, St Louis, 1993, Mosby.

National Council on Radiation Protection and Measurements (NCRP): *Exposure of the U.S. population from diagnostic medical radiation,* Report No. 100, Bethesda, Md, 1989, MCRP Publications.

National Council on Radiation Protection and Measurements (NCRP): *Medical x-ray, electron beam and gamma-ray protection for energies up to 50 MeV,* Report No. 102, Bethesda, Md, 1989, NCRP Publications.

National Council on Radiation Protection and Measurements (NCRP): *Ionizing radiation exposure of the population of the United States,* Report No. 116, Bethesda, Md, 1987, NCRP Publications.

National Council on Radiation Protection and Measurements (NCRP): R*ecommendations on limits for exposure to ionizing radiation*, Report No. 91, Bethesda, Md, 1987, NCRP Publications.

National Council on Radiation Protection and Measurements (NCRP): *Radiation protection in pediatric radiology*, Report No. 68, Washington, D.C., 1981, NCRP Publications.

National Council on Radiation Protection and Measurements (NCRP): *Medical exposure of pregnant and potentially pregnant women*, Report No. 54, Washington, D.C., 1977, NCRP Publications.

National Council on Radiation Protection and Measurements (NCRP): *Basic radiation protection criteria*, Report No. 39, Washington, D.C., 1971, NCRP Publications.

National Council on Radiation Protection and Measurements (NCRP): *Medical x-ray and gamma-ray protection for energies up to 10 MeV: equipment design and use*, Report No. 33, Washington, D.C., 1968, NCRP Publications.

Noz ME, Magture Jr GQ: *Radiation protection in the radiologic and health sciences,* Philadelphia, 1979, Lea & Febiger.

Noz ME, Maguire Jr GQ: *Radiation protection in radiologic and health sciences,* ed 2, Philadelphia, 1985, Lea & Febiger.

Olsen JO. In Ballinger PW, editor: *Merrill's atlas of radiographic positions and radiologic procedures,* ed 7, vol 3, St Louis, 1991, Mosby.

Radiation induced skin injuries can result from fluoroscopy, *ASRT Scanner* 27(2):22, Dec 1994 and Jan 1995.

Ritenour ER: *Radiation protection and biology: a self-instructional multimedia learning series, instructor manual,* Denver, Colo, 1985, Multi-Media Publishing.

Scheele RV, Wakley J: *Elements of radiation protection,* Springfield, Ill, 1975, Charles C. Thomas.

Seeram E: *Radiation protection,* Philadelphia, 1997, Lippincott-Raven.

Selman J: *The fundamentals of x-ray and radium physics,* ed 7, Springfield, Ill, 1985, Charles C. Thomas.

Selman J: *The fundamentals of x-ray and radium physics,* ed 6, Springfield, Ill, 1978, Charles C. Thomas.

Statkiewicz MA: Communication skills for the radiologic technologist, *Radiol Technol* 54:449, 1983.

Thomas CL, editor: *Taber's cyclopedic medical dictionary,* ed 13, Philadelphia, 1973, F.A. Davis.

Thompson MA et al: *Principles of imaging science and protection,* Philadelphia, 1994, W.B. Saunders.

Thompson TT: *A practical approach to modern imaging equipment,* ed 2, Boston, 1985, Little, Brown.

Thompson TT: *Cahoon's formulating x-ray techniques,* ed 9, Durham, NC, 1979, Duke University Press.

Travis EL: *Primer of medical radiobiology,* ed 2, Chicago, 1989, Year Book Medical Publishers.

US Department of Health and Human Services (HHS), Public Health Service, Food and Drug Administration, Bureau of Radiological Health: *The correlated lecture laboratory series in diagnostic radiological physics,* HHS Publication FDA 81-8150, Rockville, Md, 1981, HHS.

US Department of Health, Education, and Welfare (HEW), Public Health Service, Food and Drug Administration, Bureau of Radiological Health: *The selection of patients for x-ray examinations,* HEW Publication FDA 80-8104, Rockville, Md, Jan 1980, HEW.

US Department of Health, Education, and Welfare (HEW), Public Health Service, Food and Drug Administration, Bureau of Radiological Health: *Quality assurance programs for diagnostic radiology facilities,* HEW Publication FDA 8080-1110, Rockville, Md, Feb 1980, HEW.

US Department of Health, Education, and Welfare (HEW), Public Health Service, Food and Drug Administration, Bureau of Radiological Health: *Analysis of retakes: understanding, managing, and using an analysis of retakes program for quality assurance,* HEW Publication FDA 79-8097, Rockville, Md, Aug 1979, HEW.

US Government Printing Office: *Pre-surgical chest x-ray screening examinations,* FDA Publication 86-8265, Superintendent of Documents, Washington, D.C.

US Department of Health, Education, and Welfare (HEW), Public Health Service, Food and Drug Administration, Bureau of Radiological Health: *Gonadal shielding in diagnostic radiology,* HEW Publication FDA 75-8024, Rockville, Md, June 1975, HEW.

Webster EW et al: *A primer on low-level ionizing radiation and its biological effects,* AAPM Report No. 18, New York, 1986, American Institute of Physics (published for the American Association of Physicists in Medicine).

8

Protecting Occupationally Exposed Personnel During Diagnostic Radiologic Procedures

ALARA concept
annual occupational effective dose
beam limitation devices
Bucky slot shielding device
Compton interaction process
control-booth barrier
controlled area
diagnostic-type protective tube housing
distance
dose equivalent
fluoroscopic exposure monitor
genetically significant dose (GSD)
interventional procedures
inverse square law (ISL)
leakage radiation
mobile radiographic equipment

occupancy factor (T)
occupational risk
patient restraint
primary protective barrier
primary radiation
protective curtain or sliding panel
protective eyeglasses
protective lead apron
protective lead gloves
safe industries
scatter radiation
secondary protective barrier
secondary radiation
thyroid shield
time
uncontrolled area
use factor (U)
workload (W)

After completing this chapter, the reader will be able to perform the following:

- State the total annual occupational effective dose limit for whole-body exposure of diagnostic imaging personnel during routine operations.
- Explain the reason that occupational exposure of diagnostic imaging personnel must be limited.
- Explain the reasons for allowing a larger dose equivalent for radiation workers than for the population as a whole.
- Define *ALARA* and explain the significance of this concept for the radiation worker.
- Identify the type of x-radiation that poses the greatest occupational hazard in diagnostic radiology and explain the various ways this hazard can be reduced or eliminated.
- Explain the way various methods and techniques that reduce patient exposure during a diagnostic examination also reduce exposure for the radiographer and other diagnostic personnel.
- Discuss the responsibilities of the employer and the pregnant radiologic technologist.
- Explain the difference between a primary and a secondary protective barrier, and list examples of each.
- Describe the construction of protective structural shielding, and list the factors that govern the selection of appropriate construction materials.
- Explain the purpose of a diagnostic-type protective tube housing.
- List and describe the protective garments that may be worn to reduce whole- or partial-body exposure, and discuss the circumstances in which such garments are worn.
- Explain the various methods and devices that may be used to reduce exposure for personnel during a routine fluoroscopic examination.
- Explain the various methods and devices that may be used to reduce the radiographer's exposure during a mobile radiographic examination.
- Explain the variation in dose rate caused by scatter radiation near the entrance and exit surfaces of the patient during C-Arm fluoroscopy.

Continued

While fulfilling their professional responsibilities associated with diagnostic medical imaging, radiographers may be exposed to **secondary radiation** (scatter or leakage). Some radiologic procedures such as general fluoroscopy, interventional procedures that employ high-level–control (HLC) fluoroscopy, and mobile examinations increase the radiographer's risk of exposure. When participating in any procedure that may result in occupational exposure, the radiographer must employ appropriate methods of protection against ionizing radiation. This chapter presents an overview of methods that may be used to reduce exposure for the radiation worker during diagnostic radiologic procedures.

Annual Limit for Occupationally Exposed Personnel

Federal government standards, enforcing a recommendation of the NCRP, permit diagnostic imaging personnel to receive a total "**annual occupational effective dose** of 50 millisievert (mSv) (5 rem)"[1] for whole-body exposure during routine operations. This upper-boundary effective dose limit is greater than the annual effective dose limit allowed for individual members of the general population not occupationally exposed. That limit is 1 mSv (0.1 rem) for continuous (or frequent) exposure from artificial sources other than medical[1] and 5 mSv (0.5 rem) for infrequent annual exposure.[1] The 1 mSv (0.1 rem) annual effective dose limit "recommendation is designed to limit the exposure of members of the public to reasonable levels of risk comparable with risks from other common sources—i.e., about 10^{-4} to 10^{-6} annually"[1] (10^{-4} to 10^{-6} means an excess cancer risk of one chance in ten thousand to one chance in one million per year). The 5 mSv (0.5 rem) maximal annual effective dose limit recommendation "is made because annual exposures in excess of the 1 mSv recommendation, usually to a small group of people, need not be regarded as especially hazardous, provided it does not occur often to the same groups and that the average exposure to individuals in these groups does not exceed an average annual effective dose of about 1 mSv."[1] Both these limits "will keep the annual equivalent dose to those organs and tissues that are considered in the effective dose system below levels of concern for deterministic effects."[1]

Valid reasons exist for allowance of a larger **dose equivalent** for radiation workers. Among the most important of these reasons is that the workforce in radiation-related jobs is small when compared with the population as a whole. Thus the amount of radiation received by this workforce can be larger than the amount received by the general public without altering the **genetically significant dose (GSD),** the average annual gonadal dose equivalent to members of the population who are of childbearing age (see Chapter 7). This means that the extra amount of radiation absorbed by the radiation workforce does not significantly increase the total number of deleterious mutations in the United States. Although the radiographer and other diagnostic imaging personnel may absorb more radiation, the dose equivalent received must be minimized whenever possible. This reduces the potential for somatic and genetic damage.

ALARA Concept

In addition to the effective dose equivalent limit system, another radiation protection principle exists—the **ALARA concept.** As defined in Chapter 4, this concept holds that occupational exposure of the radiographer and other occupationally exposed persons should be kept "As Low As Reasonably Achievable." This implies that actual dose equivalent values should be kept well below their allowable maximal limits. The best way for radiologists and radiographers to do this is to employ proper radiation-control procedures such as the accurate placement and adequate collimation of the radiographic beam (Fig. 8-1). Because continual use of such radiation-awareness procedures ensures a high degree of safety from most radiation exposures, radiography is not considered a hazardous profession. The **occupational risk** for monitored diagnostic imaging personnel may be compared with the occupational risk for persons employed in other **safe industries** such as manufacturing, trade, service, and government. These safe industries have a risk of fatal accidents that is generally estimated to be about 1×10^{-4} y^{-1}.[1] The annual risk for radiation workers is unlikely to exceed this rate.

Dose Reduction Methods and Techniques

Methods and techniques that reduce patient exposure also reduce exposure for the radiographer. For example, repeat examinations should be avoided whenever

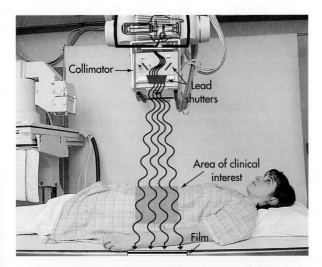

Fig. 8-1 Radiographic beam collimation (restricting the x-ray beam to the area of clinical interest) limits the production of scattered radiation. This radiation-control procedure helps keep the radiographer's occupational exposure as low as reasonably achievable.

possible to eliminate additional exposure. Other such considerations are identified in this chapter.

During a diagnostic examination the patient becomes a source of scattered radiation as a consequence of the **Compton interaction process** (see Chapter 2). At a 90-degree angle to the primary x-ray beam, at a distance of 1 meter (3.3 feet), the scattered x-ray intensity is generally approximately $\frac{1}{1000}$ of the intensity of the primary x-ray beam.

Because scattered radiation poses the greatest occupational hazard in diagnostic radiology, the use of any device or technique that minimizes the amount of scattered radiation produced decreases occupational exposure for diagnostic imaging personnel. The use of **beam limitation devices** such as the light-localizing variable-aperture rectangular collimator decreases the size of the radiographic beam so that its margins do not extend beyond the image receptor (radiographic film). This reduction in beam size results in a decrease in the number of x-ray photons available to undergo Compton scatter. Because scatter is reduced, the radiographer's exposure decreases.

When a radiographic beam is properly filtered, nonuseful low-energy photons are removed from the primary beam. Without proper filtration a relatively high percentage of the normally filtered low-energy photons interact with the tissues of the patient's body. A portion of these photons undergo Compton scatter. The radiation worker's dose equivalent could therefore increase as a result of exposure to this excess scattered radiation. Most of these low-energy photons, however, will be absorbed in the patient, increasing the patient's absorbed dose and contributing nothing to the radiographic image. Thus filtration primarily benefits the patient.

Protective lead aprons (Fig. 8-2, *A*) and shielded barriers (Fig. 8-2, *B*) function as gonadal shields for diagnostic imaging personnel. These devices protect them from scattered radiation.

Exposure factors control the quantity of scattered radiation that is produced, although this effect is not very great. Higher peak kilovoltage techniques increase the mean energy of the photons composing the radiographic beam and also require lower photon beam intensity (i.e., lower milliamperage). As the average energy of the beam increases, the percentage of radiation that is forward scatter increases. Therefore

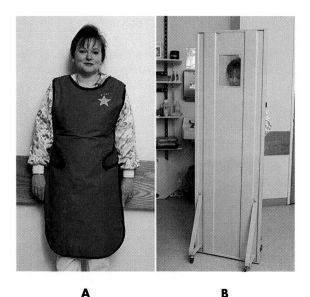

A   **B**

Fig. 8-2 A, A lead apron protects occupationally exposed personnel from scattered radiation. **B,** A lead mobile x-ray barrier of 0.5- or 1.0-mm lead equivalent provides protection from scattered radiation. It may be used during special procedures, in the operating room, and in cardiac units.

less scatter radiation is available to reach the imaging personnel, and their dose equivalent is reduced.

When high-speed image receptor systems are used, smaller radiographic exposures (less milliamperage) are required, which result in fewer x-ray photons being available to produce Compton scatter. Because of this reduction in Compton scatter, personnel exposure is decreased.

Finally, the use of good radiographic processing techniques leads to a decrease in the number of repeat examinations required, with a resultant reduction in exposure to the radiographer.

Radiation Protection for the Pregnant Radiologic Technologist

Pregnant radiologic technologists should be able to continue performing their duties without interruption of employment if they follow established radiation safety practices. Most institutions have policies for protecting pregnant personnel from radiation. Under these policies a technologist who becomes pregnant must inform her supervisor. After this declaration has been made, the institution officially recognizes the pregnancy. The institution, through its radiation safety officer, provides essential counseling and furnishes an appropriate additional monitor. This device is to be worn beneath a lead apron at waist level during all radiation procedures. The purpose of this additional monitor is to ensure that the monthly effective dose equivalent (EDE) to the embryo-fetus does not exceed 0.5 mSv (0.05 rem). This EDE excludes both medical and natural background radiation. It is designed to restrict the total lifetime risk of leukemia and other malignancies significantly in persons exposed in utero.

After receiving radiation safety counseling, the pregnant technologist must read and sign a form acknowledging that she has received instruction and understands the ways to implement appropriate measures to ensure the safety of the embryo-fetus. For additionally monitored pregnant personnel, film badge companies such as Landauer provide a monthly report that tracks the exposure to the worker and the embryo-fetus. A copy of this report is sent to the institution's radiation safety officer.

Protective Structural Shielding

Protective barriers such as the walls in an x-ray room provide radiation shielding for both imaging department personnel and the general public. This protection is necessary to ensure that occupational and nonoccupational annual effective dose equivalent limits are not exceeded. Lead sheets of appropriate thickness placed in the walls of the radiographic or fluoroscopic room are generally used to provide proper structural shielding.

Exact shielding requirements for a particular radiologic facility should be determined by a qualified medical physicist. Radiographers should understand the concept of shielding but are not responsible for determining barrier thickness.

Primary protective barrier

The purpose of a **primary protective barrier** is to prevent primary radiation from reaching personnel or members of the general public on the other side of the

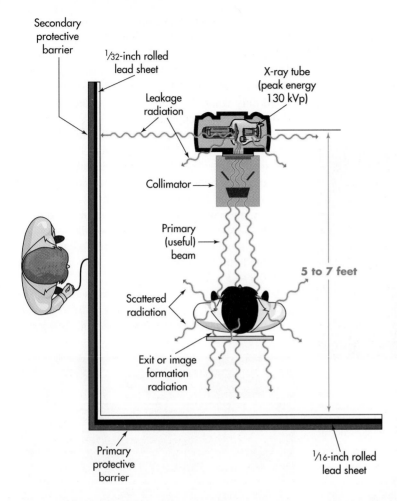

Fig. 8-3 Protective barriers are lined with lead to protect personnel and the general public from radiation. The primary protective barrier is located perpendicular to the line of travel of the primary (useful) x-ray beam. The secondary protective barrier runs parallel to the primary x-ray beam and protects diagnostic radiology personnel from secondary (leakage and scattered) radiation. The walls that are not in the direct line of travel of the primary beam are called *secondary protective barriers*, because they are designed to shield against secondary (leakage and scattered) radiation.

barrier. The primary beam is made up of the x-ray photons that follow straight-line paths between all sets of collimator shutters. Primary protective barriers are located perpendicular to the line of travel of the primary x-ray beam (Fig. 8-3). If the peak energy of the beam is 130 kVp, the primary protective barrier in a typical installation consists of $\frac{1}{16}$ inch lead and extends 7 feet (2.1 m) upward from the floor of the x-ray room when the x-ray tube is 5 to 7 feet from the wall in question.

Secondary protective barrier

Secondary radiation consists of radiation that has been deflected from the primary beam. Leakage from the tube housing (photons that pass through the housing when a defect occurs in the lead shielding around the tube) and scatter (primarily from the patient) make up the secondary radiation. A **secondary protective barrier** protects against secondary radiation (leakage and scattered radiation) only and, as such, is located parallel to the direction of travel of the x-ray beam (see Fig. 8-3). This barrier should overlap the primary protective barrier by about $\frac{1}{2}$ inch and must extend to the ceiling. In a typical installation the secondary barrier consists of $\frac{1}{32}$-inch lead.

X-ray rooms housing fixed radiographic equipment contain a stationary **control-booth barrier** for the protection of the radiographer. Because this booth intercepts leakage and scattered radiation only, it may be regarded as a secondary protective barrier. To ensure maximal protection during radiographic exposures, personnel must remain completely behind the barrier. The radiographer may observe the patient through the lead glass window in the booth (Fig. 8-4). This window typically consists of 1.5-mm lead equivalent.

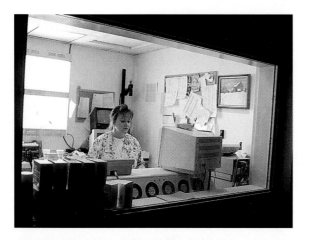

Fig. 8-4 While making a radiographic exposure with a fixed radiographic unit, the radiographer must remain completely within the control-booth barrier (behind the fixed protective barrier) for safety. The radiographer may observe the patient through the lead glass observation window in the control booth.

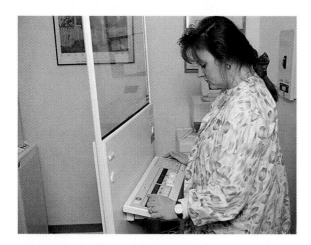

Fig. 8-5 A clear lead-plastic secondary protective barrier impregnated with approximately 30% lead lends a modern appearance to the facility.

With the appropriate lead-equivalent in the barrier, exposure of the radiographer should not exceed a maximal allowance of 1 mSv per week (100 mrem per week). For further protection, the exposure cord must be short enough so that the exposure switch can be operated only when the radiographer is completely behind the control-booth barrier.

Clear lead-plastic material impregnated with approximately 30% lead by weight may be fashioned into an effective secondary protective barrier, such as for the control booth (Fig. 8-5). This creates a modern appearance for the facility and permits a panoramic view by allowing diagnostic imaging personnel and patient to view one another. These modular x-ray barriers are shatter resistant, can extend 7 feet upward from the floor, and are available in a lead equivalency from 0.3 to 2 mm.

Clear lead-plastic protective barriers also can be used as overhead x-ray barriers (Fig. 8-6) to provide both an open view and effective protection during spe-

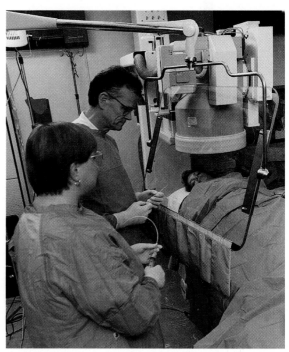

Fig. 8-6 A clear lead-plastic overhead protective barrier used during special procedures and cardiac catheterization. (Courtesy Nuclear Associates, Inc.)

cial procedures and cardiac catheterization. This shielding ensures 0.5-mm lead equivalency protection.

Diagnostic–Type Protective Tube Housing

A lead-lined metal **diagnostic-type protective tube housing** (Fig. 8-7) is required to protect both the radiographer and patient from off-focus or leakage radiation by restricting the emission of x-rays to the area of the useful or primary beam (those x-rays emitted through the x-ray tube window or port).

The housing enclosing the x-ray tube must be constructed so that leakage radiation measured at a distance of 1 m (3.3 feet) from the x-ray source does not exceed 100 mR/hr (2.58×10^{-5} C/kg/hr) when the tube is operated continuously at its highest current for its full potential (voltage). Although the x-ray tube housing is designed to protect the operator from the hazard of electric shock, the radiographer

must be careful handling this piece of equipment and its adjoining part, the collimator. When manipulating the tube housing for a radiographic examination, the radiographer should always avoid handling or severely bending the high-tension cables that connect to the positive and negative terminals of the x-ray tube. No one should touch the tube housing or high-tension cables while a radiographic exposure is in progress.

Protection During Fluoroscopic Procedures

To ensure protection from scattered radiation emanating from the patient during a fluoroscopic examination, the radiographer should stand as far away from the patient as is practical and should move closer to the patient only when assistance is required. A **protective lead apron** must be worn during all fluoroscopic procedures. **Protective lead gloves** should be worn whenever the hands must be placed in the fluoroscopic field (e.g., to assist in turning an incapacitated patient during the examination). Imaging personnel assisting during a fluoroscopic examination also should wear thyroid shields if they are standing in close proximity to the patient being examined.

Many of the methods and devices that reduce the radiographer's exposure when operating fixed radiographic equipment also reduce the dose received by the radiographer and radiologist during a fluoroscopic procedure. These methods and devices include proper beam collimation, filtration, gonadal shielding, control of exposure factors, high-speed image receptor systems, proper radiographic processing, adequate structural shielding, appropriate source-to-tabletop distance, use of a cumulative timing device, and housing of the x-ray tube in a diagnostic-type protective encasement. Some additional requirements are included in the federal government specifications for the use of fluoroscopic equipment to ensure adequate protection for the radiographer and radiologist.

Protective curtain or sliding panel

A **protective curtain or sliding panel** with a minimum of 0.25-mm lead equivalent should be positioned between the fluoroscopist and the patient to intercept scattered radiation (Fig. 8-8).

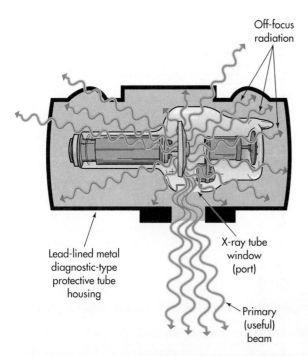

Fig. 8-7 A lead-lined metal diagnostic-type protective tube housing protects the radiographer and the patient from off-focus or leakage radiation by restricting x-ray emission to the area of the primary (useful) beam.

Bucky slot shielding device

A **Bucky slot shielding device** (Fig. 8-9) of at least 0.25-mm lead equivalent must automatically cover the Bucky slot opening in the side of the x-ray table during a fluoroscopic examination when the Bucky tray is positioned at the foot end of the table. This shielding device protects the radiologist and radiographer at gonadal level. Without this device and the protective curtain in place, the exposure rate to the fluoroscopist would exceed 100 mR per hour at a distance of 2 feet from the side of the x-ray table.

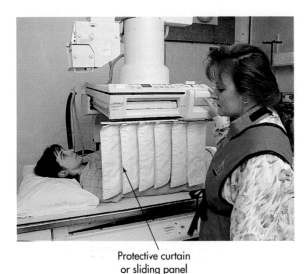

Protective curtain
or sliding panel

Fig. 8-8 Scattered radiation produced during a fluoroscopic examination can be absorbed by a protective curtain or sliding panel with a minimum of 0.25-mm lead equivalent placed between the fluoroscopist and the patient.

Fluoroscopic exposure monitor

Occupational exposure during fluoroscopic procedures may be reduced significantly through the use of a **fluoroscopic exposure monitor** (Fig. 8-10), which "provides an instantaneous audible indication of the intensity of secondary radiation."[2] This device emits "a soft chirping signal, whose frequency varies in direct proportion to the exposure rate."[2] Personnel using this monitor can select a position to stand relative to the source of radiation, thereby achieving the greatest protection. The device should be clipped to the outside of the lead apron, at the collar.

Rotational scheduling of personnel

Diagnostic imaging personnel receive the highest occupational exposure during fluoroscopy, mobile radiography, and special procedures. This exposure can be decreased by scheduling personnel to spend less time in these higher-radiation areas. Radiographers may be assigned to clinical areas in a rotational pattern. This type of scheduling uses the cardinal principle of **time** as a means of radiation protection.

Protection During Mobile Radiographic Examinations

Mobile radiographic equipment creates special radiation protection considerations for the radiographer. Suitable protective garments (lead aprons and gloves) should be worn by the radiographer whenever structural or mobile protective shielding is unavailable.

For the vast majority of mobile units, which are not equipped with a remote control exposure device, the

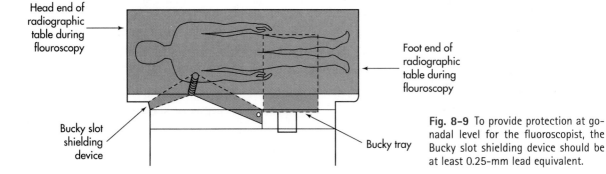

Head end of radiographic table during flouroscopy

Foot end of radiographic table during flouroscopy

Bucky slot shielding device

Bucky tray

Fig. 8-9 To provide protection at gonadal level for the fluoroscopist, the Bucky slot shielding device should be at least 0.25-mm lead equivalent.

cord leading to the exposure switch should be long enough to permit the radiographer to stand at least 2 m (approximately 6 feet, or 72 inches) from the patient, the x-ray tube, and the useful beam. This permits the radiographer to use the inverse square effect of distance to reduce exposure.

The radiographer should attempt to stand at right angles (90 degrees) to the x-ray beam scattering object (the patient) line; when the protection factors of dis-

tance and shielding have been accounted for, this is the place at which the least amount of scattered radiation is received (Fig. 8-11). However, because distance and shielding have much more influence on the reduction of the exposure of the technologist, these factors should be addressed first.

Protection During C–Arm Fluoroscopy

Safety procedures are particularly important when mobile fluoroscopy (C-Arm) systems are used. Because patterns of exposure direction are less predictable and the equipment is frequently operated by physicians whose training and experience in radiation safety may not match that of the trained radiologist, the radiographer should exercise special vigilance. For C-Arm devices with similar fields of view, the dose rate to

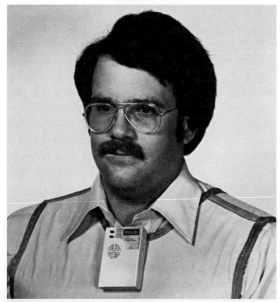

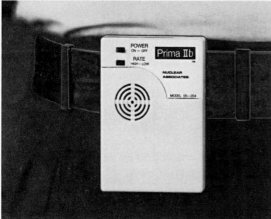

Fig. 8-10 A fluoroscopy exposure monitor can be worn outside the protective apron, at collar or waist level. (Courtesy Nuclear Associates, Inc.)

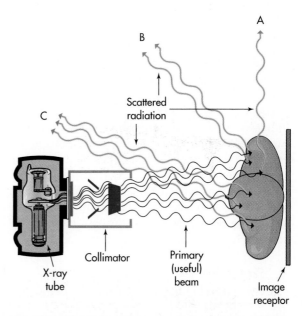

Fig. 8-11 When the protective factors of distance and shielding have been accounted for, the radiographer will receive the least amount of scattered radiation by standing at right angles (90 degrees) to the scattering object (the patient) (in position *A*). The most scattered radiation would be received at point *C* because of backscatter coming from the patient. (Intensity or quantity of x-ray exposure at any given point is indicated in this picture by the number of scattered x-rays reaching that point.)

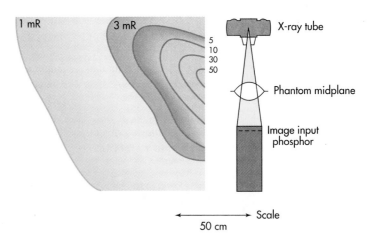

Fig. 8-12 The exposure patterns near a C-Arm fluoroscope are illustrated here as contour lines, lines along which the exposure is constant. At the side of the patient, the exposure rate is lower for locations on the image intensifier side of the beam than for locations on the x-ray tube side of the beam. This result is indicated by the bulging of the contour lines on the x-ray tube side of the patient. (From Cullings HM, Hendee WR: Radiation risks in the orthopaedic operating room, *Contemporary Orthopedics* 8(4):48-57.)

personnel located within a meter of the patient is comparable to that of routine fixed fluoroscopy—approximately several hundred centigray (cGy) per hour. Exposure of personnel is caused by scatter from the patient. During operating room procedures in which cross-table exposures are used, an understanding of the patterns of x-ray scatter is particularly useful. The dose rate caused by scatter near the entrance surface of the patient (the x-ray tube side) exceeds the dose rate caused by scatter near the exit surface of the patient (the image intensifier side) (Fig. 8-12). The difference in the scatter dose rate, typically a factor of two or three, is caused by the higher dose rate at the entrance surface of the patient. Thus the location of lower scatter dose is on the side of the patient away from the x-ray tube. Obviously, the radiographer should never encounter the actual useful beam. Outside of the beam, however, the exposure caused by scatter is lower on the image intensifier side.

Protection During High-Dose (High-Level–Control) Interventional Procedures

All the standard precautions and procedures for the reduction of dose to personnel are applicable during **interventional procedures.** These radiation safety techniques take on an increased importance in interventional procedures because of the extended length of some of these procedures (see Table 7-2), the large number of digital and cineradiographic images that are taken, and the use of high-level–control mode of oper-

ation, in which the exposure rate exceeds the rate used in routine fluoroscopy. Although the duration of the procedure and the number of exposures taken is under the control of the radiologist, the radiographer should be knowledgeable in the application of dose reduction techniques. The radiographer should verify that dose-reducing features are available and in good working order. These features include the presence of high-quality low-dose fluoroscopy mode, collimation, optimal beam filtration, removable grids, variable optical aperture, "roadmapping," time-interval differences, and "last-image-hold" features. In last-image-hold mode the last exposure remains on the viewing monitor so that the operator does not need to expose again simply to review the position of the catheter in relation to landmarks when no new information is needed. If possible, the beam entry site could be changed during the procedure to reduce total dose to any one area of skin. High-level control is to be used sparingly and only when increased resolution is necessary during a critical maneuver such as embolization or deployment of devices such as stents.[3] Records should be kept so that the cumulative fluoroscopic exposure time may be determined (as opposed to an unspecified number of resets of the 5-minute timer).

Distance

Distance is the most effective means of protection from ionizing radiation. Radiographers receive less radiation exposure by standing farther away from a

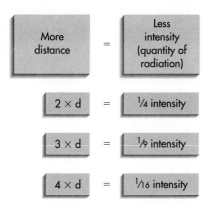

Fig. 8-13 As the distance between the source of radiation and any given measurement point increases, radiation intensity (quantity) measured at that point decreases by the square of its distance.

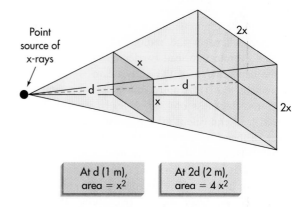

Fig. 8-14 When the distance from a point source of radiation is doubled, the radiation at the new location spans an area four times larger than the original area. However, the intensity at the new distance is only one fourth the original intensity.

source of radiation. The **inverse square law (ISL)** expresses the relationship between distance and intensity (quantity) of radiation. The law is stated as follows: "The intensity of the radiation is inversely proportional to the square of the distance." In other words, as the distance between the radiation source and a measurement point increases, the quantity of radiation measured at that point decreases by the square of its distance from the source (Fig. 8-13). This decrease in radiation intensity occurs because the area, which the same flux of x-rays at the original location now has to cover at the new location, has increased by the square of the distance. For example, when the distance from the x-ray target, a point source of radiation, is doubled, the radiation at the new location spans an area four times larger than the original area. However, because the same amount of radiation exists to cover this larger area, the intensity at the new distance consequently decreases by a factor of four (Fig. 8-14).

The inverse square law may be stated as a formula:

$$\frac{I_1}{I_2} = \frac{(d_2)^2}{(d_1)^2}$$

where I_1 expresses the exposure (intensity) at the original distance, I_2 expresses the exposure (intensity) at the new distance, d_1 expresses the original distance from the source of radiation, and d_2 expresses the new distance from the source of radiation.

Example: If a radiographer stands 1 m away from an x-ray tube and receives an exposure of 2 mR per hour, what will the exposure be if the same radiographer moves to a position located 2 m from the x-ray tube?

Answer:

$$\frac{I_1}{I_2} = \frac{(d_2)^2}{(d_1)^2}$$

$$\frac{2}{I_2} = \frac{(2)^2}{(1)^2}$$

$$\frac{2}{I_2} = \frac{4}{1} \text{ (cross-multiply)}$$

$$4I_2 = 2$$

$$I_2 = 0.5 \text{ mR/hr}$$

The inverse square law should be applied, by increasing one's distance from a source of exposure, whenever possible to reduce the radiographer's exposure from sources of x-radiation. (This law also may be applied to sources of gamma and neutron radiation.)

The inverse square law also implies that if a radiographer moves closer to a source of radiation, the radiation exposure to the radiographer dramatically increases. For example, according to the inverse square law, if the radiographer stands 2 feet away from an x-ray source instead of 6 feet, the radiographer's radiation exposure increases by a factor of nine.

Protective Devices

Protective lead aprons and gloves (Fig. 8-15) should be used whenever the radiographer cannot remain behind a protective lead barrier during an exposure. If the peak energy of the x-ray beam is 100 kVp, a protective lead (Pb) apron must be equivalent to a 0.25-mm thickness of lead. A lead apron of 0.5- or 1-mm lead equivalent affords greater protection. All three of these thicknesses are available for protective apparel. However, the 0.5-mm lead equivalent is the most widely used thickness in diagnostic radiology.

During fluoroscopic examinations the radiographer should always wear a protective apron. **Protective lead gloves** of a minimum of 0.25-mm lead equivalent should be worn whenever the hands must be protected from the beam.

Because usually no protective barrier (i.e., control booth or moveable shield) is present, lead aprons must be worn by radiographers during fluoroscopic and mobile radiographic procedures. For the latter the 6-foot-long exposure cord, when fully extended, affords a significantly reduced exposure level because of the inverse square law.

A neck and **thyroid shield** (Fig. 8-16) can protect the thyroid area of occupationally exposed people during general fluoroscopy and x-ray special procedures. It should be of 0.5-mm lead equivalent.

Scatter radiation to the lens of the eyes of diagnostic radiology personnel can be substantially reduced by wearing **protective eyeglasses** (Fig. 8-17) with optically clear lenses that contain a minimal lead equivalent protection of 0.35 mm. Side shields on the protective glasses also are available for procedures that require turning of the head. A wraparound frame containing optically clear lenses with a 0.5-mm lead equivalency is also available.

Patient Restraint

Radiographers should never stand in the primary (useful) beam to restrain a patient during a radiographic exposure (Fig. 8-18, *A*). When **patient restraint** is necessary, mechanical restraining devices should be

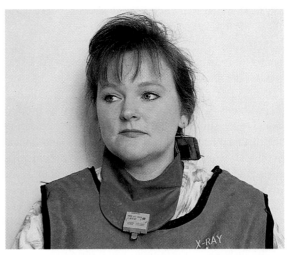

Fig. 8-16 The neck and thyroid gland can be protected from radiation exposure through the use of a 0.5-mm lead-equivalent protective shield.

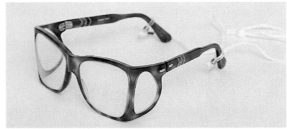

Fig. 8-17 Eyeglasses protect the lens of the eyes during general fluoroscopy and special procedures. (Shown are glasses with wrap-around frames; other styles are also available).

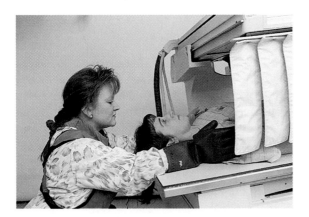

Fig. 8-15 A lead apron, gloves, and a thyroid shield protect the radiographer from scattered radiation.

used to immobilize the patient whenever possible. If mechanical means of restraint are not feasible, nonoccupationally exposed persons wearing appropriate protective apparel should perform this function. These individuals should be positioned so that their lead-protected torsos are not struck by the primary or direct beam (Fig. 8-18, *B*).

Holding patients may be necessary when they are unable to support themselves. For example, a weak elderly patient may be unable to stand alone and raise his arms above his head for a lateral chest x-ray. In this situation, a nonoccupationally exposed person may hold the patient in position during the exposure. A mechanical restraining device may be used to hold an infant in the proper upright position for chest radiographs. If

such a device is not available, the child must be held during the exposure. When nonoccupationally exposed persons such as nurses, orderlies, relatives, and friends assist in holding the patient during an exposure, suitable protective garments (lead aprons and gloves) should be worn by each person participating in the examination. This ensures maximal protection from exposure. The radiographer should take care that nonoccupationally exposed individuals do not stand in the useful beam while holding the patient during the exposure. Pregnant women should never be permitted to assist in holding a patient during an exposure because this may result in possible damage to the embryo-fetus.

Doors to X-Ray Rooms

Radiographic and fluoroscopic exposures should be made only when doors are closed. This practice affords a substantial degree of protection for persons in areas adjacent to the room door because in most facilities room doors have an attenuation for diagnostic energy x-rays equivalent to that provided by $\frac{1}{32}$ inch of lead.

Radiation Protection Design for Diagnostic X-Ray Suites

To reduce the dose equivalent to radiographers, nonoccupationally exposed personnel, and the general public to levels deemed statistically safe by both federal and international bodies, every room in which a diagnostic x-ray unit is housed must be equipped with radiation-absorbent barriers. The design of these barriers is based on the following considerations:

1. The mean energy of the x-rays that will strike the barrier
2. Whether the barrier is of a primary or secondary nature
3. The distance from the x-ray source to a position of occupancy 1 foot from the barrier
4. The workload of the unit
5. The use factor of the barrier
6. The occupancy factor behind the barrier
7. The intrinsic shielding (e.g., tube housing attenuation) of the x-ray unit
8. Whether the area beyond the barrier is "controlled" or "uncontrolled"

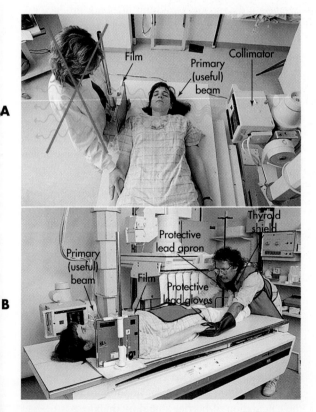

A

B

Fig. 8-18 A, The radiographer should *never* stand in the primary (useful) beam to restrain the patient. **B,** A nonoccupationally exposed person restraining a patient during a radiographic exposure should wear a lead apron, gloves, and thyroid shield and stand outside the primary beam.

The shielding designer must take all the preceding factors into account to meet necessary radiation protection standards. In addition, the designer should plan conservatively to satisfy future regulatory limits that may be more stringent. This is one reason that many diagnostic x-ray facilities are substantially overshielded. Spending some extra money up front for additional shielding is far easier and much less expensive than adding it after the suite has been completed.

Radiation shielding categories

Three categories of radiation sources can be generated in an x-ray room. They are classified as follows:

1. Primary radiation
2. Scatter radiation
3. Leakage radiation

The latter two categories are collectively known as secondary radiation.

Primary radiation

Primary radiation emerges directly from the x-ray tube collimator and moves without deflection toward a wall, door, viewing window, and so on. Because of this tendency, primary radiation also is known as direct radiation. Energy from direct radiation has not been degraded by scatter, and substantial proportions of the initial beam may not have been attenuated. Therefore a wall in the path of direct radiation requires the most radiation protection shielding to ensure the safety of personnel and the public. In a typical x-ray suite the most common primary radiation barrier is that behind the wall Bucky unit.

Scatter radiation

Scatter radiation results whenever a diagnostic x-ray beam passes through matter. Compton interactions between the x-ray photons and the electrons of atoms within the attenuating object deflect x-ray photons from their initial trajectories. As a result, photons emerge from the object in all directions. The scattered radiation is greatly reduced in intensity relative to the incident beam. It also is somewhat weakened in energy and consequently in penetrating power. The amount of shielding required to protect against scatter radiation is therefore almost always much less than for primary radiation. In general, the patient is the major source of scatter radiation.

Leakage radiation

Leakage radiation is radiation generated in the x-ray tube that does not exit from the collimator opening but rather penetrates through the protective tube-housing and, to some degree, through the sides of the collimator. Leakage radiation is therefore always present in some amount. When shielding is planned for a secondary barrier, the potential contributions from leakage radiation must be added to those from the scatter radiation reaching that barrier.

Calculational considerations

Workload (W)

Because a diagnostic x-ray unit does not produce radiation 24 hours per day, 7 days per week, a parameter must be used to reflect the unit's radiation-on time in the determination of barrier shielding requirements. The quantity that best reflects the weekly radiation usage of a diagnostic x-ray unit is called its **workload (W)**. The workload is essentially the radiation output weighted time during the week that the unit is actually delivering radiation. Workloads are specified either in units of mA-seconds per week or mA-minutes per week. The following example illustrates the concept:

Example: A radiographic x-ray suite is in operation 5 days per week. The average number of patients per day is 20, and the average number of films per patient is 3. Also the average technique factors are 90 kVp, 300 mA, 0.1 sec. Find the weekly workload.

W = (300 mA × 0.1 sec) × (5 days/wk) × (20 patients/day) × (3 films/patient)

= 9000 mA-sec/wk

= 150 mA-min/week

Please note that the kVp is not used in the workload calculation. It is, however, an important ingredient in the calculation of barrier shielding thickness.

Inverse square law (ISL)

Just as the intensity of light fades with separation from its source, so is the strength of an x-ray beam weakened as the distance from its source increases. The inverse square law (ISL) is the mathematical relation describing this property. It was introduced earlier in this chapter and serves as a fundamental component of radiation protection. As such, the ISL plays a major role in the design of radiation safety barriers. An illustration of its use for this purpose is shown in the following example:

Example: At a distance of 1 m from an x-ray tube target the exposure rate measured by a radiation survey meter was 500 milliroentgens (mR) per hour. What would that instrument read if it were moved back an extra 2 meters?

As we have already seen, ISL is mathematically given by the following proportion:

$$\frac{I_1}{I_2} = \frac{(d_2)^2}{(d_1)^2}$$

If we substitute the given data into the above relation and cross-multiply, we obtain the following result:

$$(3)^2 I_2 = 500(1)^2$$

$$I_2 = \frac{500}{9}$$

$$= 55.6 \text{ mR/hr}$$

This result demonstrates an enormous reduction in radiation intensity. Its direct consequence is a greatly reduced barrier shielding thickness requirement.

Use factor (U)

If radiation, whether primary or secondary, is never directed at a particular wall or structure, then ordinary or existing construction is sufficient. Most structures in a diagnostic x-ray suite, however, are struck by radiation to some degree for some fraction of the weekly beam-on time. The **use factor (U)** is a quantity that was introduced to select this fractional contact time.

For primary radiation, the use factor represents the portion of beam-on time during the week that the x-ray beam is directed at a primary barrier. Consider a typical radiographic suite with a wall Bucky unit. If 50% of the x-ray examinations involve this de-

vice, then the wall behind the Bucky unit has U (primary) = ½.

Because scatter and leakage radiation emerges in all directions in the x-ray room, every wall, door, viewing window, and other surface will always be struck by some quantity of radiation. Therefore U (secondary) = 1 for all radiation-accessible structures.

Table 8-1 presents the most current recommended use factor values. The use factor also may be referred to as the *beam direction factor*.

Occupancy factor (T)

Radiation barriers are installed to protect personnel and the general public from radiation that otherwise would reach them uninhibited. If no one will be present beyond an existing wall in a particular area while the x-ray unit is being operated, the addition of supplementary shielding to that wall is unnecessary. The opposite situation is an area in which someone is always present. When planning the radiation protection

Table 8-1
Use Factors Recommended by the ICRP*

Use factor	Primary barrier
Full use (U = 1)	Floors of radiation rooms except dental installations, doors, walls, and ceilings of radiation rooms exposed routinely to the primary beam
Partial use (U = ¼)	Doors and walls of radiation rooms not exposed routinely to the primary beam; also, floors of dental installations
Occasional use (U = ¹⁄₁₆)	Ceilings of radiation rooms not exposed routinely to the primary beam. Because of the low use factor, shielding requirements for a ceiling are usually determined by secondary rather than primary beam considerations

*From International Commission on Radiological Protection: *Report of Committee III on protection against x-rays up to energies of 3 MeV and beta and gamma rays from sealed sources,* ICRP Publication No. 3, New York, 1960, Pergamon Press.

shielding for a diagnostic x-ray suite, the designer must consider not only zero and full occupancy cases but also the more common partial occupancy situation. The **occupancy factor (T)** is used to modify the shielding requirement for a particular barrier by taking into account the fraction of the work week that the space beyond that barrier is occupied. Table 8-2 lists the latest recommended values for T.

Controlled and uncontrolled areas

If a region adjacent to a wall of an x-ray room is used only by occupationally exposed personnel (e.g., radiographers), that location is designated as a **controlled area.** Conversely, a nearby hall or corridor that is frequented by the general public is classified as an **uncontrolled area.** For the latter the maximal weekly permitted dose equivalent (MPDE) is equal to 20 microsievert (2 millirem); for the former, it is 1000 microsievert (100 millirem), a relatively much larger amount. The main reason for this disparity lies in the fact that the occupationally exposed population is only a tiny fraction of the overall population. Therefore the potential for detrimental radiobiologic effects to the general public as a whole as a result of the higher MPDE to occupationally exposed personnel is statistically negligible. Thus whether the area beyond a structure is designated as controlled or uncontrolled is significant in determining the amount of radiation shielding to be added to that structure.

The following sections discuss the use of these concepts in the determination of radiation shielding requirements.

Methods of determining barrier shielding requirements

For each wall, door, and other barrier in an x-ray room that is to provide protection against radiation, the product $W \cdot U \cdot T$ must be determined. The workload is generally fixed by the overall usage of the x-ray unit, whereas the use and occupancy factors are usually different among various barriers. The protection planner also must know whether the barrier is a primary or secondary one and whether the area beyond the barrier is controlled or uncontrolled.

The most common method to determine shielding requirements is to use precalculated tables for diagnostic installations. These tables are located in appendix C of NCRP Report No. 49.* One of these is reproduced in Table 8-3. The ISL reduction in radiation intensity is incorporated in the table. Separate results are listed for primary and secondary barriers and controlled and uncontrolled areas.

Primary barrier calculation

The primary radiation intensity for a selected kVp at the barrier location can be determined by making exposure measurements on the x-ray unit. This informa-

Table 8-2
Occupancy Factors Recommended by the ICRP*

Occupancy factor	Primary barrier
Full occupancy (T = 1)	Control spaces, offices, corridors, waiting spaces large enough to hold desks, darkrooms, workrooms, shops, nurse stations, rest and lounge rooms used routinely by occupationally exposed personnel, living quarters, children's play areas, and occupied space in adjoining buildings
Partial occupancy (T = 1/4)	Corridors too narrow for desks, utility rooms, rest and lounge rooms not used routinely by occupationally exposed personnel, wards and patients' rooms, elevators with operators, and unattended parking lots
Occasional occupancy (T = 1/16)	Closets too small for future occupancy, toilets not used routinely by occupationally exposed personnel, stairways, automatic elevators, pavements, and streets

*From International Commission on Radiological Protection: *Report of Committee III on protection against x-rays up to energies of 3 MeV and beta and gamma rays from sealed sources,* ICRP Publication No. 3, New York, 1960, Pergamon Press.

*NCRP Report No. 49 was published when the uncontrolled area MPDE was 0.1 mSv (10 mrem).

tion may then be used to determine the amount of shielding necessary to attenuate the radiation to permissible levels. The values in Table 8-3 are based on such output measurements averaged over many typical x-ray units. The following exercise demonstrates the way to determine the primary barrier shielding requirement in a controlled area for an average usage radiographic room.

Example: Average kVp = 100
$\qquad$ U = ½
$\qquad$ T = 1
$\qquad$ W = 15000 mA-seconds/week = 250 mA-minutes/week distance from x-ray source to occupied area = 3 m

Solution: WUT = W × U × T = (250)(½)(1) = 125 mA-min/wk

From Table 8-3, we obtain a shielding requirement of 0.65-mm lead or approximately ⅟₃₂-inch lead.

Secondary barrier calculation

Secondary barriers intercept both scatter and leakage radiation. No additional shielding against secondary radiation is needed for areas already protected against primary radiation. Because scatter and leakage radiation emerge in all directions, the use factor for these is always 1.

Scatter radiation. The intensity and energy of the scatter radiation at the location of a barrier are unknown. Therefore the following is assumed to determine barrier shielding requirements:

1. The energy of the scatter radiation is equal to the primary radiation.

Table 8-3

Minimal Shielding Requirements for Radiographic Installations

WUT* in mA min												
100 kV†	**125 kV†**	**150 kV†**	**Distance in meters from source to occupied area**									
1000	400	200	1.5	2.1	3.0	4.2	6.1	8.4	12.2			
500	200	100		1.5	2.1	3.0	4.2	6.1	8.4	12.2		
250	100	50			1.5	2.1	3.0	4.2	6.1	8.4	12.2	
125	50	25				1.5	2.1	3.0	4.2	6.1	8.4	12.2
62.5	25	12.5					1.5	2.1	3.0	4.2	6.1	8.4	12.2
Type of area	**Material**		**Primary protective barrier thickness‖**									
Controlled	Lead, mm‡	1.95	1.65	1.4	1.15	0.9	0.65	0.45	0.3	0.2	0.1	0.1
Noncontrolled	Lead, mm‡	2.9	2.6	2.3	2.05	1.75	1.5	1.2	0.95	0.75	0.55	0.35
Controlled	Concrete, cm§	18	15.5	13.5	11.5	9.5	7	5.5	4	2.5	1.5	0.5
Noncontrolled	Concrete, cm§	25	23	20.5	18.5	16.5	14	12	10	8		
			Secondary protective barrier thickness‖									
Controlled	Lead, mm‡	0.55	0.45	0.35	0.3	0	0	0	0	0	0	0
Noncontrolled	Lead, mm‡	1.3	1.05	0.75	0.65	0.45	0.35	0.3	0.05	0	0	0
Controlled	Concrete, cm§	5	3.5	2.5	2	0	0	0	0	0	0	0
Noncontrolled	Concrete, cm§	11.5	9.5	7.5	5.5	4	3	2	0.5	0	0	0

From NCRP Report #49: Structural shielding design and evaluation for medical use of x-rays and gamma rays with energies up to 10 meV, Washington D.C., 1976, Appendix C, p 66, NCRP Publications.
*W—weekly workload in mA min, U—use factor, T—occupancy factor
†Peak pulsating x-ray tube potential
‡See Table 26 for conversion of thickness in millimeters to inches or to surface density.
§Thickness based on concrete density of 2.35 g cm⁻³ (147 lb ft⁻³)
‖Barrier thickness based on 150 kV

2. The intensity of radiation scattered at 90 degrees at a distance of 1 m from its source is reduced by a factor of 1000 relative to the primary radiation for a field size of 400 cm² (about 8 inches × 8 inches).

The greater the x-ray field dimension at the source of the scatter radiation (usually the patient), the larger the amount of generated scatter radiation.

The ISL plays an important role in shielding determination, but in the case of scatter radiation the distance is measured from the center of the patient rather than from the x-ray tube target.

Example: Find the amount of lead shielding to protect a controlled area against scatter radiation for full occupancy if the area is at a distance of 2.1 m from the center of the patient. The weekly workload = 1000 mA-min and the mean kVp = 100.

Solution: U = 1
T = 1
W = 1000
W × U × T = 1000 mA-min/wk
From Table 8-3 we obtain a shielding requirement of 0.45-mm lead, which is less than $\frac{1}{32}$ inch ($\frac{1}{32}$ inch corresponds to 0.79 mm).

Leakage radiation. Leakage radiation does not emerge directly from the collimator opening but rather penetrates through the x-ray tube housing walls or through the sides of the collimator when the x-ray beam is on. Leakage radiation is therefore an additional radiation output that shielding designers must consider. Regulatory standards mandate that the maximal permissible leakage exposure rate at 1 m from the target of a diagnostic x-ray tube in all directions cannot exceed 100 mR/hr when the tube is operated continuously at its maximal permitted kVp and mA combination.

Leakage radiation is always present when the x-ray tube is "on"—even if the collimator jaws are tightly closed. Because of the attenuation that occurs when leakage radiation penetrates the tube housing walls, it is essentially a monoenergetic beam; thus the concept of half-value layers may be used at barriers to reduce

leakage radiation levels to permissible values. A long-standing rule of thumb regarding leakage radiation is stated as follows:

If the barrier shielding requirements for scatter and leakage differ by more than 3 half-value layers (HVL), install the larger shielding value; however, if the difference is less than 3 HVL, add 1 HVL to the larger shielding requirement and ignore the smaller shielding requirement.

Example: Suppose that shielding must be added to a wall that is subject only to secondary radiation to protect a controlled area. Given the following information, find the total thickness of lead needed.
HVL for scatter and leakage radiation: each is equal to 0.24-mm lead
Shielding requirement for scatter radiation alone is 0.95-mm lead
Shielding requirement for leakage radiation alone is 0.4-mm lead.

Solution: The difference in barrier shielding requirements for scatter and leakage equals 0.55-mm lead. 0.55 mm is less than 3 HVL, which amounts to 3 × 0.24-mm lead, or 0.72-mm lead. Therefore using the rule of thumb that the total shielding requirement is 0.95 mm + 1 HVL, we must install a total lead thickness equal to 0.95 + 0.24 = 1.19 mm lead.

New approaches to shielding

At the time of this writing, shielding is designed according to a report of the National Council on Radiation Protection and Measurements (NCRP Report No. 49) that is more than 20 years old. The examples given in this chapter follow those currently accepted guidelines. Some of the techniques described in this report were based on very conservative estimates and graphical data for shielding that may now be handled by computer modeling. The NCRP Report No. 49 is now being rewritten,* but the review and revision process typically takes several years. Report No. 49 is still the most appropriate guideline, but some new ap-

*For information, contact the AAPM, One Physics Ellipse, College Park, Md 20740-3846.

proaches to shielding design are expected to be adopted in the next few years. Despite the trend toward decreasing the maximal dose limits and consequently the appropriate design limits for installations, experts do not expect that retrofitting of additional shielding will be necessary in existing installations. The techniques in NCRP Report No. 49 were sufficiently conservative (in terms of overshielding) to accommodate the lower dose limits. New approaches will ensure that installations are designed in accordance with current limits.

Among the new approaches to shielding design is the use of a more rigorous analysis of workload, incorporating the range of kVps actually used. Also, the true role of leakage radiation in modern equipment will be modeled explicitly, along with scatter. The current rule of adding an HVL if leakage and scatter barrier requirements are similar will probably be abandoned in favor of exact calculations. Use factors will be estimated so that they reflect a true percentage of the time the beam is directed at various barriers. Some existing shielding that was generally ignored in older design calculations, such as the patient table, Bucky, and cassette holder, will be included in the new designs. Finally, the suggested occupancy factors are being reevaluated to approximate more closely the percentage of time that workers are expected to be present. An occupancy factor of at least $\frac{1}{16}$ is currently

assumed. Under the revised guidelines, occupancy factors for areas such as closets and stairways may be placed as low as $\frac{1}{40}$. Some changes expected in the revision of NCRP Report No. 49 are listed in Table 8-4. The interested reader should contact the National Council on Radiation Protection and Measurements for information regarding the status of the revision of Report No. 49.

Summary

In this chapter the various methods of protecting radiation workers from exposure to ionizing radiation during diagnostic radiologic procedures were described. An upper-boundary total annual occupational EDE of 50 mSv (5 rem) for whole-body exposure during routine operations and a total annual EDE limit of 1 mSv (0.1 rem) for members of the general public have been established. Radiation workers can receive this larger dose equivalent without altering the genetically significant dose. The radiologist and radiographer must always employ proper radiation control procedures to keep occupational exposure as low as reasonably achievable (ALARA). The occupational risk for those employed in diagnostic imaging may be compared with the occupational risk in other so-called safe industries. Most methods and techniques that reduce patient radiation exposure also reduce exposure for the radiographer. When scattered radiation is reduced during a diagnostic radiologic examination, the greatest occupational hazard also is reduced. Scattered radiation can be reduced through the use of beam-limitation devices, higher kVp and lower mAs, appropriate beam filtration, and adequate protective shielding. The use of appropriate protective apparel (i.e., lead aprons, gloves, and thyroid shields) also reduces the radiologist's and radiographer's exposure. Good radiographic processing techniques that reduce the number of repeat examinations are essential.

Pregnant radiologic technologists can wear an additional monitoring device at waist level to ensure that the monthly EDE to the embryo-fetus does not exceed 0.5 mSv (0.05 rem). This EDE does not include medical or natural background radiation and is designed to restrict the total lifetime risk of leukemia and other malignancies significantly in persons in utero.

Table 8-4	
Anticipated Future Approaches to Shielding Guidelines	
Item under consideration	Future approach
Workload	More realistic use of contemporary survey data
Leakage and scatter	Explicit barrier calculations
Use factor	Adjusted for beam direction data reflecting actual usage patterns
Occupancy factor	Realistic assumptions of occupancy of low-occupancy areas (e.g., stairwells)

Protective structural shielding such as primary and secondary protective barriers must be designed to ensure that occupational and nonoccupational annual EDE limits are not exceeded. For each radiologic facility a qualified medical physicist should determine the exact shielding requirements needed. To protect both the radiographer and patient from off-focus or leakage radiation, a lead-lined, metal diagnostic-type protective tube housing is required. The construction of this housing must ensure that leakage radiation measured at a distance of 1 m (3.3 feet) from the x-ray source does not exceed 100 mR/hr (2.58×10^{-5} C/kg/hr) when the tube is operated continuously at its highest current for its full potential (voltage). During routine fluoroscopy, in addition to wearing appropriate protective apparel, the radiographer should stand as far away from the patient as is practical and move closer to the patient only when assistance is required. When performing mobile radiographic examinations, the radiographer must wear protective garments and stand at least 6 feet from the patient, the x-ray tube, and the useful beam. After accounting for the protection factors of distance and shielding, the radiographer should attempt to stand at right angles to the x-ray beam–scattering object (the patient) line. During C-arm fluoroscopy, personnel exposure is caused by scatter radiation from the patient. The entrance surface of the patient has a higher dose rate to scatter than does the exit surface of the patient. Outside the useful beam the exposure caused by scatter is lower on the image intensifier side. During interventional procedures that use high-dose (high-level–control) fluoroscopy, exposure time should be limited as much as possible. Dose-reduction features such as the presence of high-quality low-dose fluoroscopy mode, collimation, optimal beam filtration, removable grids, variable optical aperture, and last-image-hold component should be available and in good working order.

Distance is the most effective means of protection from ionizing radiation. The radiographer may use the ISL to reduce radiation intensity simply by moving farther away from any source of radiation.

If a radiation worker cannot remain behind a protective barrier, a protective apron of at least 0.25-mm lead-equivalent thickness should be worn. In certain situations, lead gloves of the same lead equivalent also should be worn along with a thyroid shield. The latter is commonly used by personnel during lengthy special fluoroscopic procedures. Protective eyeglasses may be worn to reduce scattered radiation to the lens of the eyes. Radiographers should never stand in the primary beam to hold a patient during an radiographic exposure. Use of a mechanical restraining device is preferable, or a nonoccupationally exposed person with appropriate protective attire may hold the patient.

Dose equivalent to radiation workers, nonoccupationally exposed personnel, and the general public must be taken into consideration whenever diagnostic x-ray suites are constructed. These facilities must be equipped with radiation-absorbent barriers.

Review Questions

1. Because occupational exposure of the radiographer can be kept as low as reasonably achievable (ALARA) through individual monitoring and other protective measures and devices and because exposure from radiation-related jobs will not alter the _____, radiation workers may receive a larger dose equivalent than members of the general population.
   A. Mean glandular dose
   B. Genetically significant dose
   C. Mean marrow dose
   D. Tissue tolerance

2. Whenever scattered radiation decreases, the radiographer's exposure _____.
   A. Decreases
   B. Increases slightly
   C. Remains the same
   D. Increases 100 times

3. Of the devices listed below, which eliminates low-energy photons in the collimator to decrease the scattered radiation potential?
   1. Collimator light source
   2. Electronic sensors
   3. Aluminum filtration
   A. 1 only
   B. 2 only
   C. 3 only
   D. 1, 2, and 3

4. If the peak energy of the x-ray beam is 130 kVp, the primary protective barrier should consist of _____ and extend _____ upward from the floor of the x-ray room when the tube is 5 to 7 feet from the wall in question.
   A. $\frac{1}{32}$ inch lead, 10 feet
   B. $\frac{1}{32}$ inch lead, 7 feet
   C. $\frac{1}{16}$ inch lead, 10 feet
   D. $\frac{1}{16}$ inch lead, 7 feet

5. Of the following factors, which is considered when determining thickness requirements for protective barriers?
   1. Occupancy factor (T)
   2. Workload (W)
   3. Use factor (U)
   A. 1 only
   B. 2 only
   C. 3 only
   D. 1, 2, and 3

6. In terms of occupational risk, radiography may be compared with the occupational risk associated with which of the following?
   A. Extremely hazardous industries
   B. Other safe industries
   C. A nuclear war
   D. A radiation accident such as the Chernobyl nuclear power station disaster

7. For the vast majority of mobile radiographic units, which are not equipped with remote control exposure devices, the cord leading to the exposure switch should be long enough to permit the radiographer to stand *at least* _____ from the patient, the x-ray tube, and the useful beam to reduce occupational exposure.
   A. 1 m
   B. 2 m
   C. 3 m
   D. 5 m

8. When performing a mobile radiographic examination, if the protection factors of distance and shielding are equal, the radiographer should stand at a _____ to the scattering object.
   A. 30-degree angle
   B. 45-degree angle
   C. Right angle
   D. 75-degree angle

9. If a radiographer stands 6 m away from an x-ray tube and receives an exposure 4 mR per hour, what will the exposure be if the same radiographer moves to stand at a position located 12 m from the x-ray tube?
   A. 1 mR per hour
   B. 2 mR per hour
   C. 3 mR per hour
   D. 4 mR per hour

10. If the peak energy of the x-ray beam is 100 kVp, a protective lead apron must be the equivalent of which of the following measures?
    A. A 0.25-mm thickness of lead
    B. A 0.5-mm thickness of lead
    C. A 1.0-mm thickness of lead
    D. A 1.5-mm thickness of lead

11. Which of the following statements is true?
    A. If wearing a protective apron, radiographers may stand in the useful beam to restrain a patient during a difficult radiologic procedure.
    B. If wearing a protective apron, nurses, orderlies, relatives, or friends may stand in the useful beam to restrain a patient during a difficult radiologic procedure.
    C. If wearing a protective apron, pregnant women may stand in the useful beam to restrain a patient during a difficult radiologic procedure.
    D. Radiographers should never stand in the useful beam to restrain a patient during a radiographic exposure.

12. Which of the following is the *most effective* means of protection from ionizing radiation normally available to the radiographer?
    A. Decreasing the amount of time spent near a source of radiation
    B. Using protective shielding garments
    C. Placing as much distance as possible between oneself and the source of radiation
    D. Remaining behind a mobile protective shield during an exposure

13. If the intensity of the x-ray beam is inversely proportional to the square of the distance, how does the intensity change when the distance from a point source of radiation is tripled?
    A. It increases by a factor of 3 at the new distance
    B. It increases by a factor of 9 at the new distance
    C. It decreases by a factor of 9 at the new distance
    D. It decreases by a factor of 3 at the new distance

14. A Bucky slot shielding device of at least _____ must automatically cover the Bucky slot opening in the side of the x-ray table during a fluoroscopic examination when the Bucky tray is positioned at the foot end of the table.
    A. 0.25-mm aluminum equivalent
    B. 0.25-mm lead equivalent
    C. 0.5-mm aluminum equivalent
    D. 0.5-mm lead equivalent

15. Protective shielding for a controlled area must ensure that the exposure rate remains below _____ mR per week.
    A. 1000
    B. 100
    C. 2
    D. 10

16. What is the term for the proportional amount of time during which the x-ray beam is energized or directed toward a particular barrier?
    A. Occupancy factor
    B. Workload factor
    C. Distance factor
    D. Use factor

17. A diagnostic-type protective tube housing must be constructed so that leakage radiation measured at a distance of 1 m from the x-ray source does *not* exceed _____ when the tube is operated continuously at its highest current for its full potential.
    A. 500 mR per hour (500 mR/hr $\times$ 10^{-5} C/kg/hr)
    B. 300 mR per hour (300 mR/hr $\times$ 10^{-5} C/kg/hr)
    C. 100 mR per hour (100 mR/hr $\times$ 10^{-5} C/kg/hr)
    D. 50 mR per hour (50 mR/hr $\times$ 10^{-5} C/kg/hr)

18. Which of the following methods and devices reduce(s) the radiographer's exposure during a fluoroscopic examination?
    1. Proper beam collimation
    2. Control of exposure factors
    3. Gonadal shielding of the patient
    A. 1 only
    B. 2 only
    C. 3 only
    D. 1 and 2

19. Which of the following adjustments in exposure techniques decrease the production of scattered radiation?
    A. Decrease kVp and increase mAs in compensation
    B. Decrease kVp and decrease mAs
    C. Increase kVp and decrease mAs in compensation
    D. Increase kVp and increase mAs

20. A protective curtain or sliding panel of a minimal thickness of 0.25-mm lead equivalent should be positioned between the fluoroscopist and the patient to intercept which of the following?
    A. Primary radiation
    B. Scattered radiation
    C. Remnant radiation
    D. Useful radiation

21. When a radiologic technologist becomes pregnant, which of the following is likely?
    A. Her employer terminates her employment until after her child is born.
    B. She is able to continue her employment but not permitted to perform any radiologic procedures during her pregnancy.
    C. Her employer terminates her employment until after the completion of the first trimester.
    D. She continues to perform her duties without interruption of employment, provided that she follows established radiation safety practices.

22. Units of either mA-seconds/week or mA-minutes/week are used to determine the _____ for a specific x-ray room.
    A. Workload
    B. Use factor
    C. Occupancy factor
    D. Distance factor

23. The lead glass window of the control-booth barrier in a fixed radiographic installation typically consists of which of the following?
    A. 0.25-mm lead equivalent
    B. 0.5-mm lead equivalent
    C. 1.0-mm lead equivalent
    D. 1.5-mm lead equivalent

24. Which of the following equivalents for protective gloves provide the radiographer with the most protection from ionizing radiation?
    A. 0.25-mm lead equivalent
    B. 0.1-mm lead equivalent
    C. 0.3-mm lead equivalent
    D. 0.5-mm lead equivalent

25. Diagnostic imaging personnel may receive a total annual occupational effective dose limit of _____ for whole-body exposure during routine operations.
    A. 1 mSv (0.1 rem)
    B. 5 mSv (0.5 rem)
    C. 25 mSv (2.5 rem)
    D. 50 mSv (5 rem)

26. Members of the general public *not* occupationally exposed have an annual effective dose limit of _____ for continuous (or frequent) exposure from artificial sources other than medical and _____ for infrequent annual exposure.
    A. 50 mSv (5 rem), 25 mSv (2.5 rem)
    B. 1 mSv (0.1 rem), 5 mSv (0.5 rem)
    C. 3 mSv (0.3 rem), 5 mSv (0.5 rem)
    D. 5 mSv (0.5 rem), 3 mSv (0.3 rem)

27. Which part(s) of a diagnostic x-ray unit should a radiographer avoid touching while a radiographic exposure is in progress?
    A. Control panel
    B. Exposure switch
    C. Kilovoltage control on the control panel only
    D. Tube housing, collimator, and high-tension cables

28. Which of the following is a tenet of the ALARA concept?
    A. The radiographer's occupational exposure should not exceed the maximal annual effective dose equivalents established for members of the general public.
    B. The radiographer's occupational exposure should be as high as necessary to allow for radiographers to hold patients during diagnostic radiographic procedures.
    C. The radiographer's occupational exposure should be kept as low as reasonably achievable.
    D. The radiographer's occupational exposure should be as high as necessary to allow radiographers to hold patients during diagnostic fluoroscopic procedures.

29. Which of the following is another term for use factor (U)?
    A. Workload factor
    B. Occupancy factor in controlled and uncontrolled areas
    C. Beam direction factor
    D. Protective barrier thickness consideration factor

30. During which of the following radiologic examinations should a radiographer wear a thyroid shield?
    A. Fluoroscopy and x-ray special procedures
    B. Mobile radiographic procedures
    C. General diagnostic radiographic procedures
    D. Computed tomographic procedures

31. At a 90-degree angle to the primary x-ray beam, at a distance of 1 m (3.3 feet), the scattered radiation is what fraction of the intensity of the primary beam?
    A. $\frac{1}{10}$
    B. $\frac{1}{100}$
    C. $\frac{1}{1000}$
    D. $\frac{1}{10,000}$

32. The annual effective dose limit established for the general public is designed to do which of the following?
    A. Limit exposure to the same level of risk compared with risk incurred by radiation workers during routine operations
    B. Limit exposure to reasonable levels of risk compared with risk from other common sources
    C. Permit exposure to a higher level of risk than the risk incurred by radiation workers during routine operations
    D. None of the above

33. While standing behind the control-booth barrier, a radiographer makes a radiographic exposure. The x-rays scattered from the patient's body should _____.
    A. Not reach the control-booth barrier
    B. Scatter only once before reaching any area behind the control-booth barrier
    C. Scatter a minimum of two times before reaching any area behind the control-booth barrier
    D. Scatter a minimum of ten times before reaching any area behind the control-booth barrier

34. If the Bucky slot shielding device and protective curtain or sliding panel were *not* in proper position during a routine fluoroscopic examination, what would the fluoroscopist do?
    A. Exceed an exposure rate of 100 mR per hour at a distance of 2 feet from the side of the x-ray table
    B. Not exceed an exposure rate of 100 mR per hour at a distance of 2 feet from the side of the x-ray table
    C. Exceed an exposure rate dose of 250 mR per hour at a distance of 2 feet from the side of the x-ray table
    D. Exceed an exposure rate of 500 mR per hour at a distance of 2 feet from the side of the x-ray table

35. Which of the following are radiation sources that can be generated in an x-ray room?
1. Primary radiation
2. Scatter radiation
3. Leakage radiation

A. 1 only
B. 2 only
C. 3 only
D. 1, 2, and 3

References

1. National Council on Radiation Protection and Measurements (NCRP): NCRP Report No. 116, *Limitation of exposure to ionizing radiation,* Bethesda, Md, 1993, NCRP.
2. Catalog G-5, *Instruments and accessories for improved imaging and safety in diagnostic radiology, CT and MRI,* Carle Place, NY, 1988, Victoreen.
3. Marx MV: *Interventional procedures: risks to patients and personnel, in radiation risk,* Reston, Va, 1996, American College of Radiology, Commission on Physics and Radiation Safety.

Bibliography

Ballinger PW: *Merrill's atlas of radiographic positions and radiologic procedures,* ed 5, vol 1, St Louis, 1982, Mosby.

Ballinger PW, editor: *Merrill's atlas of radiographic positions and radiographic procedures,* ed 7, vol 1, St Louis, 1991, Mosby.

Bushong SC: *Radiologic science for technologists: physics, biology and protection,* ed 6, St Louis, 1997, Mosby.

Bushong SC: *Radiologic science for technologists: physics, biology and protection,* ed 5, St Louis, 1993, Mosby.

Bushong SC: *Radiologic science for technologists: physics, biology, and protection,* ed 2, St Louis, 1980, Mosby.

Carlton RR, Adler AM: *Principles of radiographic imaging: an art and a science,* Albany, New York, 1992, Delmar.

Christensen EE, Curry III TS, Dowdey JE: *An introduction to the physics of diagnostic radiology,* ed 2, Philadelphia, 1978, Lea & Febiger.

Curry III TS, Dowdey JE, Murry Jr RC: *Christensen's introduction to the physics of diagnostic radiology,* ed 3, Philadelphia, 1984, Lea & Febiger.

Dowd SB: *Practical radiation protection and applied radiobiology,* Philadelphia, 1994, W.B. Saunders.

Donohue DP: *Analysis of radiographic quality: lab manual and workbook,* Baltimore, 1980, University Park Press.

Donohue DP: *An analysis of radiographic quality: lab manual and workbook,* ed 2, Rockville, Md, 1984, Aspen.

Frankel R: *Radiation protection for radiologic technologists,* New York, 1976, McGraw-Hill.

Hendee WR, Ritenour ER: *Medical imaging physics,* ed 3, St Louis, 1992, Mosby.

Malott JC, Fodor III J: *The art and science of medical radiography,* ed 7, St Louis, 1993, Mosby.

National Council on Radiation Protection and Measurements (NCRP): *Medical x-ray and gamma-ray protection for energies up to 10 MeV: equipment design and use,* Report No. 33, Washington, D.C., 1968, NCRP Publications.

National Council on Radiation Protection and Measurements (NCRP): *Structural shielding design and evaluation for medical use of x-ray and gamma rays with energies up to 10 MeV,* Report No. 49, Washington, D.C., 1976, NCRP Publications.

National Council on Radiation Protection and Measurements (NCRP): *Recommendations on limits for exposure to ionizing radiation,* Report No. 91, Bethesda, Md, 1987, NCRP Publications.

National Council on Radiation Protection and Measurements (NCRP): *Ionizing radiation exposure of the population of the United States,* Report No. 93, Bethesda, Md, 1987, NCRP Publications.

National Council on Radiation Protection and Measurements (NCRP): *Limitation of exposure to ionizing radiation,* Report No. 116, Bethesda, Md, 1993, NCRP Publications.

Ritenour ER: *Radiation protection and biology: a self-instructional multimedia learning series, instructor's manual,* Denver, 1985, Multi-Media Publishing.

Scheele RV, Wakley J: *Elements of radiation protection,* Springfield, Ill, 1975, Charles C. Thomas.

Seeram E: *Radiation protection,* Philadelphia, 1997, Lippincott-Raven Publishers.

Selman J: *The fundamentals of x-ray and radium physics,* ed 6, Springfield, Ill, 1978, Charles C. Thomas.

Selman J: *The fundamentals of x-ray and radium physics,* ed 7, Springfield, Ill, 1985, Charles C. Thomas.

9

Radiation Monitoring

Chapter Outline

characteristic curve
control badge
deep, eye, and shallow oc-
    cupational exposure
densitometer
extremity dosimeter
film badge dosimeter
film badges
Geiger–Müller (G-M) detec-
    tors
ionization chamber-type
    survey meter (cutie pie)
monitoring

optical density
personnel dosimeter
personnel dosimetry
personnel monitoring report
pocket ionization chambers
    (pocket dosimeters)
protective lead apron
proportional counters
radiation-dosimetry film
radiation survey instruments
thermoluminescent dosime-
    ter (TLD)
TLD analyzer

After completing this chapter, the reader will be able to perform the following:

- State the reason that a radiation worker should wear a personnel dosimeter.

- Explain the function of a personnel dosimeter.

- Identify the appropriate location on the body where the dosimeter should be worn during the following:

    Routine radiographic procedures

    Fluoroscopic procedures

    Special radiographic procedures

- List the characteristics of a personnel dosimeter.

- Describe the various components of the film badge, and explain the use of the device as a personnel monitor.

- Describe the pocket ionization chamber, and explain the use of the device as a personnel monitor.

- Describe the thermoluminescent dosimeter, and explain the use of the device as a personnel monitor.

- Explain the function of radiation survey instruments.

- List three gas-filled radiation survey instruments.

- Explain the requirements for radiation survey instruments.

- Explain the function of the following:

    Ionization chamber-type survey meter

    Proportional counter

    Geiger–Müller detector

- Identify the radiation survey instrument that can be used to calibrate radiographic and fluoroscopic x-ray equipment.

Some means of **monitoring** personnel exposure must be employed to ensure that occupational radiation exposure levels are kept well below the annual total effective dose equivalent limit. The radiographer and other occupationally exposed persons must be aware of the various personnel and area radiation exposure monitoring devices and their functions. This chapter provides an overview of personnel and area monitoring.

Personnel Monitoring

Monitoring of radiation exposure to any person occupationally exposed on a regular basis to ionizing radiation is recommended. Exposure monitoring is accomplished through the use of **personnel dosimetry.** Exposure monitoring of personnel is required whenever radiation workers are likely to risk receiving 10% or more of the annual total effective dose equivalent (TEDE) limit of 50 mSv (5 rem) in any single year. In keeping with the ALARA concept, most institutions issue dosimetry devices when personnel might receive about 1% of the annual TEDE limit in any month, or approximately 0.5 mSv (50 mrem).

The **personnel dosimeter** provides some indication of the working habits and working conditions of diagnostic imaging personnel. It indicates occupational exposure by detecting and measuring the quantity of ionizing radiation to which the dosimeter has been exposed over a period of time. This instrument, however, does not protect the wearer from exposure.

Because this monitoring device records only the exposure received in the area where it is worn, it should be anatomically located so that it will indicate the exposure received by the body trunk. During routine radiographic procedures, when a protective apron is not being worn, the **film badge dosimeter** (Fig. 9-1, *A*) can be attached to the clothing on the front of the body at waist level (Fig. 9-1, *B*) or chest level (Fig. 9-1, *C*).

Fluoroscopy and special radiographic procedures produce the highest occupational radiation exposure for diagnostic imaging personnel. When a **protective**

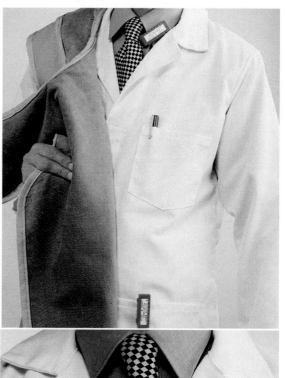

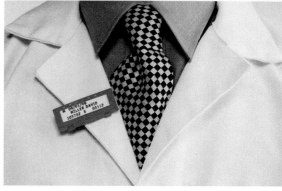

A

B

C

Fig. 9-1 A, Film badge dosimeter used in personnel monitoring. The film badge dosimeter should be worn on the body front at waist level **(B)** or at chest level **(C)** during routine radiographic procedures.

lead apron is worn during such procedures, the dosimeter should be worn outside of the apron at collar level on the anterior surface of the body (Fig. 9-2) because the unprotected head, neck, and lenses of the eye receive 10 to 20 times more exposure than the protected body trunk. When the personnel dosimeter is located at collar level, it can provide a reading of the approximate dose equivalent to the thyroid gland and eyes of the occupationally exposed person.

If the lead apron's shielding integrity is not compromised, a dosimeter reading that is within acceptable limits outside the apron ensures a minimal reading under the apron.

During special radiographic procedures, some institutions may prefer to have diagnostic imaging personnel wear two separate film badge dosimeters, one located beneath a wraparound lead apron at waist level and the other outside the protective apparel at collar level to monitor the approximate dose equivalent to the thyroid gland and eyes. When two separate film badge dosimeters are worn, each badge should be color coded to prevent confusion.

A second film badge dosimeter should be assigned to pregnant occupationally exposed persons to monitor the abdomen during gestation. An additional monitoring device should also be used when performing a radiographic procedure that requires the hands to be near the primary x-ray beam. In this situation, employees may wear an **extremity dosimeter** (Fig. 9-3) to monitor the dose equivalent to the hands.

A record of exposure should become part of the employment record of all radiation workers. Table 9-1 gives occupational exposure values (gathered from film badge readings) for a typical year. The values represent the average annual effective dose equivalent to the whole body.

Characteristics of Personnel Dosimeters

A personnel dosimeter must be lightweight and easy to carry. It should be made of materials durable enough to tolerate normal daily use. The dosimeter must be able to detect and record both small and significant exposures in a consistent, reliable manner. Outside influences such as heat, humidity, and mechanical shock should not affect the performance of the instrument. Because many employees may be required to wear a radiation monitor, it should be reasonably inexpensive. This permits institutions to accommodate large numbers of radiation workers in a cost-effective manner.

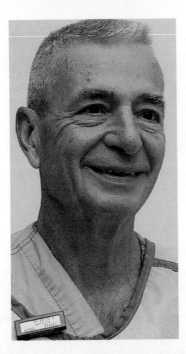

Fig. 9-2 When a protective lead apron is worn during fluoroscopy or special radiographic procedures, the dosimeter should be worn outside of the apron at collar level on the body front. (From Gurley LT, Callaway W: *Introduction to radiologic technology,* ed 4, St Louis, 1996, Mosby.)

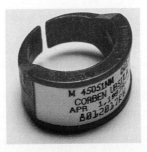

Fig. 9-3 Extremity dosimeter (TLD ring badge) can be used to monitor the dose equivalent to the hands. (Courtesy of RS Landauer Jr & Co.)

Table 9-1				
Occupational Exposure Values for a Typical Year				
	Number of workers (thousands)		Average annual effective dose equivalent (mSv)		Collective effective dose equivalent (person-Sv)*
Category	All	Exposed	All	Exposed	
Medicine	584	277	0.7	1.5	416
Industry	350	156	1.2	2.4	380
Nuclear power	151	91	3.6	5.6	550
Flight crews/flight attendants	97	97	1.7	1.7	165
Other†					789
				Total:	2300

Compiled from data found in NCRP Report No. 101, Tables 4.1-4.3, pp. 65-70.
*Refer to Chapter 3, page 44.
†Other = US Government (Dept. of Energy, US Public Health Service), Uranium Mining, Well Logging, Miscellaneous Workers, Visitors to Facilities, etc..

Types of Personnel Dosimeters

Three types of personnel dosimeters are used to measure individual exposure to ionizing radiation: film badges, pocket ionization chambers, and thermoluminescent dosimeters (TLDs).

Film badges

Film badges (Fig. 9-4) are the most widely used and economical type of personnel dosimeter. In general, these devices record whole-body radiation exposure accumulated at a low rate over a long period of time.

The film badge consists of three parts: a durable, lightweight plastic film holder; an assortment of metal filters; and a film packet. The film holder should be made of a plastic material of a low atomic number to filter low energy x and gamma radiation as well as beta radiation. Inside the plastic holder are metal filters of aluminum or copper that are secured in a permanent position. These filters allow the measurement of the approximate energy of the radiation reaching the dosimeter. Penetrating radiations cast a faint shadow of the filters on the processed dosimetry film, whereas soft radiations cast a more pronounced image of the filters. The density of the image cast by the filters permits estimation of the energy of the radiation. From this data the radiation dose can be evaluated as deep (penetrating) or shallow (nonpenetrating). In addition, the direction from which the radiation reached

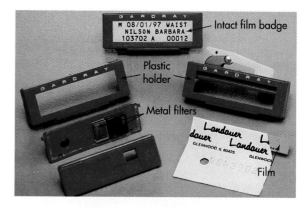

Fig. 9-4 Disassembled film badge, demonstrating badge components: plastic holder, metal filters, and film packet. (Courtesy of RS Landauer Jr & Co.)

the film (from front to back or from back to front) can be estimated from the filter shadows imaged on the processed dosimetry film. The filter images may also be used to determine whether the exposure was due to excessive amounts of scattered radiation or to a single exposure from a primary beam. Excessive exposure to scatter, such as that produced by poor working habits (e.g., radiographer standing too close to a patient during an exposure) or poor facility design, results in a relatively fuzzy image of the filters because the film badge was irradiated from many different angles. A single exposure from a primary beam, such as that which would result if a radiographer inadvertently left the film badge on a table during an exposure (the badge may have fallen off while the radiographer was positioning the patient and gone unnoticed), results in a sharply defined image.

The **radiation-dosimetry film** contained in the radiographic film packet is similar to dental film. This film is sensitive to doses ranging from as low as 0.1 mSv (10 mrem) to as high as 5000 mSv (500 rem). Dose equivalents less than 0.1 mSv (10 mrem) are not usually detected and will be reported as minimal (M). The outside of the film packet forms a light-free envelope for the dosimetry film. Inside the envelope a sheet of lead foil backs the film to absorb scatter radiation coming from behind the dosimeter. Radiation interacting with the film in the badge causes the film to darken once it is developed. After processing, the density or degree of blackening of the image of the filters recorded on the dosimetry film is proportional to the amount of radiation received and the energy of the radiation. An instrument called a **densitometer** (Fig. 9-5) is used to measure this density. It measures the intensity of light transmitted through a given area of the dosimetry film (**optical density**) and compares it with the intensity of light incident on the anterior side of the film. The amount of radiation to which the film was exposed is determined by locating the exposure value of a control film of a similar optical density on a **characteristic curve** (Fig. 9-6). For example, in the characteristic curve in Fig. 9-6, if the optical density of the dosimetry film is determined to be 0.5, the film badge has received slightly more than 0.1 mSv (10 mrem).

The monitoring company that supplies an institution with film badges provides a **control badge** with each batch of badges. This control badge serves as a basis of comparison with the remaining film badges after they have been returned to the monitoring company for processing. Because the control badge is supposed to be kept in a radiation-free area within an imaging facility, its optical density reading should be zero. After processing, if a control badge reading above zero is indicated, then the batch of badges may have been exposed while in transit to or from the institution. To ensure that false readings are not re-

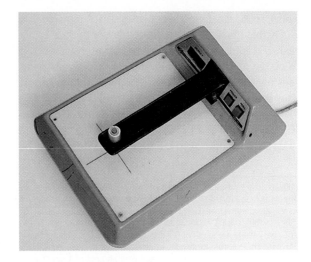

Fig. 9-5 The densitometer, an instrument that measures occupational exposure by comparing optical densities of exposed film badge (dosimetry) films.

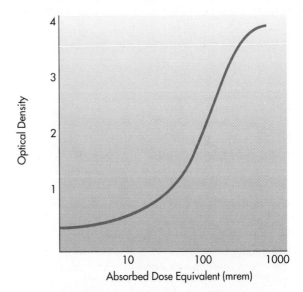

Fig. 9-6 Typical characteristic curve.

ported, the control badge reading is reported to the institution. This reading, if different from zero, must be subtracted from each of the remaining film badges in the batch to ensure accuracy in exposure reporting.

Results from personnel monitoring programs must be recorded accurately and maintained for review to meet state and federal regulations. To comply with such requirements, institutions frequently use established dosimetry services. These monitoring services process film badges and other types of personnel dosimeters and prepare a written **personnel monitoring report** (Fig. 9-7, *A*) for the health care facility. This report lists the **deep, eye, and shallow occupational exposure*** of each person in the institution as measured by the exposed monitors. Information on

the report is arranged in a series of columns. These columns include the following:
1. Personal data listing each participant's identification number (the number on the front of each person's personnel dosimeter), name, Social Security number, birth date, and sex
2. Type of dosimeter: *G* representing a film badge and *U* representing a finger badge used to monitor x, gamma, and beta radiation.
3. Radiation quality (e.g., x-ray, beta particle, neutron, combined radiation exposure)
4. Dose equivalent data, including current deep and shallow recorded dose equivalents (millirems) for the time indicated on the report (e.g., from the first day of a given month to the last day of that month)

---

*Deep dose equivalent, as described by Landauer on the back of the report seen in Fig. 9-7, "applies to external whole-body exposure and is the dose equivalent [DE] at a tissue depth of 1 cm. Eye [DE] applies to the external exposure of the lens of the eye and is taken as the [DE] at a tissue depth of 0.3 cm. Shallow [DE], which applies to the external exposure of the skin or an extremity, is taken as the [DE] at a tissue depth of 0.007 cm averaged over an area of 1 cm². "

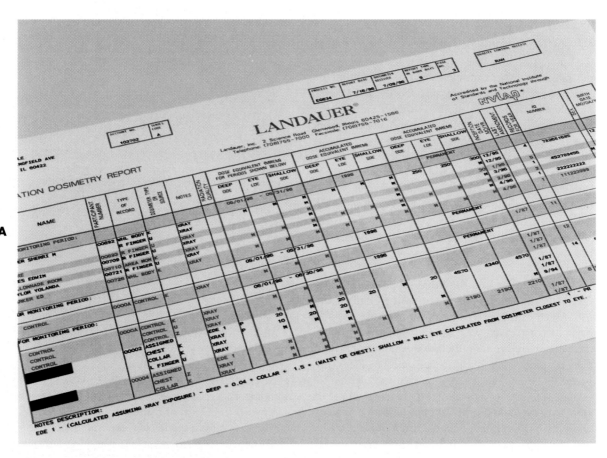

Fig. 9-7 A, Personnel monitoring report must include the items of information shown here. (Courtesy Landauer, Inc., Glenwood, Illinois.)

5. Cumulative dose equivalents for deep, eye, and shallow radiation exposures for the calendar quarter (3 months), the year to date, and lifetime radiation. The cumulative columns provide a continuous audit of actual absorbed radiation dose equivalent. These totals can be compared with allowable values established by regulatory agencies. Whenever the letter *M* appears under the current monitoring period or in the cumulative columns, it signifies that a dose equivalent below the minimum measurable radiation quantity recorded during that time. According to Landauer, Inc., for x-rays and gamma rays, *M* can represent a value up to 0.1 mSv (10 mrem), for energetic beta particles a value up to 0.4 mSv (40 mrem), for fast and moderate energy neutrons up to 0.2 mSv (20 mrem), and up to 0.1 mSv (10 mrem) for thermal neutrons.

When changing employment, the radiation worker must convey the data pertinent to accumulated permanent dose equivalent to the new employer so that this information can be placed on file. Fig. 9-7, *B* provides an example of an appropriate summary of occupational exposure report. A copy of such a report should be received by the radiation worker on termination of employment.

The main advantage of the film badge dosimeter is that the film itself, which is maintained by the monitoring company, constitutes a permanent, legal record of personnel exposure. In many institutions that have a well-structured radiation safety program, personnel monitoring reports are received and reviewed by the radiation safety officer (RSO). Film badge readings that exceed a trigger level set by the institution are investi-

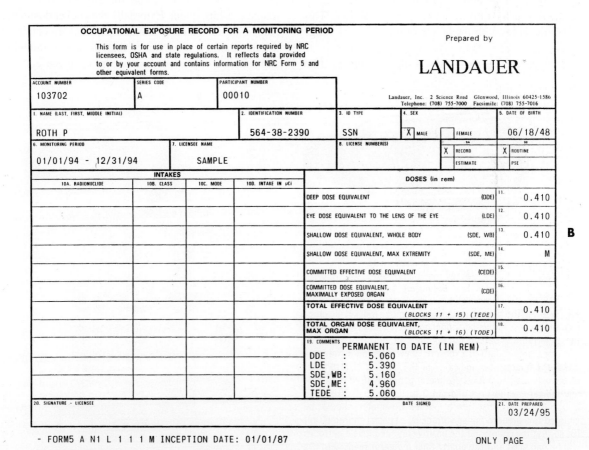

Fig. 9-7—cont'd B, Report showing a summary of occupational exposure. (Courtesy RS Landauer Jr. & Co.)

gated to ascertain the cause of that reading. Such a process should be an integral component of the institution's radiation safety programs. This practice is compatible with the ALARA policy (i.e., keeping radiation exposures to personnel *as low as reasonably achievable*).

The film badge dosimeter also has other benefits. This monitoring device is reasonably economical, costing only a few dollars per unit per month. The film badge can be used to monitor x, gamma, and all but very-low-energy beta radiation in a reliable manner. Moreover, the film badge can discriminate between the types of radiation and the energies of each of these radiations. Another advantage of the film badge dosimeter is that it has mechanical integrity. For example, the dosimeter will not be damaged if the badge is accidently dropped.

The film badge does have some objectionable characteristics. Temperature and humidity cause fogging of the dosimetry film over long periods of time. This effect increases with the length of time that the badge is worn and can result in a substantially inaccurate high exposure reading. Film badge dosimetry film

must be shipped to the monitoring company for processing and exposure determination. Because this takes time, a radiation worker's exposure cannot be determined on the day of occurrence. Manufacturers recommend 1 month as the maximum period of time that a film badge should be worn for personnel monitoring before being read.

Other types of personnel dosimeters are more sensitive to ionizing radiation and are therefore more effective monitors in some situations. The film badge dosimeter is most sensitive to photons having an energy of 50 keV; above and below this energy range, dosimetry film sensitivity decreases.

Pocket ionization chambers (pocket dosimeters)

Pocket ionization chambers (pocket dosimeters) (Fig. 9-8) are the most sensitive personnel dosimeters. However, the use of these monitors in diagnostic imaging is infrequent. Externally the pocket dosimeter resembles an ordinary fountain pen, but it contains a thimble ionization chamber that measures radiation exposure. A clip is present on the eyepiece end, al-

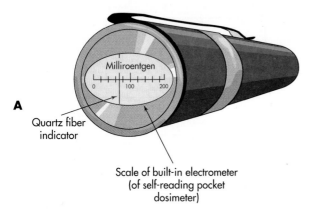

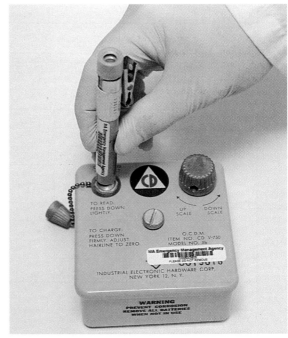

Fig. 9-8 A, The pocket ionization chamber (pocket dosimeter), the most sensitive personnel dosimeter, looks like a fountain pen from the outside but contains an ionization chamber that measures radiation exposure. Viewed through an eyepiece, the quartz fiber indicator of the built-in electrometer of the self-reading pocket dosimeter generally used in radiology indicates exposures of from 0 to 5.2×10^{-5} C/kg (0 to 200 mR). Before use, each pocket dosimeter should be charged to a predetermined voltage by a special charging unit **(B)** so that the charges of the positive and negative electrodes will be balanced and the quartz fiber indicator reads zero (0).

lowing the dosimeter to be attached to an individual's apparel (e.g., like a pen in a lab coat pocket).

Two types of pocket ionization chambers exist: the self-reading type, which contains a built-in electrometer (a device that measures electrical charge), and the non–self-reading type, which requires a special accessory electrometer to read the device. The non–self-reading type has largely been replaced by the self-reading type. The operating principle of both self-reading and non–self-reading pocket dosimeters is similar to that of the gold leaf electroscope, which detects the presence and sign of an electric charge.

The pocket ionization chamber contains two electrodes, one positively charged (the central electrode) and one negatively charged (the outer electrode). A quartz fiber may form part of the positive electrode and function as the indicator of the transparent reading scale; in such a system the quartz fiber casts a shadow onto a scale so that the amount of charge on the positively charged electrode determines the position of the shadow along the scale and is equivalent to the scale reading at that position. When the charged electrodes in the device are exposed to gamma or x-radiation, the air surrounding the central electrode (+) becomes ionized and discharges the mechanism in direct proportion to the amount of radiation to which it has been exposed.

A special charging unit is required for pocket ionization chambers. Each dosimeter must be charged to a predetermined voltage before use so that the quartz fiber indicator of the reading scale indicates zero (0). As the dosimeter is exposed to ionizing radiation, it discharges and the fiber indicator shows the exposure in milliroentgen. Pocket chambers generally used in medical imaging are sensitive to exposures ranging from 0 to 5.2×10^{-5} C/kg (0 to 200 mR).

The primary advantage to the use of pocket ionization chambers is that they provide an immediate exposure readout for radiation workers who work in high exposure areas (e.g., a cardiac catheterization laboratory). Such individuals can read the dosimeter on site to determine the dose received at the completion of a given assignment and, if necessary, alter their working habits. Furthermore, pocket ionization chambers are compact units that are easy to carry and convenient to use. Reasonably accurate and sensitive, they are ideal

monitoring devices for procedures that last for relatively short periods of time.

Some disadvantages are associated with the use of pocket ionization chambers. They are fairly expensive, costing $150.00 or more per unit. If not read each day, the dosimeter may give an inaccurate reading because the electric charge tends to escape (i.e., the fiber indicator drifts with time; thus a false high reading might be obtained from a dosimeter read too late). Pocket dosimeters can also discharge if subjected to mechanical shock, which again would result in a false high reading. Because pocket dosimeters provide no permanent, legal record of exposure, institutions that use this method to record personnel exposure must delegate someone to keep such a record. This task is generally the responsibility of the RSO.

Thermoluminescent dosimeters

The exterior of a **thermoluminescent dosimeter (TLD)** badge (Fig. 9-9) may look similar to that of a film badge. However, the interior of this monitoring mechanism differs completely. This light-free device usually contains a crystalline form (powder or small chips) of lithium fluoride (LiF), which functions as the sensing material of the TLD.

Ionizing radiation causes the LiF crystals in the TLD to undergo changes in some of their physical properties. When irradiated, some of the electrons in

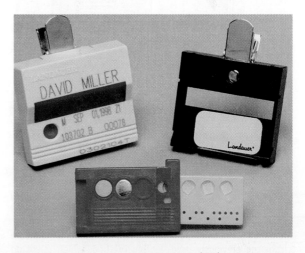

Fig. 9-9 Thermoluminescent dosimeter (TLD) badge containing the sensing material lithium flouride.

the crystalline lattice structure of the LiF molecule absorb energy and are "excited" to higher energy levels or bands. The presence of impurities in the crystal causes these electrons to become trapped within these bands. When the LiF crystals are passed through a special heating process, however, these trapped electrons receive enough energy to rise above their present locations into a region called the conduction band. From here the electrons can return to their original or normal state with the emission of energy in the form of visible light. The energy emitted is equal to the difference between the electron-binding energy of the two orbital levels. The intensity of the light is proportional to the amount of radiation that interacted with the crystals. A device called a **TLD analyzer** (Fig. 9-10) measures the amount of ionizing radiation to which a TLD badge has been exposed by first heating the crystals to free the trapped, highly energized electrons and then recording the amount of light emitted by the crystals (which is proportional to the TLD badge exposure).

The TLD has several advantages over the film badge. The LiF crystals interact with ionizing radiation as human tissue does;* hence this monitor determines dose more accurately. Exposures as low as 1.3×10^{-6} C/kg (5 mR) can be measured precisely. Humidity, pressure, and normal temperature changes do not affect the TLD. Unlike the film in the film badge, which can fog if worn for more than 1 month, the TLD may be worn up to 3 months. After the TLD reading has been obtained, the crystals can be reused. This makes the device somewhat cost-effective, even though the initial cost is high (approximately twice the cost of a film badge service).

TLDs have some disadvantages other than their high cost. A TLD can be read only once. The readout process destroys the stored information; the TLD may be reused, but once the crystal is heated, the record of any previous exposure is gone. The necessity of using calibrated dosimeters (which must be prepared and read with each group of these monitoring devices when they are processed) with TLDs is also a disadvantage.

Table 9-2 provides a summary of the advantages and disadvantages of the personnel monitoring devices covered in this chapter.

Radiation Survey Instruments for Area Monitoring

Radiation survey instruments are area monitoring devices that detect and measure radiation. The detection system indicates the presence or absence of radiation, whereas the dosimeter system measures only cumulative radiation intensity.

When in contact with ionizing radiation, survey instruments respond to the charged particles that are produced as radiation interacts with and ionizes the gas (usually air) in the detector. These instruments measure either the total quantity of electrical charge resulting from the ionization of the gas or the rate at which the electrical charge is produced. The ionization chamber-type survey meter (cutie pie), the proportional counter, and the Geiger-Müller detector are three different gas-filled radiation detectors that serve as field survey instruments. They detect the presence of radiation and, when properly calibrated, give a reasonably accurate measurement of the exposure. Each

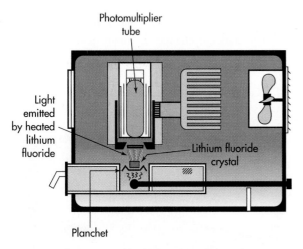

Fig. 9-10 Diagram of a typical analyzer. The analyzer measures the amount of ionizing radiation to which a badge has been exposed by heating the irradiated lithium fluoride (liF) crystals of the exposed badge with linearly rising temperatures produced by hot gas steam. This represents a departure from the previously used heating method, which relied on physical contact between the crystals and a heated plate. The new method is a technical improvement because it eliminates any need for contact readjustments.

---

*The effective atomic number of LiF is equal to 8.2, which is similar to that of soft tissue (7.4).

Table 9-2
Advantages and Disadvantages of Personnel Dosimeters

Personnel monitoring device	Advantages	Disadvantages
Film badge	It is lightweight, durable, and easy to carry	It records only the exposure received in the body area where it is worn
	It provides cost-efficient monitoring for large numbers of people	It is not effective as a monitoring device if it is not worn
	It records radiation exposure accumulated at a low rate over a long period of time	Temperature and humidity can cause film in the badge to fog over long periods of time, causing inaccurate exposure reading
	It provides a permanent, legal record of personnel exposure	Film sensitivity is decreased above and below 50 keV
	It detects and records small and large exposures in a consistent, reliable manner	Exposure cannot be determined on day of occurrence
	Instrument performance is usually not affected by outside influences such as heat and humidity fluctuations and nonextreme mechanical shock	Accuracy is limited to + or −20%
	Filters contained in the badge make it possible to estimate the direction from which the radiation came	
	Filters can indicate whether exposure was due to excessive amounts of scattered radiation as opposed to a single exposure from the primary beam	
	Control badge can indicate if badges in the group were exposed in transit to and/or from an institution	
	It can be used to monitor x-, gamma, and all but very-low-energy beta radiation in a reliable manner	
	It can discriminate between type of radiation and energy of x-, gamma, and beta radiation	
Pocket ionization chamber	Small, compact unit is easy to carry and convenient to use	Fairly expensive, it is not cost-effective for large numbers of imaging professionals
	It is reasonably accurate and sensitive	Readings must be carefully obtained, or they may be lost
	It can be used as a monitor for procedures that last relatively short periods of time	Dosimeter must be read each day it is used to prevent inaccurate reading.
	Self-reading chambers provide an immediate exposure readout for radiation workers in high exposure areas	If subjected to mechanical shock, the unit can discharge and give a false high reading
		No permanent, legal record of exposure is provided
		It records only the exposure received in the body area in which it is worn
Thermoluminescent dosimeter (TLD)	Crystals contained in TLD interact with ionizing radiation as human tissue does; hence TLD determines dose more accurately	The initial cost is greater than that of a film badge service

Continued

Table 9-2
Advantages and Disadvantages of Personnel Dosimeters—cont'd

Personnel monitoring device	Advantages	Disadvantages
Thermolumines-cent dosimeter (TLD)—cont'd	It is not affected by humidity, pressure, or normal temperature changes It can be worn up to 3 months After reading has been obtained, TLD crystals can be reused, making the device somewhat cost-effective	Readouts must be carefully obtained, or results can be lost Readout process destroys information stored in TLD, which prevents the "read" TLD from serving as a permanent, legal record of exposure Calibrated dosimeters must be prepared and read with each group of TLDs as they are processed It records only the exposure received in the body area in which it is worn It is not effective as a monitoring device if it is not worn

of these instruments has its own special use, and they are not all equally sensitive in the detection of ionizing radiation.

Radiation Survey Instrument Requirements

Radiation survey instruments for area monitoring should meet certain requirements. First, these devices must be easy to carry so that one person can operate the device in an efficient manner for a period of time. Second, survey instruments must be durable enough to withstand normal use, including routine handling that occurs during standard operating procedures. Third, area monitors must be reliable; only in such a case can radiation exposure or exposure rate in a given area be accurately assessed. Fourth, area monitoring devices should interact with ionizing radiation in a manner similar to the way human tissue reacts. This permits dose to be determined more accurately. Fifth, a radiation survey instrument should be able to detect all common types of ionizing radiation. Such a capability increases the usefulness of an area monitoring device. Sixth, the energy of the radiation should not affect the response of the detector, and the direction of the inci-

dent radiation should not affect the performance of the unit. Such characteristics ensure consistency in unit operation among individual users. Seventh, survey equipment should be cost-effective. The initial cost and subsequent maintenance charges should be as low as possible.

Types of Gas-Filled Radiation Survey Instruments

As mentioned, three types of gas-filled radiation survey instruments exist: the ionization chamber-type survey meter (cutie pie), the proportional counter, and the Geiger-Müller detector.

Ionization chamber–type survey meter (cutie pie)

The ionization chamber–type survey meter, or "**cutie pie,**" (Fig. 9-11) is both a rate meter device (measures exposure rate) used for area surveys and an accurate integrating or cumulative exposure instrument. This device measures x or gamma radiation and, if equipped with a suitable window, can also record beta radiation.

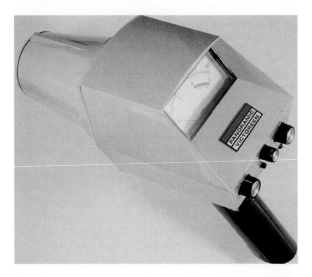

Fig. 9-11 Ionization chamber-type survey meter, or "cutie pie." (Courtesy Victoreen, Inc.)

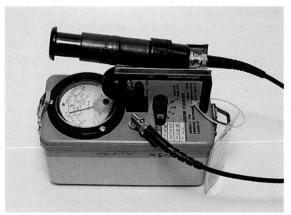

Fig. 9-12 Geiger-Müller detector.

In the rate mode the cutie pie can measure radiation intensity ranging from 1 mR per hour to several thousand roentgens per hour and in the integrate mode can sum exposures from as little as 0.1 mR to 1 R. This device can be used to monitor diagnostic x-ray installations when exposure times of a second or more are chosen and to measure fluoroscopic scatter radiation exposure rate, exposure rate from patients containing therapeutic doses of radioactive materials, exposure rate in radioisotope storage facilities, and the cumulative exposures received outside protective barriers.

The advantage of using the cutie pie is that it can measure a wide range of radiation exposures within a few seconds. The delicate construction and relatively large size of the unit, however, may be considered a disadvantage. Another disadvantage is that without adequate warm-up time, its meter will drift and produce an inaccurate reading. This device cannot be used to measure exposures produced by typical diagnostic procedures because the exposure times are too short to permit the meter to respond. Instead, it is most commonly used to measure the exposure rates (mr/hr) at various distances from a patient who has received radioactive materials for diagnostic or therapeutic purposes.

Proportional counter

Proportional counters serve no useful purpose in diagnostic imaging. They are generally used in a laboratory setting to detect alpha and beta radiation and small amounts of other types of low-level radioactive contamination. The proportional counter can discriminate between alpha and beta particles. Because alpha radiation travels only a short distance in air, the operator of the proportional counter must hold the unit's probe close to the surface of the object being surveyed to obtain an accurate reading of the alpha radiation emitted by the object.

Geiger-Müller (G-M) detector

Geiger-Müller (G-M) detectors (Fig. 9-12) serve as the primary radiation survey instrument for area monitoring in nuclear medicine facilities. With the exception of alpha particle emission, the unit is sensitive enough to detect individual particles (e.g., electrons emitted from certain radioactive nuclei) or photons. Hence it can easily detect any area contaminated by radioactive material. Because the G-M detector allows for rapid monitoring, it can be used to locate a lost radioactive source or low-level radioactive contamination.

The G-M detector has an audible sound system (an audio amplifier and speaker) that alerts the operator to the presence of ionizing radiation. Metal encloses the counter's gas-filled tube or probe, which is the unit's sensitive ionization chamber. When the shield covering the probe's sensitive chamber is open, beta and very-low-energy x- and gamma radiation can be detected. Meter readings are usually obtained in milliroentgen per hour. Because G-M tubes tend to lose their calibration, the instrument generally has a "check source" of a weak, long-lived radioisotope located on one side of its external surface.

The meter reading of a G-M detector is not independent of the energy of the incident photons. This means that photons of widely different energies cause the instrument to respond quite differently, which is a disadvantage in diagnostic imaging usage. The cutie pie ionization chamber survey meter exhibits a much flatter or more constant response with varying photon energies. Also, the G-M detector is likely to saturate or jam when placed in a very high-intensity radiation area, thereby giving a false reading.

Calibration Instruments

Ionization chambers can be used to calibrate radiographic and fluoroscopic x-ray equipment. We have seen previously that a cutie pie ionization chamber is used for radiation protection surveys. If this instrument were to be placed in the beam of an x-ray tube during a radiographic exposure, the electrical signal produced by the cutie pie during the very brief radiographic exposure would be too small to be recorded and measured reliably. An ionization chamber specifically designed for calibration purposes is connected to an electrometer, a device that can measure tiny electrical currents with high precision and accuracy. (Such a combination is shown in Fig. 9-11.) Both parts of the ionization chamber and electrometer system must be calibrated periodically to meet state and federal requirements for patient dose evaluation. Several regional calibration laboratories offer this service. A current listing of calibration laboratories is available from the American Association of Physicists in Medicine.* Ionization chambers con-

*One Physics Ellipse, College Park, MD 20740-3846 or http://www.aapm.org

nected to electrometers are used to perform the standard measurements that are required by state, federal, and health care accrediting organizations for radiographic and fluoroscopic devices. These measurements include x-ray output in mR/mAs, reproducibility of output, timer accuracy, half-value layer, tabletop exposure rates for fluoroscopy units, and in-air exposure measurement, which are required for the calculation of average glandular dose for mammography units.

Summary

In this chapter the subject of radiation monitoring was introduced. The operating principles of the various personnel and area monitoring devices and instruments have been discussed in detail. Personnel monitoring ensures that occupational radiation exposure levels are kept well below the annual total effective dose equivalent limit. Such monitoring is required whenever radiation workers are likely to risk receiving 10% or more of the annual TEDE limit of 50 mSv (5 rem) in any 1 year. To keep radiation exposure as low as reasonably achievable, most health care facilities issue dosimetry devices when personnel might receive about 1% of the annual TEDE limit in any month, or approximately 0.5 mSv (50 mrem).

The working habits and conditions of diagnostic imaging personnel can be assessed over a designated period of time by determining occupational exposure through the use of a personnel dosimeter that detects and measures the quantity of ionizing radiation received. A radiation worker should wear a monitoring device such as a film badge dosimeter to indicate the exposure received by the body trunk. During routine radiographic procedures the device may be attached to the clothing on the front of the body at waist or chest level. During high-level radiation procedures such as fluoroscopy and special radiographic studies, imaging professionals should wear a protective lead apron, with the dosimeter worn outside of the garment at collar level on the front of the body. During special radiographic procedures, two separate film badge dosimeters may be worn, one beneath a wraparound lead apron at waist level and the other outside the protective garment at collar level. Pregnant radiation workers should wear a second film badge dosimeter to monitor the abdomen during gestation. Extremity dosimeters are worn under certain conditions to monitor and determine the dose equivalent to the hands when they are near the primary beam.

Institutions must maintain a record of exposure recorded by personnel dosimeters as part of each radiation worker's employment record. In general, personnel dosimeters must be portable, durable, and cost-efficient. Three types of personnel monitoring devices exist: film badges, pocket ionization chambers, and thermoluminescent dosimeters (TLDs). Of these, the film badge is the most economical and widely used. It records whole-body radiation exposure accumulated at a low rate over a long period of time (usually 1 month). Radiation interacting with the film in the badge causes the film to darken once it is developed.

A densitometer is used to measure the density, or degree of blackening, of the image of the filters recorded on the dosimetry film. This density is proportional to the amount of radiation received and the energy of the radiation. It is necessary to locate the exposure value of a control film of a similar optical density on a characteristic curve to determine the amount of radiation to which the film was exposed. To meet state and federal regulations, results from personnel monitoring programs must be recorded accurately and maintained by each institution. The radiation safety officer (RSO) in an institution receives and reviews personnel film badge monitoring reports to assess compliance with ALARA guidelines.

A pocket ionization chamber (pocket dosimeter) can be worn to monitor radiation workers who work in high exposure areas such as cardiac catheterization laboratories. Resembling an ordinary fountain pen externally, this very sensitive device contains a thimble ionization chamber that measures radiation exposure. The chambers generally used in the healing arts are sensitive to exposures from 0 to 5.2×10^{-5} C/kg (0 to 200 mR). In health care facilities the RSO generally assumes responsibility for maintaining a record of personnel exposure recorded with pocket dosimeters.

TLDs contain the sensing material lithium fluoride, which interacts with ionizing radiation as human tissue does. Exposures as low as 1.3×10^{-6} C/kg (5 mR) can be measured precisely. These monitors can be read only once because the readout process destroys the stored information. However, they can be recalibrated and reused. (Table 9-2 provides a summary of the advantages and disadvantages of the film badge, pocket dosimeter, and the TLD.)

Area monitoring can be accomplished through the use of radiation survey instruments designed to detect and measure radiation. In such instruments the detection system indicates the presence or absence of radiation, whereas the dosimeter system measures only cumulative radiation intensity. Radiation survey instruments for area monitoring must be durable and easy to carry. They should be able to detect all common types of ionizing radiation and not be affected by the energy of the radiation or the direction of the incident radiation. The ionization chamber-type survey meter (cutie pie), the proportional counter, and the Geiger-Müller detector are the three types of gas-filled radiation survey instruments. The ionization chamber-type survey meter measures x- or gamma radiation and, if equipped with a suitable window, can also measure beta radiation. Uses for this device include (1) monitoring of x-ray installations when exposure times of a second or more are chosen, (2) measuring exposure rate from patients containing therapeutic doses of radioactive materials, (3) measuring exposure rate in radioisotope storage facilities, and (4) measuring cumulative exposures received outside protective barriers. In a laboratory setting a proportional counter is used to detect alpha and beta radiation and small amounts of other types of low-level radioactive contamination. In nuclear medicine facilities the Geiger-Müller detector serves as the primary radiation survey instrument. It can detect any area contaminated by radioactive material and can be used to locate a lost radioactive source or low-level radioactive contamination.

Radiographic and fluoroscopic units can be calibrated with ionization chambers. When used for this purpose, the ionization chamber is connected to an electrometer that can measure tiny electrical current with high precision and accuracy.

Review Questions

1. Which of the following chemicals function as the sensing material in a thermoluminescent dosimeter?
   A. Calcium tungstate
   B. Sodium iodide
   C. Lithium fluoride
   D. Barium sulfate

2. Which of the following items is *not* a basic component of the film badge?
   A. Radiographic film packet
   B. Plastic film holder
   C. Charged electrodes
   D. Assortment of metal filters

3. Which of the following personnel dosimeters resembles an ordinary fountain pen externally?
   A. Pocket dosimeter
   B. Film badge
   C. Thermoluminescent dosimeter
   D. None of the above

4. Of the following, which are advantages of using the film badge as a personnel dosimeter?
   1. It is economical
   2. It provides a permanent, legal record of personnel exposure
   3. It can be used to monitor x-, gamma, and all but very-low-energy beta radiation
   A. 1 only
   B. 2 only
   C. 3 only
   D. 1, 2, and 3

5. Which of the following statements is *not* true?
   A. Personnel monitoring becomes necessary whenever radiation workers are likely to risk receiving 10% or more of the annual total effective dose equivalent limit
   B. Personnel dosimeters protect the radiographer or other diagnostic imaging personnel from exposure to ionizing radiation
   C. A personnel dosimeter records only the exposure received in the body area where it is worn
   D. Personnel dosimeters measure the quantity of ionizing radiation to which they have been exposed over a period of time

6. Where should nonpregnant occupationally exposed persons wear a personnel dosimeter when performing a fluoroscopic procedure or special radiographic procedure?
   A. Outside of the protective apron, at hip level on the anterior surface of the body
   B. Under the protective apron, at hip level on the anterior surface of the body
   C. Under the protective apron, at the level of the sternal angle
   D. Outside of the protective apron, at collar level on the anterior surface of the body

7. The metal filters contained in the film badge are generally composed of which of the following materials?
   A. Aluminum or copper
   B. Aluminum or lead
   C. Zinc or copper
   D. Lead or zinc

8. When radiation interacts with the radiographic film contained in the film badge, the film after development _____.
   A. Turns green
   B. Darkens in proportion to the exposure
   C. Remains unchanged in terms of density
   D. Lightens in proportion to the exposure

9. What is the suggested maximum period of time that a film badge should be worn as a personnel dosimeter?
   A. 1 week
   B. 2 weeks
   C. 1 month
   D. 3 months

10. Which of the following personnel dosimeters allows a radiation worker to determine exposure received immediately on completion of a specific radiologic procedure?
    A. Film badge
    B. Pocket dosimeter
    C. Thermoluminescent dosimeter
    D. None of the above

11. Film badges are *most sensitive* to a photon energy of which of the following?
    A. 200 keV
    B. 100 keV
    C. 50 keV
    D. 25 keV

12. When the negatively and positively charged electrodes in the pocket ionization chamber are exposed to ionizing radiation, the mechanism does which of the following?
    A. It charges in direct proportion to the amount of radiation to which it has been exposed
    B. It discharges in direct proportion to the amount of radiation to which it has been exposed
    C. It heats the central electrode
    D. It heats the outer electrode

13. Before a pocket dosimeter is used to record radiation exposure, the quartz fiber indicator of the transparent reading scale should indicate which of the following?
    A. Zero
    B. 100 mR
    C. 150 mR
    D. 200 mR

14. The film badge holder should be made of a (an) _____ to filter x- and gamma radiation as well as beta radiation.
    A. Aluminum material of a low atomic number
    B. Lead-impregnated material of a high atomic number
    C. Plastic material of a high atomic number
    D. Plastic material of a low atomic number

15. Of the following, which are disadvantages of using pocket ionization chambers as personnel dosimeters?
    1. Mechanical shock causes pocket chambers to discharge
    2. A permanent record of personnel exposure cannot be obtained with a pocket dosimeter
    3. False high readings may be obtained if the pocket dosimeter is not read each day
    A. 1 only
    B. 2 only
    C. 3 only
    D. 1, 2, and 3

16. Which of the following devices is used to measure the visible light emitted by the sensing material contained in the thermoluminescent dosimeter after exposure to ionizing radiation and heating?
    A. X-ray tube
    B. Densitometer
    C. Photomultiplier tube
    D. Sensitometer

17. When the sensing crystals contained in the thermoluminescent dosimeter are exposed to ionizing radiation, which of the following occurs:
    A. The protons in the crystalline lattice structure of the LiF molecule absorb energy and are excited to a higher energy level
    B. The neutrons in the crystalline lattice structure of the LiF molecule absorb energy and are excited to higher energy levels
    C. The electrons in the crystalline lattice structure of the LiF molecule absorb energy and are excited to higher energy levels
    D. The freed electrons are trapped at a lower energy level

18. Of the following, which are disadvantages of using a thermoluminescent dosimeter as a personnel monitoring device?
    1. Only one readout may be obtained
    2. Readout or results can be lost if the readout procedure is not carefully conducted
    3. There is a greater initial cost than with film badge service
    A. 1 only
    B. 2 only
    C. 3 only
    D. 1, 2, and 3

19. What is the maximum period of time that a TLD may be worn as a personnel dosimeter?
    A. 1 hour
    B. 1 week
    C. 1 month
    D. 3 months

20. Exposure from 2.58×10^{-6} C/kg to 5.2×10^{-5} C/kg (10 to 200 mR) can be recorded by using the following dosimeter(s):
    1. Film badge
    2. Thermoluminescent dosimeter
    3. Pocket ionization chamber
    A. 1 only
    B. 2 only
    C. 3 only
    D. 1, 2, and 3

21. Which of the following personnel dosimeters possesses the most mechanical integrity?
    A. Thermoluminescent dosimeters
    B. Pocket ionization chambers
    C. Film badges
    D. None of the above

22. A densitometer is used to measure which of the following?
    A. The density on the processed film from a film badge
    B. The light emitted from the sensing material of the thermoluminescent dosimeter after exposure
    C. The freed electrons
    D. The discharged electricity

23. Of the following types of personnel dosimeters, which device is least sensitive to ionizing radiation?
    A. Film badge
    B. Thermoluminescent dosimeter
    C. Pocket dosimeter
    D. Sensitivity in personnel dosimeters a, b, and c is equal

24. In the characteristic curve in Fig. 9-6, if the optical density of the dosimetry film is determined to be 1.0, the film badge has been exposed to which of the following?
    A. 1 mSv (100 mR)
    B. 0.5 mSv (50 mR)
    C. 0.15 mSv (15 mR)
    D. 0.1 mSv (10 mR)

25. The image densities cast by the filters in the film badge permit which of the following?
    A. The percentage of visible light emission to be determined
    B. The film to be reused
    C. The energy of the radiation to be estimated
    D. The electrical discharge to be determined

26. Radiation survey instruments measure which of the following?
    A. The total quantity of electrical charge resulting from ionization of the gas
    B. The rate at which an electrical charge is produced
    C. A or B
    D. None of the above

27. The detection system of a radiation survey instrument does which of the following?
    A. It only measures cumulative radiation intensity
    B. It indicates the presence of radiation
    C. It counts uncharged particles
    D. A and B only

28. Which of the following instruments is used to calibrate radiographic and fluoroscopic x-ray equipment?
    A. Proportional counter
    B. Geiger-Müller detector
    C. Ionization chamber with electrometer
    D. Pocket ionization chamber

29. Which of the following requirements should radiation survey instruments fulfill?
    1. Instruments must be reliable by accurately recording exposure or exposure rate
    2. Instruments must be durable enough to withstand normal use
    3. Instruments should interact with ionizing radiation in a manner similar to the way in which human tissue interacts
    A. 1 only
    B. 2 only
    C. 3 only
    D. 1, 2, and 3

30. Which of the following instruments should be used in an x-ray installation to assess fluoroscopic scatter radiation exposure rate?
    A. Geiger-Müller detector
    B. Ionization chamber with electrometer
    C. Proportional counter
    D. Thermoluminescent dosimeter

31. Which of the following instruments should be used to locate a lost radioactive source or detect low-level radioactive contamination?
    A. Geiger-Müller detector
    B. Proportional counter
    C. Ionization chamber-type survey meter
    D. Thermoluminescent dosimeter analyzer

32. Which of the following instruments should be used in a laboratory setting to detect alpha and beta radiation and small amounts of other types of low-level radioactive contamination?
    A. Ionization chamber-type survey meter
    B. Proportional counter
    C. Geiger-Müller detector
    D. Pocket ionization chamber

33. Which of the following instruments is called a *cutie pie?*
    A. Geiger-Müller detector
    B. Film badge dosimeter
    C. Ionization chamber-type survey meter
    D. Proportional counter

34. What do ionization chamber-type survey meters, proportional counters, and Geiger-Müller detectors have in common?
    A. These instruments all measure x- and beta radiation only
    B. These instruments can all be used to calibrate radiographic and fluoroscopic x-ray equipment
    C. These instruments can all be used to measure the dose received outside protective barriers
    D. Each of these units contains a gas-filled chamber

35. Which component(s) of the Geiger-Müller detector alert(s) the operator to the presence of ionizing radiation?
  A. The shield covering the probe's sensitive chamber
  B. An audio amplifier and speaker
  C. The metal that encloses the counter's gas-filled tube
  D. The meter scale

36. Which of the following instruments generally has a check source of weak, long-lived radioisotope located on one side of its external surface?
  A. Pocket dosimeter
  B. Proportional counter
  C. Geiger-Müller detector
  D. Ionization chamber-type survey meter

37. If a radiographer leaves his or her film badge in a closed car, where it is exposed to sunlight for a considerable period of time, the dosimetry film in the badge will respond in which of the following ways?
  A. It will become fogged as a result of increased temperature and humidity causing a false high reading
  B. It will decrease in sensitivity and not provide an accurate reading
  C. It will turn bright orange and melt
  D. It will not be affected by increased temperature and humidity and will continue to provide an accurate reading

38. Which of the following is the most cost-effective personnel dosimeter for continual monitoring of a large number of radiography team members employed in a busy hospital imaging department?
  A. Thermoluminescent dosimeter
  B. Film badge
  C. Pocket dosimeter
  D. A, B, and C all cost the same

39. When performing a routine radiographic procedure without wearing a protective apron, a radiographer may wear a film badge dosimeter attached to which of the following?
  1. Clothing on the front of the body at chest level
  2. Clothing on the front of the body at waist level
  3. Wristwatch band
  A. 1 only
  B. 2 only
  C. 3 only
  D. 1 and 2 only

40. In keeping with the ALARA concept, most institutions issue personnel dosimetry devices when personnel might possibly receive about _____ of the annual total effective dose equivalent limit in any one month.
  A. 1%
  B. 5%
  C. 10%
  D. 25%

Bibliography

Ballinger PW, Bushong SC: *Merrill's atlas of radiologic positions and radiologic procedures,* ed 7, vol 1, St Louis, 1991, Mosby.

Ballinger PW: *Merrill's atlas of radiographic positions and radiologic procedures,* ed 5, vol 1, St Louis, 1982, Mosby.

Bushong S: *Radiologic science for technologists: physics, biology, and protection,* ed 2, St Louis, 1980, Mosby-Year Book.

Bushong SC: *Radiologic science for technologists: physics, biology, and protection,* ed 6, St Louis, 1997, Mosby.

Bushong SC: *Radiologic science for technologists: physics, biology, and protection,* ed 5, St Louis, 1993, Mosby.

Dowd SB: *Practical radiation protection and applied radiobiology,* Philadelphia, 1994, WB Saunders.

Early PJ, Sodee DB: *Principles and practice of nuclear medicine,* ed 2, St Louis, 1995, Mosby.

Frankel R: *Radiation protection for radiologic technologists,* New York, 1976, McGraw-Hill.

Hendee WR, Ritenour ER: *Medical imaging physics,* ed 3, St Louis, 1992, Mosby.

Moscovitch M et al: A TLD system based on gas heating with linear time-temperature profile, *Radiat Protect Dosimetry* 34:361, 1990.

Moscovitch M et al: Mixed field personnel dosimetry using a nearly tissue-equivalent multi-element thermoluminescence dosimeter, *Radiat Protect Dosimetry* 34:145, 1990.

National Council on Radiation Protection and Measurements (NCRP): *Exposure of the U.S. population from occupational radiation,* Report No. 101, Bethesda, Md, 1989, NCRP Publications.

National Council on Radiation Protection and Measurements (NCRP): *Recommendations on limits for exposure to ionizing radiation,* Report No. 91, Bethesda, Md, 1987, NCRP Publications.

Noz ME, Maguire Jr GQ: *Radiation protection in radiologic and health sciences,* ed 2, Philadelphia, 1985, Lea & Febiger.

Noz ME, Maguire Jr GQ: *Radiation protection in the radiologic and health sciences,* Philadelphia, 1979, Lea & Febiger.

Scheele RV, Wakley J: *Elements of radiation protection,* Springfield, Ill, 1975, Charles C Thomas.

Seeram E: *Radiation protection,* Philadelphia, 1997, Lippincott-Raven Publishers.

Selman J: *The fundamentals of x-ray and radium physics,* ed 6, Springfield, Ill, 1978, Charles C Thomas.

Thompson MA et al: *Principles of imaging science and protection,* Philadelphia, 1994, WB Saunders.

Travis EL: *Primer of medical radiobiology,* ed 2, St Louis, 1989, Mosby.

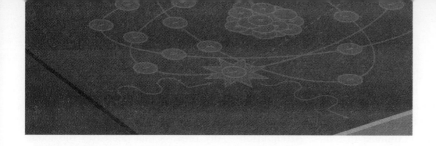

Glossary

Aberration Deviation from normal development or growth.

Absolute risk Model predicting that a specific number of excess cancers will occur as a result of exposure to ionizing radiation.

Absorbed dose The amount of energy per unit mass absorbed by the irradiated object. This absorbed energy is responsible for whatever biologic damage occurs as a result of tissues being exposed to x-radiation. The gray (Gy) is the SI unit of this radiation quantity.

Absorption Transference of energy from an x-ray beam to the atoms or molecules of the matter through which it passes.

Acid–base balance State of equilibrium or stability between acids and bases.

Acids Hydrogen-containing compounds that can attack and dissolve metal (e.g., HNO_3, nitric acid).

Acute Something that begins suddenly and runs a short but rather severe course (e.g., an acute disease).

Acute radiation syndrome (ARS) Radiation sickness that occurs in humans after whole-body reception of large doses of ionizing radiation (1 Gy [100 rad] or more) delivered over a short period of time.

Acute somatic effects (See *Early somatic effects.*)

Added filtration Sheets of aluminum (or its equivalent) of appropriate thickness interposed outside the glass window of the x-ray tube housing above the collimator shutters.

Adenine (A) One of two purine bases found in both DNA and RNA.

Adenosine triphosphate (ATP) High-energy–releasing phosphate compound essential for life.

Agreement states Individual states of the United States that have entered into an agreement with the Nuclear Regulatory Commission (NRC) to assume responsibility for enforcing radiation protection regulations through their respective health departments.

ALARA concept Precept holding that occupational exposure of the radiographer and other occupationally exposed persons should be kept "As Low As Reasonably Achievable."

Alkali A member of a group of elements that includes lithium, sodium, and potassium.

Alkaline earth A member of a group of elements including calcium, magnesium, and strontium.

Alpha particle A particulate form of radiation. This particle is positively charged and consists of two protons and two neutrons. Alpha particles are ejected by certain radioactive elements.

Aluminum (Al) The metal most frequently selected as filter material because it effectively removes low energy (soft) x-rays from a polyenergetic x-ray beam.

American Association of Physicists in Medicine (AAPM) Professional organization responsible for accrediting calibration laboratories that measure radiation exposure in medical radiography.

American College of Radiology (ACR) Major professional organization of American radiologists.

Amino acids The structural units of protein.

Ampere The SI unit of electric charge. One ampere represents the flow of electrons amounting to a charge of 1 coulomb crossing unit area per second.

Anaphase The phase of mitosis during which two chromatids repel each other and migrate along the mitotic spindle to opposite sides of the cell.

Anemia A condition characterized by a lack of vitality and caused by a decrease in the number of red blood cells in the circulating blood.

Anion A negatively charged ion.

Annihilation radiation Two 0.511-keV gamma rays emitted in opposite directions. It occurs as a result of the destructive interaction of a positron and an electron. This type of radiation is emitted from patients who have been injected with a radiopharmaceutical containing atoms that decay by the process of positron decay.

Annual total effective dose equivalent (TEDE) limit A radiation protection term that specifies the maximum allowable total dose (the sum of any internal and external dose) that may accumulate over a year for a certain category of individual. Different categories include the occupationally exposed, general public, embryo-fetus, and radiography students.

Anode The positively charged target in the x-ray tube.

Antibodies Materials developed by the body in response to the presence of foreign antigens such as bacteria or a flu virus. They provide a primary defense mechanism against such antigens.

Antimatter Matter composed of the counterparts of ordinary matter that does not exist freely in the universe and is unstable in the presence of ordinary matter.

Aperture diaphragm A simple beam limitation device that consists of a flat piece of lead with a hole of a designated size and shape cut in its center.

Aplastic anemia Anemia resulting from bone marrow failure.

Apoptosis A nonmitotic or nondivision form of cell death that occurs when cells die without attempting division during the interphase portion of the cell life cycle.

Artificial radiation (See *Man-made radiation.*)

Atom The smallest portion of an element that has all of its chemical properties.

Atomic Energy Commission (AEC) (See *Nuclear Regulatory Commission* [NRC].)

Atomic number The number of protons contained within the nucleus of an atom.

Atrophy A wasting caused by lack of nutrition in any part.

Attenuation Any process that decreases the intensity of the primary photon beam directed toward some destination.

Audible sound system An audio amplifier and speaker. Geiger-Müller detectors contain an audible sound system.

Auger electron Monoenergetic electrons occasionally emitted from atoms undergoing photoelectric interactions with x-rays. Essentially an "internal" photoelectric effect in which the characteristic radiation released within an atom by an inner shell transition is delivered to another electron of that atom, thereby ejecting it from the atom.

Axon Nerve cell process that extends out from the cell body and conducts impulses away from the cell body.

Backscatter Photons that have interacted with the atoms of an object and as a result are deflected backward (toward the x-ray tube).

Bases Alkali or alkaline earth OH compounds that can neutralize acids (e.g., $Mg(OH)_2$, otherwise known as *milk of magnesia*).

Beam direction factor (See *Use factor.*)

Beam limiting device A device that limits the parameters of the useful beam to a designated size and shape before it enters the area of clinical interest.

Becquerel The SI unit of radioactivity. It is equal to 1 disintegration per second.

Beta particles High-speed electrons or positrons.

Binding energy Force that holds an atom together.

Biologic dosimetry A method of dose assessment in which biologic markers or effects of radiation exposure are measured and the dose to the organism is inferred from previously established dose-effect relationships. Examples of such biologic markers include white blood cell counts and chromosomal aberrations.

Biologic damage Damage in living tissue.

Biologic radiation Radiation from radionuclides deposited in the human body via natural processes.

Biology A science that explores living things and life processes.

Birth effects (See *Embryologic effects.*)

Bone marrow dose (See *Mean active bone marrow dose.*)

Bone marrow syndrome (See *Hematopoietic syndrome.*)

Bragg–Gray theory Relates the ionization produced in a small cavity in an irradiated medium or object to the energy absorbed in that medium as a result of its radiation exposure.

Brems radiation (See *Bremsstrahlung.*)

Bremsstrahlung Ionizing electromagnetic radiation that is nonuniform in energy and wavelength and that is produced when a bombarding beam of electrons in an x-ray tube undergoes deceleration by interaction with the nuclei of the x-ray tube target atoms.

Bucky slot shielding device A protective device of at least 0.25-mm lead equivalent that automatically covers the Bucky slot opening in the side of the x-ray table during a fluoroscopic examination when the Bucky tray is positioned at the foot end of the table. This device protects the radiographer and radiologist from radiation exposure at the gonadal level.

Bureau of Radiological Health (BRH) (See *Center for Devices and Radiological Health.*)

Calibration instrument A device used to measure the expected output of a piece of equipment so that a comparison may be made with expected values. In radiography an ionization chamber is used to measure the x-ray output of radiographic equipment.

Candela per square meter Unit used to describe luminance. One candela corresponds to 3.8 million billion photons per second being emitted from a light source through a unit conelike field of view.

Carbohydrates Compounds composed entirely of carbon, hydrogen, and oxygen. There are always twice as many atoms of hydrogen as of oxygen. Carbohydrates are involved in the chief energy-releasing processes in animals and plants. Sugars and starches are examples of carbohydrates.

Carbon Nonmetallic element that is the basic constituent of all organic matter.

Carcinogenesis The production or origin of cancer.

C-Arm fluoroscope A portable device for producing real-time (motion) images of a patient. The opposite ends of the C-shaped support arm hold the x-ray tube and the image intensifier.

Catalyst Agent that affects the speed of a chemical reaction without being altered itself.

Catalytic failure The inability to influence the speed of a required chemical reaction (e.g., during protein synthesis).

Cataractogenesis The production or origin of cataracts.

Cataracts Opacity of the eye lens.

Cathode The negatively charged source of the high-speed electrons in an x-ray tube.

Cation A positively charged ion.

Cell division The multiplication process whereby one cell divides to form two or more cells.

Cell membrane A very frail structure encasing and surrounding the cell.

Cell metabolism Chemical reactions that modify foods for cellular use.

Cells The basic units of all living matter.

Cell survival curve Method of displaying the radiation sensitivity of a particular type of cell.

Cellular damage Injury on the cellular level resulting from sufficient exposure to ionizing radiation at the molecular level.

Center for Devices and Radiological Health (CDRH) Known before 1982 as the Bureau of Radiological Health (BRH), this agency is responsible for conducting an ongoing electronic product radiation control program.

Centigray One one-hundredth of a gray (1/100 Gy).

Centrioles A pair of small, hollow, cylindric structures located adjacent to the nucleus that are believed to play a part in the formation of the mitotic spindle during cell division.

Centromere A clear region on a chromosome where its two—or four—arms join.

Centrosomes Structures located in the center of the cell near the nucleus that contain the centrioles.

Cerebrovascular syndrome   Form of acute radiation syndrome that results from the central nervous system and the cardiovascular system receiving doses of 50 Gy (5000 rad) or more of ionizing radiation. Death may occur from a few hours to several days (2 or 3) after exposure.

Characteristic curve   A graph that represents the response of an image receptor to some probe. A film-screen characteristic curve plots the optical density of the developed film on the vertical axis as a function of the exposure (actually the logarithm of the exposure compared with a reference exposure—the "log relative exposure") on the horizontal axis.

Characteristic photon   A quantum or quantity of radiant energy given off by the parent atom when an electron from an outer shell drops down to fill an inner shell vacancy after the atom has interacted with an x-ray photon and lost an inner shell electron as a result. The energy of a characteristic photon is equivalent to the difference in energy level between the two electron shells.

Characteristic radiation   Radiation released as a result of the photoelectric effect that consists of photons whose energies represent the electron energy level structure of the atom with which it interacts. Characteristic radiation comprises about 10% of primary radiation, between 80 and 100 kVp.

Chromatid   A highly coiled strand; one of the two duplicate portions of DNA that appear during cell division.

Chromatid aberrations   Lesions that result when irradiation of individual chromatids occurs later in interphase, after DNA synthesis has taken place.

Chromosome aberrations   Lesions that result when irradiation occurs early in interphase, before DNA synthesis takes place.

Chromosome breakage   The breaking of one or both of the sugar-phosphate chains of a DNA molecule, which can be caused by exposure of the molecule to ionizing radiation.

Chromosomes   Small, rod-shaped bodies that contain genes.

Chronic   Something that continues for a long time (e.g., a chronic disease).

Cinefluorography   An imaging technique in which serial radiographic images are recorded over a short period of time (typically less than 30 seconds) on a strip of 16- or 35-mm film. During the recording the x-ray tube is operated continuously or near-continuously (pulsed rapidly on and off). The images are played back through a projector to allow study of motion within the patient, such as the spread of contrast material through vessels or the motion of structures within the heart.

Classical scattering   (See *Coherent scattering.*)

Clear lead   Transparent lead-plastic material that has been impregnated with approximately 30% lead by weight.

Cleaved chromosome   Broken chromosome.

Code of Standards for Diagnostic X-Ray Equipment   Effective as of August 1, 1974, this code established equipment performance standards for complete systems and major components manufactured after that date.

Coherent scattering   The process wherein a low-energy photon (less than 100 keV) interacts with an atom as a whole and the atom responds by releasing the excess energy it has received in the form of a scattered photon that has the same wavelength and energy as the original incident photon but emerges from the atom moving in a slightly different direction. This process is also known as *Rayleigh scattering, classical scattering,* and *unmodified scattering.*

Collective effective dose equivalent (S_E)   Used to describe radiation exposure of a population from different sources.

Compensating filter   A material such as aluminum or lead-acrylic inserted between the x-ray source and the patient to modify the quality (penetrating power, spectrum) of the beam across the field of view.

Compton scattered electron   An energetic electron dislodged from the outer shell of an atom of the irradiated object as a result of interacting with an incoming x-ray photon.

Compton scattering An interaction between an incoming x-ray photon and a loosely bound outer shell electron of an atom in the irradiated object in which the photon surrenders a portion of its kinetic energy to dislodge the electron from its outer shell orbit and then continues in a new direction. This process accounts for most of the scattered radiation produced during diagnostic procedures.

Computed tomography (CT) Process of creating a cross-sectional tomographic plane (slice) of any part of the body. The image is reconstructed by a computer using x-ray absorption measurements collected at multiple points around the periphery of the part being scanned.[1]

Cone A circular metal tube that attaches to the x-ray tube housing or variable rectangular collimator to limit the beam to a predetermined size and shape.

Congenital abnormalities Defects existing at birth that are not inherited but rather acquired during development in utero.

Contrast media A substance consisting of a high atomic solution (e.g., barium or iodine based) that is either ingested or injected into the biologic tissues or structures to be visualized.

Consumer–Patient Radiation Health and Safety Act of 1981 Provides federal legislation requiring the establishment of minimum standards for the accreditation of educational programs for persons who administer radiologic procedures and the certification of such persons.

Control badge Film badge provided by the monitoring company with each batch of badges to serve as a basis for comparison with the remainder of the film badges after the batch has been returned to the monitoring company for processing. The control badge determines whether the batch of badges has been exposed to radiation while in transit to or from the institution.

Controlled area A hospital area occupied by workers who have been trained in radiation safety procedures and who wear radiation monitoring devices.

Cosmic radiation (cosmic rays) Very-high-speed particles, mainly protons, that are generated as a result of extreme reactions within stars.

Coulomb (C) SI unit of electric charge equal to 1 ampere-second (the quantity of electric charge transferred across unit area by a current of 1 ampere in 1 second).

Coulomb per kilogram (C/kg) SI unit of radiation exposure: 1 coulomb per kilogram (C/kg) of air equals 1 SI unit of exposure, or $1/(2.58 \times 10^{-4})$ R = 3.88×10^3 R.

Covalent bond A chemical union between atoms that arises as a result of the sharing of one or more pairs of electrons.

Covalent cross-links (See *Covalent bond.*)

Cross-over Process occurring during meiosis wherein the chromatids exchange some chromosomal material (genes).

Cumulative effect (1) An effect that increases with additional exposure to ionizing radiation. (2) An effect that results from several different causes or repeated or long-term application of one or more agents.

Cumulative timing device A required device on a fluoroscopic x-ray unit that times the x-ray exposure and sounds an alarm or temporarily interrupts the exposure after the fluoroscope has been activated for 5 minutes.

Cumulative whole-body effective dose equivalent (EDE) limit The sum of effective dose from occupational exposure over a number of years (e.g., an entire career). The National Council on Radiation Protection and Measurement suggests that the value of the cumulative EDE not exceed the workers age in years multiplied by 10 mSv.

Curie The standard unit of radioactivity in use before the SI system of units was established. One curie is equal to 3.7×10^{10} disintegrations per second.

Cutie pie Nickname for an ionization chamber-type survey meter.

Cyclotrons Units that produce high-energy particles such as protons.

Cytoplasm The protoplasm that exists outside of the cell's nucleus.

Cytoplasmic organelles Small structures present in the cytoplasm of the cell.

Cytosine (C) One of two pyrimidine bases found in both DNA and RNA.

Daughter cell   A cell resulting from division of an individual parent cell.

Dead-man-type fluoroscopic exposure switch   A fluoroscopic exposure switch (operated by foot pressure) that requires continuous pressure from the operator. The exposure automatically terminates if the operator becomes incapacitated.

Deep dose   The dose equivalent from all types of radiation at a depth of 1 cm in soft tissue (as defined by Landauer, Inc.). This number is regarded as the dose equivalent to the whole body.

Deletion   A part of the chromosome or chromatid is lost at the next cell division, creating an aberration known as an *acentric fragment.*

Dendrites   Nerve cell processes that extend outward from the cell body and conduct impulses toward the cell body.

Densitometer   An instrument that can be used to determine the amount of radiation to which a film badge dosimeter has been exposed. It measures the degree of blackening or density of the radiographic film.

Deoxyribonucleic acid (DNA)   A type of nucleic acid that carries the genetic information necessary for cell replication and directs the building of proteins.

Deoxyribose   A five-carbon sugar molecule.

Desquamation   Shedding of the outer layer of skin.

Deterministic effects   (See *Nonstochastic effects.*)

Diagnostic efficacy   The degree to which the diagnostic study reveals the presence of disease in the patient when it is present and the absence of disease when it is absent.

Diagnostic-type protective tube housing   The lead-lined metal housing enclosing the x-ray tube that protects both the radiographer and the patient from leakage radiation by restricting the emission of x-rays to the area of the useful or primary beam (those x-rays emitted through the x-ray tube window or port).

Dicentric chromosomes   Chromosomes having two centromeres.

Diffusion   The motion of liquid, gas, or solid particles from an area of relatively high concentration to an area of lower concentration.

Direct action   Biologic damage occurring as a result of radiation interacting without an intermediary on master, or key, molecules (DNA). This interaction causes molecules to become either inactive or functionally altered.

Direct radiation   (See *Primary radiation.*)

DNA synthesis   The building-up of DNA macromolecules.

Dominant mutation   A genetic mutation that will probably be expressed in offspring.

Dose   The amount of radiant energy absorbed by an irradiated object per unit mass.

Dose commitment   The dose that could ultimately be delivered from a given intake of radionuclide.[2]

Dose equivalent (H)   The product obtained by multiplying the absorbed dose (AD) times the quality factor (QF). This quantity considers the biologic effects of various types of radiation on humans.

Dose equivalent limits   Established guidelines for occupational and nonoccupational radiation exposure.

Dose limitation   Restricting the amount of ionizing radiation received during a period of time to a specified limit.

Double-emulsion x-ray film   Film with emulsion coated on both sides.

Double-strand break   The ionization of a DNA macromolecule that results in the rupture of one or more of its chemical bonds and thereby creates one or more breaks in each of the two sugar-phosphate chains of the DNA ladderlike molecular structure.

Doubling dose   The radiation dose that causes the number of spontaneous mutations occurring in a given generation to increase to two times their original number.

Dry air   Air without humidity.

Early somatic effects   Effects of ionizing radiation that appear within minutes, hours, days, or weeks of the time of exposure; also called *acute effects.*

Effective atomic number   A composite atomic number for the many different chemical elements composing a material.

Effective communication   Communication between the radiographer and the patient in which verbal and nonverbal messages are understood as intended.

Effective dose Sometimes called *effective dose equivalent,* this dosimetry term attempts to specify the overall risk of harm to an organism. The term implies that the type of radiation (e.g., x-, gamma, neutron) and also the organ or body parts irradiated have been taken into account through the use of appropriate weighting factors.

Effective dose equivalent (H$_E$) The sum or total of both internal and external equivalent dose. It is used to relate the absorbed dose to different organs of the body when radiation exposure is localized.

Effective dose equivalent limit The upper boundary dose of ionizing radiation that will result in a negligible risk of bodily injury or genetic damage to the recipient.

Effective dose equivalent-limiting (EDE) system A method to determine the various risks of cancer and genetic effects to tissues or organs exposed to radiation.

Elective examinations Radiologic procedures not considered urgent by the referring physician. These examinations can be booked at an appropriate time to meet patient needs and safety.

Electrical potential difference (voltage difference) The change in electrical potential energy per unit electrical charge experienced by a charged particle as it moves from one position to another. The unit of electrical potential difference is called a *volt.*

Electrical potential energy The electrical energy acquired by a charged particle as a result of its position relative to other charged particles. The unit of electrical potential energy is the joule.

Electrolytes (See *Salts.*)

Electromagnetic radiation Composed of interacting, varying electric and magnetic fields that propagate through space at the speed of light. Electromagnetic radiation originates as a result of energy changes that occur within an atom or result from an interaction between an atom and some incident particle. Examples of electromagnetic radiation are radio waves, microwaves, visible light, ultraviolet rays, x-rays, and gamma rays.

Electrometer A device used to measure electrical charge.

Electron volt (eV) A unit of energy equivalent to the quantity of kinetic energy an electron acquires as it moves through a potential difference of 1 volt.

Electrons Negatively charged atomic particles.

Element A substance made up of atoms that all have the same atomic number and hence the same chemical properties.

Emaciation The state of being extremely thin.

Embryologic effects Damage to an organism that occurs as a result of exposure to ionizing radiation during the embryonic stage of development. These effects are also known as *birth effects.*

Endoplasmic reticulum A vast, irregular network of tubules and vesicles spreading and interconnecting in all directions throughout the cytoplasm.

Energy The ability to do work.

Entrance exposure Quantity of radiation, given in SI units of coulombs per kilogram or in traditional units of roentgens, incident upon an object. Backscatter radiation is excluded.

Enzymatic proteins Proteins that control the cell's various physiologic activities by functioning as catalysts.

Epidemiologic studies Observations and statistical analysis of data, such as incidence of disease within groups of people.

Epilation Loss of hair.

Epithelial tissue A substance that lines and covers body tissue; the cells that compose this tissue are highly radiosensitive.

Erg A unit of energy and work.

Erythema Diffused redness over an area of skin after irradiation.

Erythroblasts Red blood stem cells.

Erythrocytes Red blood cells.

Excess cancers Cancers that would not have occurred in a population without the exposure to ionizing radiation.

Excitation The addition of energy to a system, transforming it from a calm, or low-energy, state to an excited, or higher, energy state.

Exit or image formation radiation All of the x-ray photons that reach their destination (the film) after passing through the object being radiographed. This radiation was previously referred to as *remnant radiation.*

Exposure   The total electric charge per unit mass that x-ray and gamma ray photons with energies up to 3 Mev generate in air only. Exposure may be viewed as the amount of ionizing radiation that may strike an object, such as the human body, when in the vicinity of a radiation source. The SI unit of exposure is the coulomb per kilogram (C/kg). The traditional unit of exposure is the roentgen (R).

Exposure linearity   Consistency in radiation intensity stated in milliroentgens per milliampere-seconds (mR/mAs) when changing from one milliampere station to another with a variance of not more than 10%.

Exposure reproducibility   Consistency in output of radiation intensity from an individual exposure to other subsequent exposures.

Extension cylinder   A cylindric metal tube that possesses a 10- to 20-inch metal extension at the far end of the barrel to limit the size of the useful beam.

Extrapolate   To infer from known information.

Extremity dosimeter   A device that monitors the dose equivalent to the hands.

Fallout   Radiation produced as a consequence of nuclear weapons testing and chemical explosions in nuclear power plants.

Fats   Compounds composed of carbon, hydrogen, and oxygen, with the ratio of hydrogen atoms to oxygen atoms being very much greater than 2 to 1, the ratio that exists in carbohydrates. Fats are a rich energy source, yielding gram for gram over twice as much energy as carbohydrates.

Fatty acids   When the sugar glucose is broken down in the body during respiration, fats are among the generated intermediate products. When some of these fats combine with an acidic group of atoms (e.g., the carboxyl group: COOH), an acid is formed. It is called a *fatty acid*. An example is CH_3COOH, which is commonly known as *acetic acid*. Fatty acids are constituents of amino acids, from which proteins are built.

Fetus   A developing human in utero.

Fiber   A protracted, threadlike structure.

Fibril   A minute fiber or strand that is frequently part of a compound fiber.

Fibrosis   Abnormal formation of fibrous tissue.

Film badge dosimeter   The most widely used and economical type of personnel monitoring device, it records radiation exposure accumulated at a low rate over a long period of time.

Filtration   Elements that are part of or added to the x-ray tube to reduce exposure to the patient's skin and superficial tissue. Filtration elements function by absorbing most of the lower-energy photons from the heterogeneous beam, thereby increasing its mean energy.

First trimester   The first 3 months of gestation.

Fission   The splitting of the nuclei of atoms whereby some mass is converted into energy.

Fixed radiographic equipment   Radiologic equipment that is installed in and cannot be moved from a specific place in an imaging facility.

Flat contact shield   Uncontoured lead strip or lead-impregnated material placed directly over the patient's reproductive organs to provide protection from exposure to ionizing radiation.

Fluorescent radiation   (See *Characteristic radiation*.)

Fluorescent yield   Refers to the number of characteristic x-rays emitted per K-shell vacancy.

Fluoroscopic exposure monitor   A device that "provides an instantaneous audible indication of the intensity of secondary radiation."[3] It emits "a soft chirping signal, whose frequency varies in direct proportion to the exposure rate."[4]

Fluoroscopic exposure switch (foot pedal)   A deadman type of switch that causes the fluoroscopic tube to emit x-radiation as long as the operator continues to apply pressure to the foot pedal.

Focal spot   The area on the anode of the x-ray tube from which the x-rays appear to emanate.

Forward scatter   Photons that have interacted with the atoms of an object and consequently are deflected forward (toward the radiographic film). (See also *Small angle scatter*.)

Free air ionization chamber   An instrument used in a calibration laboratory to obtain a precise measurement of exposure to x radiation.

Free radical   (1) A solitary atom or most often a combination of atoms that behaves as an extremely reactive single entity. (2) A configuration of either one or more atoms having no net electrical charge.

Frequency   The number of vibrations or waves per second (crests or cycles per second).

Gadolinium   A rare-earth phosphor used in rare-earth intensifying screens.

Gamma rays   Short-wavelength, high-energy electromagnetic waves emitted by the nuclei of radioactive substances. Although generally shorter in wavelength than x-rays and with a different point of origin, their other characteristics are identical to those of diagnostic x-rays.

Gastrointestinal (GI) syndrome   A form of acute radiation syndrome that appears in humans at a whole-body threshold dose of approximately 6 Gy (600 rad) and peaks after a dose of 10 Gy (1000 rad).

Geiger–Müller (G–M) detector   A device that detects individual radioactive particles (e.g., electrons emitted from certain radioactive nuclei) or photons and that serves as the primary radiation survey instrument for area monitoring in nuclear medicine facilities.

Genes   The basic units of heredity.

Genetic cells (germ cells)   Cells of the human body associated with reproduction.

Genetic damage   Radiation damage to generations yet unborn.

Genetic effects   Biologic effects of ionizing radiation on generations yet unborn.

Genetically significant dose (GSD)   The dose equivalent to the reproductive organs that, if received by every human, would be expected to cause an identical gross genetic injury to the total population as does the sum of the actual doses received by exposed individual population members. For the population of the United States, this dose is estimated to be about 0.20 mSv (20 mrem).

Germ cells   Reproductive cells.

Glucose   The primary energy source for the cell.

Glycerine   A sweet, colorless, odorless, syrupy liquid obtained from fats that are soluble in water. It is often used as a moistening agent.

Golgi apparatus   Tiny sacs located near the cell nucleus, the Golgi apparatus synthesizes glycoproteins and transports enzymes and hormones through the cell membrane.

Gonadal shielding devices   Used during radiologic procedures to protect the reproductive organs from exposure to the useful beam when they are in or within approximately 5 cm of a properly collimated beam, unless this would compromise the diagnostic value of the examination.

Gonads   Male and female reproductive organs.

Gram   A unit of mass of the metric system. An object near the earth's surface that has a mass of 454 grams will weigh 1 pound.

Granule   A small particle such as the insoluble nonmembranous particles found in cytoplasm.

Granulocyte   A scavenger type of white blood cell that fights bacteria.

Gray (Gy)   SI unit of absorbed dose. An energy absorption of 1 joule (J) per kilogram (kg) in the irradiated object.

Guanine (G)   One of two purine bases found in both DNA and RNA.

Half–life   Statistical quantity equal to the amount of time associated with a 50% decrease in the radioactivity of a sample containing a very large number of radioactive atoms.

Half–value layer (HVL)   The thickness of a designated absorber (customarily a metal such as aluminum) required to decrease the intensity of the primary beam by 50% of its initial value.

Hematopoietic syndrome (bone marrow syndrome)   A form of acute radiation syndrome that occurs when humans receive whole-body doses of ionizing radiation ranging from 1 to 10 Gy (100 to 1000 rad) and in which the reduction of the number of blood cells in the circulating blood results in a loss of the body's ability to clot blood and fight infection.

Hemoglobin   A protein; the oxygen-carrying pigment of the red blood cells (erythrocytes).

Hemorrhage   Abnormal escape of blood; heavy bleeding.

Hibakusha   Japanese atomic bomb survivors.

High–LET radiation   Includes particles that possess substantial mass and charge such as alpha particles, ions of heavier nuclei, and charged particles released from interactions between neutrons and atoms. Low-energy neutrons, which carry no electrical charge, are also a high-LET radiation.

High–level control (HLC) fluoroscopy An operating mode of fluoroscopic equipment in which exposure rates are higher than normally allowed for routine fluoroscopic procedures. The higher exposure rate allows visualization of smaller and lower-contrast objects than are normally visible during fluoroscopy. It is used for interventional procedures in which visualization of fine catheters or other structures is of critical importance. An audible signal constantly reminds personnel that the high-level control is being used.

Highly differentiated cells Mature or more specialized cells.

High resolution The ability of a system to make two adjacent objects visually distinguishable.

High–speed image receptor system A relative term that describes an image receptor that requires less exposure to obtain a response, such as storage of a digital image or a chemical change such as an increase in optical density (darkening) of film.

Holistic approach to patient care Treating the whole person rather than just the area of concern.

Homeostasis A state of equilibrium between the different elements of an organism or a tendency toward such a state; the ability of the body to return to and maintain normal functioning despite the changes it has undergone.

Hormones Chemical secretions manufactured by various endocrine glands and carried by the bloodstream to influence activities of other parts of the body. Hormones regulate body functions such as growth and development.

Hydrocephaly Abnormal fluid in the brain.

Hydrogen peroxide A cellular poison that can result from the radiolysis of water.

Hydroperoxyl radical A substance toxic to the cell that can result from the radiolysis of water.

Hyperbaric oxygen High-pressure oxygen sometimes used in radiotherapy treatment of certain types of cancerous tumors to increase their radiosensitivity.

Hypoxic cells Cells that lack an adequate amount of oxygen.

Image intensification fluoroscopy Use of an image intensifier to increase the brightness of the real-time image produced on a fluorescent screen during fluoroscopy. Virtually all modern fluoroscopy is image intensification fluoroscopy.

Image intensifier A device that increases the brightness of an image. An image is produced on a fluorescent screen by x-rays at the input end (input phosphor). The bright image at the output end (output phosphor) is viewed by a television camera, film, or other recording device.

Image receptor Radiographic film or phosphorescent screen.

Incident photon Incoming photon.

Incoherent scattering (See *Compton scattering.*)

Indirect action Involves the effects of reactive free radicals created by the interaction of radiation with water molecules. These agents can cause substantial disruption to master molecules, resulting in cell death.

Inelastic scatter The interaction of an incident photon with a loosely bound outer shell electron of the target atom in which the photon surrenders some of its kinetic energy to free the electron from its orbit and then continues on its way in a new direction.

Inherent filtration The glass envelope encasing the x-ray tube, the insulating oil surrounding the tube, and the glass window in the tube housing. It amounts to approximately 0.5-mm aluminum equivalent.

Inorganic compounds Compounds that do not contain carbon. The inorganic compounds found in the human body occur in nature independent of living things.

Instant cell death Immediate death of large numbers of cells occurring when a volume is irradiated with an x-ray or gamma ray dose of about 1000 Gy (100,000 rad) in a period of seconds or a few minutes.

Intensifying screens By amplifying the exit or image formation radiation reaching the radiographic film, intensifying screens enhance the action of x-rays on the film. They convert x-ray energy into visible light. Light forms more than 99% of the latent image, and x-ray photons contribute less than 1%. The visible light enhancement produced by the intensifying screens greatly aids in reducing patient dose.

Intensity (of radiation) Quantity or amount (of radiation) crossing unit area per unit time.

Interference of function Permanent or temporary interference of cellular function independent of the cell's ability to divide can be brought about by exposure to ionizing radiation.

Intermittent fluoroscopy Periodic activation of the fluoroscopic tube by the operator.

International Commission on Radiological Protection (ICRP) Evaluates information on biologic effects of radiation and provides radiation protection guidance through general recommendations regarding occupational and public dose limits.

International system of units (SI) System of units that allows an interchange of units among all branches of science throughout the world.

Interphase The period of cell growth that occurs before actual cell division.

Interphase death (See *Apoptosis.*)

Interslice scatter Radiation that scatters from the CT slice being scanned into adjacent slices.

Interstrand cross-link A cross-link formed between complementary DNA strands or between entirely different DNA molecules.

Intrastrand cross-link A cross-link formed between two places on the same DNA strand.

Interventional procedures Medical procedures performed by a physician during an imaging procedure such as fluoroscopy. The interventional physician, usually a radiologist or cardiologist, inserts catheters into vessels or tissues for the purpose of drainage, biopsy, or alteration of vascular occlusions or malformations.

Inverse square falloff of radiation intensity with distance A consequence of this decrease in radiation intensity as the square of the distance from the radiation source is that when a small source-skin distance is employed, patient entrance exposure is significantly greater than the exit exposure. This results in the entrance surface receiving an unnecessary high exposure. When the source-to-object distance is increased, a more uniform exposure throughout the patient is maintained.

Inverse square law (ISL) The intensity of the radiation at any location decreases with the square of its distance from the source of radiation. Thus tripling a person's separation from a radiation source causes the exposure received by that person to decrease by a factor of 3^2, or 9.

Involuntary motion Motion that cannot be willfully controlled. It is caused by muscle groups such as those of the digestive organs and heart.

Ionization The conversion of atoms to ions.

Ionization chamber A device that measures the amount of electrical charge resulting from the presence of all the ions of one sign produced during the irradiation of a specific volume of air.

Ionization chamber–type survey meter (cutie pie) Both an exposure rate meter normally used for area surveys as well as an accurate integrating or cumulative exposure device for x- or gamma radiation. If equipped with a suitable window, it can also measure beta radiation.

Ionize To remove electrons.

Ionizing radiation Radiation that on passing through matter produces positively and negatively charged particles (ions).

Ion pair Two oppositely charged particles.

Ions Positively and negatively charged particles.

Isotope An atom that contains a different number of neutrons but the same number of protons in its nucleus as does the reference atom (e.g., helium-3 and helium-4, whose nuclei contain one and two neutrons respectively). Radioactive isotopes of atoms that make up biologic materials may be used in medical imaging nuclear medicine studies.

Joule (J) A unit of energy. It is the work done or energy expended when a force of 1 newton acts on an object along a distance of 1 meter.

Key molecule (See *Master molecule.*)

Kiloelectron volt (keV) A unit used to measure the kinetic energy of an individual electron in the high-speed electron stream within the x-ray tube; it is equivalent to 1000 electron volts (1 keV = 1000 eV). This unit is also used to measure the energies of x-rays. The keV and kVp for x-ray beams differ. An x-ray beam with a broad spectrum of photon energies 100 kVp corresponds approximately to an effective energy of 35 keV.

Kilogram (kg) 1000 grams.

Kilovolt (kV) Electrical potential equal to 1000 volts.

Kinetic energy Energy of motion.

Lanthanum A rare-earth phosphor used in rare-earth intensifying screens.

Last-frame-hold feature An optional equipment feature in which the most recent fluoroscopic image remains in view as a guide to the radiologist when the x-ray beam is off.

Late somatic effects Nongenetic effects that appear after a period of months or years following exposure to ionizing radiation.

Latent period The period after the prodromal stage of acute radiation syndrome during which no visible effects or symptoms of radiation exposure occur.

Law of Bergonié and Tribondeau The radiosensitivity of cells is directly proportional to their reproductive activity and inversely proportional to their degree of differentiation.

LD 50/30 A quantitative measurement signifying the whole-body dose of radiation that can be lethal to 50% of the exposed population within 30 days. For adult humans, LD 50/30 is about 3.0 Gy (300 rad).

LD 50/60 A quantitative measurement signifying the whole-body dose of radiation that can be lethal to 50% of the exposed population within 60 days.

Lead-equivalent Thickness of radiation-absorbing material that produces an attenuation equivalent to that which would be accomplished by a specified amount of lead (Pb).

Leakage radiation Photons that instead of coming out of the collimator opening with the useful beam emerge in multiple directions through the protective housing of the x-ray tube. Regulatory standards require that the leakage radiation exposure rate at 1 meter from the tube target should not exceed 100 mR per hour when the x-ray unit is run at maximum operating conditions.

Leukemia A neoplastic overproduction of white blood cells.

Leukemogenesis The production or origin of leukemia.

Leukocytes White blood cells.

Leukopenia An abnormal decrease of white blood corpuscles usually below 5000/mm^3.

Light-localizing variable-aperture rectangular collimator A versatile device for defining the size and shape of the radiographic beam. It is box-shaped and contains the radiographic beam-defining system, which consists of two sets of adjustable lead shutters mounted within the device at different levels, a light source to illuminate the x-ray field and permit it to be centered over the area of clinical interest, and a mirror to deflect the light toward the object to be radiographed.

Linear dose-response curve A model used to calculate the occurrence of cancer by extrapolating from information associated with high levels of radiation to determine the risk associated with low doses. The linear dose-response curve describes current high-dose information satisfactorily but exaggerates the actual risk or danger at low doses and dose rates.

Linear energy transfer (LET) The average energy deposited per unit path length to a medium by ionizing radiation as it passes through that medium.

Linear, nonthreshold dose-response relationship The relationship between dose and response is such that the chance of sustaining biologic damage and the amount of that biologic damage are directly proportional to the magnitude of the ionizing radiation exposure; even the most minuscule radiation dose has the potential to cause some damage.

Linear-quadratic dose-response curve A model used to calculate the occurrence of cancer by extrapolating from information associated with high levels of radiation to determine the risk associated with low doses. This model fits current high-dose information satisfactorily but may underestimate risk at low doses.

Linear, threshold dose-response relationship The relationship between dose and response is such that a biologic response does not occur below a specified level of radiation dose.

Lipids Water-insoluble organic macromolecules that consist only of carbon, hydrogen, and oxygen. Among other functions, lipids store energy for the body for long periods of time.

Lithium fluoride (LiF) The sensing material of the thermoluminescent dosimeter (TLD).

Log, or logarithmic, scale A method used to graph data that cover several orders of magnitude (the powers of ten; e.g., 1, 10, 100, 1000). The scale itself is compressed so that the first section of the scale covers one range of powers of ten, such as 0.1 to 1, the next section covers 1 to 10, the next 10 to 100, and so on.

Long scale of radiographic contrast Radiographic contrast in which there are many shades of gray. A wide range of exposures will produce a wide range of shades of gray when a long scale image receptor or display is used.

Low-LET radiations External electromagnetic radiations such as x-rays and gamma rays that have neither mass nor charge.

Low-level radiation "An absorbed dose of [0.1 Sv] 10 rem or less delivered over a short period of time" or "a larger dose delivered over a long period of time, for instance, [0.5 Sv] 50 rem in 10 years."[5]

Luminance A scientific term that refers to the brightness of a surface. Luminance quantifies the intensity of a light source (i.e., the amount of light per unit area coming from its surface).

Lymphocyte A type of white blood cell that plays an active role in producing immunity for the body by producing antibodies to combat disease. Lymphocytes are the most radiosensitive blood cells in the human body.

Lysosomes Small pealike sacs containing digestive enzymes.

M On a personnel monitoring report, this letter signifies that a dose equivalent below the minimum measurable quantity of radiation has been received during the interval of time covered by the report.

Macromolecule Large molecule built up from smaller chemical structures.

Mammography Radiographic study of the breast.

Manifest illness The stage of acute radiation syndrome during which symptoms become visible.

Man-made radiation Ionizing radiation created by humans for various uses, including nuclear fuel for generation of power, consumer products containing radioactive material, and medical radiation. It also is called *artificial radiation.*

Man-rem Traditional radiation unit for the quantity collective effective dose equivalent (S_E).

mAs (See *Milliampere-seconds.*)

Mass density Quantity of matter per unit volume. It is generally specified in units of kilograms per cubic meter (kg/m^3) or grams per cubic centimeter (gm/cc).

Master molecule A molecule vital to the survival of the cell. It maintains normal cell function. It is also referred to as a *key molecule.*

Matter-antimatter annihilation reaction The destructive interaction between matter and antimatter. In pair production the combining of a positron with an electron, resulting in the mutual elimination of the electron and the positron and the transformation of their masses into energy that is carried by two photons of 0.511 MeV each. These photons emerge in opposite directions from the annihilation site. In this process, mass has been converted into energy.

Maximum permissible dose (MPD) A term used in the past to indicate the maximum dose equivalent of ionizing radiation that an occupationally exposed person could absorb in a specified time period without sustaining appreciable bodily injury.

Mean energy The average energy of an x-ray beam.

Mean active bone marrow dose "The average radiation dose to the entire active bone marrow."[6]

Medical exposure Exposure to ionizing radiation incurred for the purpose of obtaining medical diagnosis or undergoing treatment.

Megakaryocytes Platelet stem cells.

Meiosis The process of germ (genetic) cell division, which reduces the chromosomes in each daughter cell to half the number of chromosomes in the parent cell.

Mesons Penetrating, unstable, subatomic particles that are components of cosmic radiation.

Metabolism Chemical reactions that modify foods for cellular use.

Metaphase That phase of cell division during which the mitotic spindle is completed.

Milliampere-seconds (mAs) The product of x-ray electron tube current and the amount of time in seconds that the x-ray is on.

Milligray (mGy) One one-thousandth of a gray (1/1000 Gy).

Millirad (mrad) One one-thousandth of a rad (1/1000 rad).

Millirem (mrem)   One one-thousandth of a rem (1/1000 rem).

Millisievert (mSv)   One one-thousandth of a sievert (1/1000 Sv).

Mitochondria   Large bean-shaped structures containing highly organized enzymes, which function as "powerhouses" for the cell.

Mitosis   The process of somatic cell division wherein a parent cell divides to form two daughter cells identical to the parent cell.

Mitotic death (genetic death)   Cell death occurring after one or more divisions following irradiation.

Mitotic delay   The failure of a cell to start dividing on time; can occur when a cell is exposed to as little as 0.01 Gy (1 rad) of ionizing radiation just before it would begin to divide.

Mitotic spindle   The delicate fibers attached to the centrioles and extending from one side of the cell to the other.

Mobile radiographic equipment   Manually portable radiologic equipment.

Modified scattering   (See *Compton scattering.*)

Molecular change   An alteration in the basic structure of a molecule caused by some type of destructive process, such as exposure to ionizing radiation.

Molecular damage   Injury on the molecular level resulting from exposure to ionizing radiation.

Molecular lesions   (See *Point lesions.*)

Molecule   The smallest unit of a specific substance composed of one or more atoms.

Molten   Melted or liquefied by heat.

Muscle tissue   Contains fibers that affect movement of an organ or part of the body; muscle tissue does not divide and is relatively insensitive to radiation.

Mutagenesis   Birth defects caused by irradiation of reproductive cells (sperm and ova) before conception.

Mutagens   Agents that can increase the frequency of occurrence of mutations, such as elevated temperatures, ionizing radiations, viruses, and chemicals.

Mutation frequency   The number of spontaneous or mutagen-caused mutations that occur in a given generation.

Mutations   Changes in genes caused by the loss or change of a base in the DNA chain.

Myeloblasts   Precursors of granulocytes, a type of white blood cell.

National Academy of Science/National Research Council Committee on the Biological Effects of Ionizing Radiation (NAS/NRC–BEIR)   Reviews studies of the biologic effects of ionizing radiation and risk assessment and provides the information to organizations for evaluation.

National Council on Radiation Protection and Measurements (NCRP)   Reviews regulations formulated by the ICRP and decides how to include them in U.S. radiation protection criteria.

National Institute of Standards and Technology (NIST)   Professional organization responsible for accrediting calibration laboratories that measure radiation exposure in medical radiography.

Natural background radiation   Ionizing radiation from environmental sources, including radioactive materials in the earth, cosmic radiation from space, and radionuclides deposited in the human body.

Necrosis   Death of areas of tissue or bone surrounded by healthy parts.

Negatron   A normal electron carrying a negative charge.

Neonatal death   Death at birth.

Nervous tissue   Found in the brain and spinal cord, this tissue is highly specialized in the adult and does not divide. If damaged but not destroyed by exposure to radiation, nerve cells may still be able to function, but their function may be impaired. Very high doses of radiation will cause severe damage to the central nervous system. Nerve tissue in the embryo-fetus is more radiation sensitive. Irradiation can lead to CNS anomalies.

Neutrino   An electrically neutral particle that according to current theory has almost negligible mass. Thus the neutrino shows an exceedingly small tendency to interact with any type of matter.

Neutron   An electrically neutral particle, one of the fundamental constituents of the atom; located within the nucleus of the atom. The mass of the neutron is just slightly greater than that of the proton.

Neutrophils   Leukocytes that fight infection.

Newton   Unit of force in the meter-kilogram-second system of physical units. One newton corresponds to approximately one quarter of a pound.

Nit   (See *Candela per square meter.*)

Nitrogen   A tasteless, odorless, colorless gaseous chemical element found free in the air. Because nitrogen is an integral part of protein and nucleic acids and thus found in every living cell, it is important biologically.

Nitrogenous bases Organic bases that contain the element nitrogen.

Nonagreement states Individual states in the United States in which both the state Department of Environmental Protection and the Nuclear Regulatory Commission (NRC) enforce radiation protection regulations.

Nonoccupational exposure Radiation exposure received by members of the general population who are not employed as radiation workers.

Nonoccupational persons Any persons not employed as radiation workers.

Non–image–intensified fluoroscopy A procedure that employs a fluoroscopic screen made of zinc cadmium sulfide that produces a fluoroscopic image of the area of clinical interest of a very low brightness level. This technique is considered outmoded and has been superseded by image-intensified fluoroscopy.

Non–self-reading pocket dosimeter A pocket ionization chamber that requires a special accessory electrometer to read the device and is used for personnel monitoring in areas of low radiation exposure when immediate readout is not necessary.

Nonspecific life span shortening Life span shortening that results from premature but not peculiar diseases. Radiation-induced life span shortening is nonspecific.

Nonstochastic effects Biologic effects of ionizing radiation that demonstrate the existence of a threshold and the severity of the biologic damage increases as a consequence of increased absorbed dose. These effects are also known as *deterministic effects.*

Nonverbal messages Unconscious actions or body language.

Nuclear medicine procedure The administration, either orally or intravenously, of a radioactive isotope for the purpose of conducting a diagnostic study of a body area. The isotope is associated with a chemical compound that preferentially concentrates in the body area of interest.

Nuclear reactor A mechanism for creating and continuing a controlled nuclear chain reaction in a fissionable fuel for the production of energy or supplementary fissionable material.

Nucleic acids Large, complex macromolecules made up of nucleotides.

Nucleotides Units formed from a nitrogenous base such as adenine, guanine, cytosine or thymine, a five-carbon sugar molecule, deoxyribose, and a phosphate molecule. Several nucleotides make up a nucleic acid.

Nucleus The center of the cell; a spherical mass of protoplasm containing the genetic material (DNA), which is stored in its molecular structure. The nucleus also contains a rounded body called the *nucleolus,* which holds a large amount of RNA.

Occupancy factor (T) A factor used to modify the shielding requirement for a particular barrier by taking into account the fraction of the x-ray unit's workload for which there is occupancy beyond that barrier.

Occupational and nonoccupational dose equivalent limits Upper boundary doses of ionizing radiation that will result in a negligible risk of bodily injury or genetic damage.

Occupational exposure Radiation exposure received by radiation workers in the course of exercising their professional responsibilities.

Occupationally exposed person Individuals employed as radiation workers.

Off-focus radiation X-rays emitted from parts of the tube other than the focal spot. This is also called *stem radiation.*

Oogonium Female germ cell.

Optimization (See *ALARA concept.*)

Optical density The intensity of light transmitted through a given area of the medical imaging film.

Organic acids Organic compounds containing the carboxyl (COOH) group (e.g., acetic acid, the distinctive component of vinegar, has the chemical formula CH_3COOH).

Organic compounds All carbon compounds, both natural and artificial.

Organic damage Genetic or somatic changes in the organism, such as mutations, cataracts, and leukemia, which result from sufficient radiation-induced damage at the cellular level.

Organogenesis (1) Period of gestation from the second to the eighth week after conception during which the nerve cells in the brain and spinal cord of the fetus develop and the fetus is most susceptible to radiation-induced congenital abnormalities. (2) The stage in which the undifferentiated cells are implanted in the uterine wall.

Organ-weighing factor (W$_T$) A factor that "indicates the ratio of the risk of stochastic effects attributable to irradiation of a given organ or tissue to the total risk when the whole body is uniformly irradiated."[7]

Osmotic pressure The force created when a semipermeable membrane separates two solutions of different concentration.

Osteogenic sarcoma Bone cancer.

Osteoporosis Decalcification of the bone.

Oxidation Most simply, the combining of a substance with oxygen. The oxidation of iron leads to iron oxide, commonly known as *rust*. The definition of oxidation, however, has been broadened to include reactions in which electrons are lost by an atom.

Oxygen enhancement ratio (OER) A ratio of the radiation dose required to cause a particular biologic response of cells or organisms in an oxygen-deprived environment to the radiation dose required to cause an identical response under normally oxygenated conditions.

Pair production Interaction between an incoming photon of at least 1.022 MeV and an atom of the irradiated object in which the photon approaches, strongly interacts with the nucleus of the atom of the irradiated material, and disappears. In the process the energy of the incoming photon is transformed into two new particles, a negatron and a positron, after which these particles exit from the atom in opposite directions.

Particulate radiation As opposed to x-rays and gamma rays, examples of particulate radiation are electrons, protons, neutrons, alpha particles (nuclei of helium), and so forth.

Patient restraint Immobilization of the patient by mechanical device or human restraint during a radiologic procedure.

Peak voltage Maximum voltage directed across an x-ray tube.

Peptic bond Chemical bond connecting two amino acids.

Permeable Penetrable.

Personnel dosimeter A device that provides an indication of the exposure received by radiation workers as a result of their working habits and working conditions.

Personnel dosimetry Monitoring of radiation exposure to any person occupationally exposed on a regular basis.

Personnel monitoring report A written report of occupational radiation exposure of personnel prepared by a monitoring company.

Person-sievert SI radiation unit for the quantity collective effective dose equivalent (S$_E$).

Photoelectric absorption An interaction between an x-ray photon and an inner shell electron in which the photon surrenders all its kinetic energy to the orbital electron and ceases to exist. As a result, the electron escapes its inner shell and leaves the atom. Characteristic x-radiation is also emitted from the atom when an outer shell electron fills the inner shell vacancy. Photoelectric absorption is the process most responsible for the contrast between bone and soft tissue in diagnostic radiographs.

Photoelectron The electron ejected from its inner shell orbit during the process of photoelectric absorption.

Photon A particle associated with electromagnetic radiation that has neither mass nor electric charge.

Photopic vision Cone vision.

Picocurie A very small quantity of radioactivity equivalent to one trillionth (10^{-12}) of a curie.

Platelets Circular or oval disks found in the blood of all vertebrates. Platelets initiate blood clotting and prevent hemorrhage.

Pocket ionization chamber (pocket dosimeter) A personnel monitoring device that contains a positively charged electrode and a negatively charged electrode; when these electrodes are exposed to ionizing radiation, the air around the positively charged electrode is ionized and discharges the mechanism in direct proportion to the amount of radiation to which it has been exposed.

Point lesions (molecular lesions) Injured areas in molecules caused by the breaking of a single chemical bond.

Point mutations Genetic mutations in which the chromosome is not broken but the DNA within it is damaged. (See *Single-strand break.*)

Portable radiographic equipment (See *Mobile radiographic equipment.*)

Positive beam limitation (PBL) A feature of current radiographic collimators that automatically adjusts the collimators so that the radiation field size matches the film size.

Positron A positively charged electron, which is a form of antimatter.

Potential difference The difference in electrical potential or voltage between two points in a circuit.

Potential risk The possibility of inducing a radiogenic cancer or genetic defect after irradiation.

Precursor cells (see *Stem cells.*)

Preimplantation stage About 0 to 9 days after conception.

Primary beam (See *Useful beam.*)

Primary protective barrier (1) A barrier designed to prevent primary or direct radiation from reaching personnel or members of the general public on the other side of the barrier. (2) A barrier located perpendicular to the line of travel of the primary x-ray beam.

Primary radiation Radiation that emerges directly from the x-ray tube collimator and moves without deflection toward a wall, door, viewing window, and so on. It is also called *direct radiation.*

Probabilistic effects (See *Stochastic effects.*)

Prodromal syndrome The first stage of acute radiation syndrome, prodromal syndrome occurs within hours after a whole-body absorbed dose of 1 Gy (100 rad) or more. The stage is characterized by nausea, vomiting, diarrhea, fatigue, and leukopenia.

Programmed cell death (See *Apoptosis.*)

Prophase The phase of cell division during which the nucleus and the chromosomes enlarge and the DNA begins to take structural form.

Proportional counter A radiation survey instrument generally used in a laboratory setting to detect alpha and beta radiation and small amounts of other types of low-level radioactive contamination.

Protective apparel Special garments such as aprons, gloves, and thyroid shields that are conventionally made of lead-impregnated vinyl and worn during fluoroscopic and certain selective radiographic procedures. In the diagnostic x-ray energy range, they attenuate ionizing radiation to provide a significantly higher degree of radiation protection for the wearer.

Protective barrier Any medium of adequate composition and thickness that absorbs primary and/or secondary radiation, thereby reducing exposure of persons located on the other side of the barrier.

Protective curtain A sliding panel with a minimum of 0.25-mm lead equivalent attached to the front of the spot film device of a fluoroscopic x-ray unit for the purpose of intercepting scattered radiation before it reaches the fluoroscopist.

Protective eyeglasses Eyeglasses with optically clear lenses that contain a minimum lead-equivalent protection of 0.35 mm. Side shields on the protective glasses are also available for procedures that require turning of the head. A wrap-around frame containing optically clear lenses with a 0.5-mm lead equivalency is also available.

Protective lead apron (See *Protective apparel.*)

Protective lead gloves (See *Protective apparel.*)

Protein Amino acids linked in various patterns and combinations. They contain carbon, hydrogen, nitrogen, oxygen, and occasionally other elements, such as sulfur.

Protein synthesis The making of new proteins.

Proton One of the three main constituents of an atom, the other two being electrons and neutrons. The proton carries a positive electrical charge equal in magnitude to that of an electron. The proton, which is located within the central core or nucleus of the atom, has a mass in excess of 1800 times that of an electron. The combination of one proton and one electron constitutes the simplest atom.

Protoplasm The building material of all living things, protoplasm consists of inorganic substances, such as water and mineral salts, and organic substances, including proteins, carbohydrates, lipids, and nucleic acids.

Purines A class of nitrogenous bases found in DNA or RNA. These bases include adenine (A) and guanine (G).

Pyrimidines A class of nitrogenous bases found in DNA and/or RNA. These bases include cytosine (C), thymine (T), or uracil (U).

Quality factor (Q or QF) A modifying factor used in the calculation of the dose equivalent to determine the ability of a dose of any kind of ionizing radiation to cause biologic damage.

Quantum mottle Faint blotches in the recorded radiographic image produced by an intrinsic fluctuation in the incident photon intensity. This effect is more noticeable when very-high-speed rare-earth systems are used.

Rad ("radiation–absorbed–dose") The unit that indicates the amount of radiant energy transferred to an irradiated object by any type of ionizing radiation. One rad is equivalent to an energy transfer of 100 erg per gram of irradiated object. It also is equivalent to $1/_{100}$ J/kg. Because 1 joule equals 10^7 ergs and 1 kilogram equals 10^3 grams, 100 erg/g $= 100 \times 10^{-7}$ J/10^{-3} kg $= 10^{-2}$ J/kg $= 1/_{100}$ J/kg.

Radiant energy Energy that moves in the form of a wave and is transmitted by radiations such as x-rays and gamma rays.

Radiation A transfer of energy that results from either a change occurring naturally within an atom (see *radiation decay*) or a process caused by the interaction of a particle with an atom.

Radiation biology The science concerned with the effects of ionizing radiations on living systems.

Radiation Control for Health and Safety Act of 1968 Law passed by Congress (Public Law 90-602) to protect the public from the hazards of unnecessary radiation exposure resulting from electronic products such as microwave ovens, color televisions, and diagnostic x-ray equipment.

Radiation decay A naturally occurring process in which atoms with unstable nuclei relieve that instability by various types of nuclear spontaneous emissions, including charged particles, uncharged particles, and photons.

Radiation dose–response curve A graph that maps out the effects of radiation observed in relation to the dose of radiation received.

Radiation hormesis effect A beneficial consequence of radiation for populations continuously exposed to moderately higher levels of radiation.

Radiation dosimetry film Radiographic film that is sensitive to doses ranging from as low as 0.1 mSv (10 mrem) to as high as 5000 mSv (500 rem). It is contained in the film badge dosimeter packet.

Radiation monitoring device A device worn by diagnostic radiology personnel to indicate occupational exposure by measuring the quantity of radiation to which it has been exposed over time.

Radiation permeability The ability of a structure to be penetrated by radiation.

Radiation protection Tools and techniques employed by radiation workers to protect patients and personnel from exposure to ionizing radiation.

Radiation safety officer (RSO) A qualified individual such as a medical physicist, health physicist, or radiologist designated by an institution and approved by the Nuclear Regulatory Commission and the state to ensure that internationally accepted guidelines for radiation protection are followed by the institution. The RSO is responsible for developing an appropriate radiation safety program for the institution and maintaining radiation monitoring records for all personnel.

Radiation survey instruments Area monitoring devices that detect and/or measure radiation.

Radiation therapy treatment Use of x- or gamma rays, usually with energies much greater than those employed for diagnostic purposes, to destroy the cells composing a tumor while sparing the surrounding nontumor tissues.

Radicals Groups of atoms that remain together during a chemical change and behave almost like a single atom. Atoms in a radical are held together by covalent bonding.

Radioactive nuclides (radionuclides) Unstable atomic species that change naturally into other atomic species by altering their nuclear structure. They give off ionizing radiation during their disintegration (radioactive decay) process.

Radiogenic malignancies Cancerous neoplasms induced by exposure to ionizing radiation.

Radiographer A person qualified through formal education and certification to practice medical imaging procedures and provide related patient care.

Radiographic beam–light beam coincidence Means that both physical size (length and width) and alignment between the radiographic beam and the localizing light beam must correspond to within 2% of the source-image distance (SID).

Radiographic contrast Differences in density level between the radiographic images of objects in a radiograph.

Radiographic grid A device (made of parallel radiopaque lead strips alternated with low attenuation strips of aluminum, plastic, or wood) placed between the patient and the film to remove scattered x-ray photons that emerge from the object being radiographed before they reach the film. Use of a grid improves image quality.

Radiologist A qualified physician who specializes in diagnosis and treatment through the use of radiant energy.

Radiolucent Transparent to radiation; a material that allows radiation to pass through.

Radiolysis of water Interaction of radiation with water.

Radionuclide Any atom that emits radiation.

Radiosensitive Capable of being damaged or destroyed by ionizing radiation.

Radon The first decay product of radium; a colorless, odorless, chemically inert heavy radioactive gas that along with its decay products is always present to some degree in the air. It decays with a half-life of 3.8 days by way of alpha particles emission.

Rayleigh scattering (see *Coherent scattering.*)

Recessive mutation A genetic mutation that will probably not be expressed for a number of generations because both parents must possess the same mutation. If only one parent possesses the mutation, it will not be expressed.

Recoil electron (See *Compton scattered electron.*)

Relative biologic effectiveness (RBE) Describes the relative capability of radiations with differing LETs to produce a particular biologic reaction. Simply defined, it is the dose of a reference radiation quality (conventionally, 250 kVp x-rays) necessary to produce the same biologic reaction in a given experiment as that produced by a dose of the test radiation delivered under the same conditions.

Relative risk Model predicting that the number of excess cancers will increase as the natural incidence of cancer increases in a population with age.

Rem ("rad-equivalent-man") The traditional radiation quantity unit for dose equivalent, *rem* was defined as the dose equivalent of any type of ionizing radiation that produces the same biologic effect as one rad of x-radiation.

Remnant radiation (See *Exit or image formation radiation.*)

Repair enzymes Enzymes that can mend damaged molecules.

Repeat analysis program An important part of an overall quality control program in medical imaging, repeat analysis is an attempt to record the various causes of inadequate quality on occasions when an image had to be retaken.

Repeat radiograph Any radiograph that must be performed more than once because of a human or mechanical error in the process of producing the initial radiograph. Radiation exposure for the patient and the radiation worker increases when a radiograph must be repeated.

Reproductive cells Male and female germ cells; relatively radiosensitive.

Reproductive death On average, this effect results from exposure of cells to moderate doses of ionizing radiation (1 to 10 Gy, or 100 to 1000 rad). The cell does not die but permanently loses its ability to procreate.

Restitution A process whereby chromosome breaks rejoin in their original configuration with no visible damage.

Retina The rod- and cone-containing area of the eye; the retina receives the image formed by the lens.

Ribonucleic acid (RNA) Type of nucleic acid that carries the genetic information from the DNA in the cell nucleus to the ribosomes located in the cytoplasm.

Ribosomes Small, spherical cytoplasmic organelles that attach to the endoplasmic reticulum. They are the cell's "protein factories."

Right-To-Know Act (Employee) A series of statutes passed by the individual states requiring that employees be made aware of the hazards in the workplace. The act covers hazardous substances, infectious agents, ionizing radiation, and nonionizing radiation. The act requires employers to evaluate their workplaces for hazardous agents and to provide training and written information to their employees.

Risk The possibility of inducing a radiogenic cancer or genetic defects after irradiation.

Roentgen (R) Internationally accepted unit for measurement of exposure to x- and gamma radiation. One roentgen is the photon exposure that produces under standard conditions of pressure and temperature a total positive or negative ion charge of 2.58×10^{-4} coulombs per kilogram of dry air.

Rung A step in the DNA ladderlike structure composed of a pair of nitrogenous bases.

Saccharides (See *Carbohydrates.*)

Safe industries Industries that have a risk of fatal accidents generally estimated to be about $1 \times 10^{-4} \, y^{-1}$[8]. Safe industries include manufacturing, trade, service, and government.

Salts (electrolytes) Chemical compounds that result from the action of an acid and a base on each other.

Scattered radiation All the radiation that arises from the interactions of an x-ray beam with the atoms of an object in the path of the beam.

Scattering The process wherein x-ray photons undergo a change in direction after interacting with the atoms of an object.

Secondary protective barrier A barrier that affords protection from secondary radiation (leakage and scattered radiation) only and, as such, is not designed to intercept the direct x-ray beam and provide adequate attenuation of it.

Secondary radiation The radiation that results from the interaction between primary radiation and the atoms of the irradiated object and the off-focus or leakage radiation that penetrates the x-ray tube protective housing. Secondary radiation consists of scattered radiation and leakage radiation.

Self-reading pocket dosimeter A pocket ionization chamber that contains a built-in electrometer and provides an immediate exposure readout for radiation workers who work in high-exposure areas.

Semipermeable membrane A film that permits the passage of a pure solvent such as water but does not allow materials dissolved by the solvent to pass through.

Shadow shield A shield of radiopaque material suspended from above the radiographic beam-defining system; this shield hangs over the area of clinical interest to cast a shadow in the primary beam over the patient's reproductive organs.

Shallow dose Defined, for example, by Landauer, Inc., 2 Science Road, Glenwood, Illinois, 60425, in their *Radiation Dosimetry Report* as "the dose equivalent from all radiations at approximately 0.007-cm depth in soft tissue." This dose is considered by Landauer as "equivalent to the dose to the skin of the whole body."

Shaped contact shield A cup-shaped radiopaque shield that encloses the scrotum and penis to protect the male reproductive organs from exposure to ionizing radiation.

Short-term somatic effects (early or acute effects) Somatic effects that appear within minutes, hours, days, or weeks of the time of radiation exposure.

Side scatter Photons that interact with the atoms of an object and consequently are deflected to the side.

Sievert (Sv) The SI radiation quantity unit for dose equivalent. One sievert equals 1 joule of energy absorbed per kilogram of tissue (for x-radiation, QF = 1). This unit is used only for radiation protection purposes. It provides a common scale whereby varying degrees of biologic damage caused by equal absorbed doses of different types of ionizing radiation can be compared with the degree of biologic damage caused by the same amount of x or gamma radiation.

Signal-to-noise ratio (SNR) The comparison of the average CT number in a region with the statistical variation of CT number in that region.

Single-strand break The ionization of a DNA macromolecule resulting in a break of one of its chemical bonds, thereby severing one of the sugar-phosphate chain side-rails or strands of the ladderlike DNA molecular structure.

Skin dose The absorbed radiation dose, stated in gray or rads, delivered to the most superficial layers of the skin as a result of a radiation exposure. Backscatter radiation contribution is included.

Skin erythema dose The received quantity of radiation (corresponding roughly to a modern dose of several gray [several hundred rads]) that causes diffused redness over an area of skin after irradiation.

Small-angle scatter Photons that pass through the object being radiographed, interact with the atoms of the object, and are deflected only at a small enough angle so that they reach the film, thereby degrading the radiographic image by producing small amounts of radiographic fog.

Somatic cells   All the cells in the human body with the exception of the germ cells.

Somatic damage   Biologic damage to the body of the exposed individual.

Somatic effects   Biologic damage sustained by living organisms (such as human beings) as a consequence of exposure to ionizing radiation.

Source–image distance (SID)   The distance from the anode focal spot to the radiographic film.

Source–skin distance (SSD)   The distance from the anode focal spot to the skin of the patient.

Source-to-tabletop distance   The distance from the anode focal spot to the top of the radiographic table.

Specific area shielding   The use of protective lead or lead-impregnated material to protect selective body areas from exposure to ionizing radiation.

Spiral CT   Also known as *helical CT,* this is a technique in computed tomography in which the patient couch moves in or out of the bore of the scanner while the x-ray tube rotates around the patient.

Spermatogonium   The male germ cell.

Spontaneous mutations   A natural phenomenon involving alterations in genes and DNA. These mutations occur at random and without a known cause.

Stationary control-booth barrier   A nonmoveable enclosure where x-ray equipment controls are located. This booth is designed to intercept leakage and scattered radiation only; it may be regarded as a secondary protective barrier.

Stem cells   Immature or precursor cells.

Stem radiation   (See *Off-focus radiation.*)

Stochastic effects   Nonthreshold, randomly occurring biologic effects of ionizing radiation in which their probability of occurrence (rather than their severity) is proportional to the dose. Examples of stochastic processes are cancer and genetic effects. They are also called *probabilistic events.*

Structural proteins   Those proteins from which the body acquires its shape and form.

Syndrome   A collection of symptoms.

Target theory   The theory that the cell will die if inactivation of the master molecule occurs as a result of exposure to ionizing radiation.

Telangiectasis   Dilatation of capillaries and sometimes of terminal arteries of an organ.

Telophase   The phase of mitosis during which cell division is completed with the formation of two new daughter cells, each of which contains exactly the same genetic material as the parent cell. Telophase in meiosis involves not only division of the parent cell into two daughter cells but also division of these daughter cells into two granddaughter cells each. Because this second division does not involve DNA replication, the result of these two successive divisions is the formation of four granddaughter cells, each of which contains only half the genetic material of the original parent cell.

Ten-day rule   A rule based on the low degree of probability that a woman would be pregnant during the first 10 days after the onset of menstruation. The rule suggests that abdominal x-rays of fertile women be postponed until sometime during the first 10 days after the onset of the next menstruation if the results of the examination are not relevant to an immediate illness. This rule is now obsolete.

Teratogenesis   Birth defects induced by irradiation in utero.

Terrestrial radiation   Radiation resulting from radioactive minerals found in natural deposits within the earth.

Thermal neutron   Nominally classified as a neutron whose kinetic energy is approximately less than or equal to 1 eV. Typically, these are neutrons whose kinetic energy has been significantly degraded as a result of multiple energy loss collisions.

Thermoluminescent dosimeter (TLD) badge   A personnel monitoring device that most often contains a crystalline form (powder or chips) of lithium fluoride as its sensing material. When the device is placed in a TLD analyzer and heated, the crystals emit visible light in proportion to the amount of radiation to which the TLD badge was exposed. This device is most frequently used to directly measure skin dose.

Threshold   (1) The point at which a response or reaction to an increasing stimulation first occurs. (2) A dose below which an individual has a negligible chance of sustaining specific biologic damage.

Thrombocytes   (See *Platelets.*)

Thymine (T)   A pyrimidine base found only in DNA.

Thymus gland   An organ of the lymphatic system, located in the mediastinal cavity anterior to and above the heart. It plays a critical role in the body's defense against infection.

Thyroid gland   A gland located in the neck just below the larynx. The hormone produced by this gland helps regulate the body's metabolic rate and the process of growth.

Thyroid shield   (See *Protective apparel.*)

Tissue weighting factor (W_T)   A value denoting the percentage of the summed stochastic (cancer plus genetic) risk stemming from irradiation of tissue to the all-inclusive risk, in which the entire body is irradiated in a uniform fashion. This factor assigns risk for potential biologic responses from various types of ionizing radiation on a common scale.

TLD analyzer   A device that measures the amount of ionizing radiation to which a TLD badge has been exposed.

Total effective dose (TED)   A radiation dosimetry term that indicates a summation of interest effective dose and external effective dose.

Total effective dose equivalent (TEDE) limit   A radiation protection term that specifies the maximum allowable total dose (the sum of any internal and external dose) that may accumulate over a specified period of time, such as yearly or quarterly, for a certain category of individual. Different categories include the occupationally exposed, general public, embryo-fetus, and radiography students.

Total filtration   Inherent filtration plus added filtration.

Tubule   A small tube.

Tungsten   A metal with a high melting point (greater than 3400° C) and high atomic number (Z = 74). The anode in the x-ray tube is usually made primarily of this metal.

Ulceration   The process of pus formation on a free surface, such as the skin or a mucous membrane, to form an ulcer.

Umbra   (See *Useful beam.*)

Uncontrolled area   Area in which members of the general public (i.e., individuals who are not trained to work with radiation) may be found.

Undifferentiated cells   Immature or nonspecialized cells.

Unit   A fixed amount of some property or characteristic (e.g., distance-meter, time-second, energy-joule) used as a measure for which other amounts of that property or characteristic can be described.

United Nations Scientific Committee on the Effects of Atomic Radiation (UNSCEAR)   Evaluates human and environmental ionizing radiation exposure and derives radiation risk assessments from epidemiologic data and research conclusions. It provides information to organizations such as the ICRP for evaluation.

United States Environmental Protection Agency (EPA)   Facilitates the development and enforcement of regulations pertaining to the control of radiation in the environment.

United States Food and Drug Administration (FDA)   Conducts an ongoing electronic products radiation control program regulating the design and manufacture of products such as x-ray equipment.

United States Nuclear Regulatory Commission (NRC)   Formerly known as the Atomic Energy Commission [AEC], this federal agency oversees the nuclear energy industry. It also enforces radiation protection standards and publishes its rules and regulations in Title 10 of the United States Code of Federal Regulations.

United States Occupational Safety and Health Administration (OSHA)   Functions as a monitoring agency in places of employment, predominantly in industry.

Unmodified scattering   (See *Coherent scattering.*)

Unnecessary exposure   Any radiation exposure that does not benefit a person in terms of diagnostic information obtained or any radiation exposure that does not enhance the quality of the study.

Unnecessary radiologic procedure   Radiologic examination for which there is no sufficient justification to subject a patient to the minimal risk of the absorbed radiation dose resulting from the procedure.

Uracil (U)   A pyrimidine base found only in RNA. It replaces thymine (T) as the nitrogenous base in ribonucleic acid.

Use factor (U)   The proportional amount of time during which the x-ray beam is energized or directed toward a particular barrier. It is also referred to as the *beam direction factor.*

Useful beam Primary beam or umbra.

Variable rectangular collimator A box-shaped device containing the radiographic beam-defining system; the device most often used to define the size and shape of the radiographic beam.

Vesicle A small cavity or sac containing liquid.

Volt (V) SI unit of electric potential and potential difference.

Voltage Electric potential at a point or position relative to ground potential.

Voluntary motion Motion controlled by will (i.e., skeletal muscle).

Wavelength Distance between two consecutive crests or troughs in a wave.

Workload (W) Essentially the radiation output weighted time during the week that the unit is actually delivering radiation. It is specified either in units of mA-seconds per week or mA-minutes per week.

X-ray photons Particles associated with electromagnetic radiation that have neither mass nor electric charge.

X-rays Electromagnetic radiation that emerges from the anode of an x-ray tube after bombardment of this target by high-speed electrons in a highly evacuated glass tube.

Yttrium A rare-earth phosphor used in rare-earth intensifying screens.

References

1. Johnson KC, Rowberg AH. In Ballinger PW: *Merrill's atlas of radiographic positions and radiologic procedures,* ed 7, vol 3, St Louis, 1991, Mosby.
2. National Council on Radiation Protection and Measurements (NCRP): *Ionizing radiation exposure of the population of the United States,* Report No. 93, Bethesda, Md, 1987, NCRP Publications.
3. *Instruments and accessories for improved imaging and safety in diagnostic radiology, CT and MRI,* Catalog G-5, Carle Place, NY, 1988, Victoreen.
4. *Instruments and accessories for improved imaging and safety in diagnostic radiology, CT and MRI,* Catalog G-5, Carle Place, NY, 1988, Victoreen.
5. Ritenour ER. In Hendee WR, editor: *Health effects of low-level radiation,* Norwalk, Conn, 1984, Appleton-Century-Crofts.
6. Bushong SC: *Radiologic science for technologists: physics, biology and protection,* ed 6, St Louis, 1997, Mosby.
7. National Council on Radiation Protection and Measurements (NCRP): *Recommendations on limits for exposure to ionizing radiation,* Report No. 91, Bethesda, Md, 1987, NCRP.
8. National Council on Radiation Protection and Measurements (NCRP): *Limitation of exposure to ionizing radiation,* Report No. 116, Bethesda, Md, 1993, NCRP.

Answers to Review Questions

Chapter 1
1. C
2. B
3. C
4. A
5. D
6. B
7. B
8. D
9. B
10. D
11. B
12. D
13. A
14. A
15. C
16. C
17. D
18. C
19. D
20. B
21. D
22. A
23. D
24. D
25. C
26. C
27. B
28. C
29. B
30. A

Chapter 2
1. B
2. D
3. C
4. A
5. B
6. B
7. A
8. A
9. B
10. C
11. C
12. C
13. A
14. D
15. A
16. A
17. B
18. D
19. B
20. B
21. D
22. B
23. B
24. C
25. A
26. C
27. D
28. D
29. D

Chapter 3
1. C
2. B
3. D

4. B
5. A
6. D
7. B
8. C
9. D
10. A
11. B
12. D
13. D
14. B
15. D
16. C
17. A
18. D
19. D
20. D
21. C
22. A
23. C
24. C
25. D
26. B
27. C
28. C
29. D
30. C
31. B
32. C
33. A

Chapter 4
1. B
2. D
3. B

4. D
5. D
6. A
7. A
8. B
9. A
10. A
11. B
12. B
13. C
14. D
15. A
16. C
17. C
18. D
19. D
20. A
21. B
22. B
23. D
24. B
25. A

Chapter 5
1. C
2. C
3. B
4. B
5. D
6. B
7. B
8. D
9. B
10. D
11. D

12. C	42. D	37. A	32. B
13. D	43. A	38. D	33. C
14. B	44. A	39. A	34. A
15. B	45. C	40. D	35. D
	46. C	41. A	
Chapter 6	47. D	42. C	**Chapter 9**
1. B	48. C	43. D	1. C
2. A	49. C	44. D	2. C
3. B	50. D	45. B	3. A
4. C		46. C	4. D
5. A	**Chapter 7**	47. A	5. B
6. D	1. D	48. C	6. D
7. C	2. A	49. D	7. A
8. B	3. B	50. D	8. B
9. B	4. B		9. C
10. B	5. B	**Chapter 8**	10. B
11. A	6. D	1. B	11. C
12. B	7. C	2. A	12. B
13. A	8. C	3. C	13. A
14. C	9. B	4. D	14. D
15. D	10. D	5. D	15. D
16. D	11. A	6. B	16. C
17. A	12. B	7. B	17. C
18. D	13. D	8. C	18. D
19. D	14. D	9. A	19. D
20. B	15. C	10. A	20. D
21. D	16. C	11. D	21. D
22. C	17. D	12. C	22. A
23. C	18. B	13. C	23. A
24. B	19. B	14. B	24. B
25. C	20. A	15. B	25. C
26. D	21. B	16. D	26. C
27. D	22. A	17. C	27. B
28. A	23. C	18. D	28. D
29. D	24. D	19. C	29. D
30. D	25. B	20. B	30. C
31. D	26. B	21. D	31. A
32. D	27. C	22. A	32. B
33. C	28. D	23. D	33. C
34. D	29. A	24. D	34. D
35. B	30. D	25. D	35. B
36. D	31. C	26. B	36. C
37. B	32. A	27. D	37. A
38. D	33. D	28. C	38. B
39. C	34. B	29. C	39. D
40. A	35. B	30. A	40. A
41. A	36. C	31. C	

Appendix A

Chance of a 50 KeV photon to interact with atoms of tissue as it travels through 5 cm of soft tissue

Let N_0 be the number of x-ray photons incident on a uniform slab of tissue of thickness "y". The probability that there will be an interaction of any sort between a photon and an atom within the slab is, in the simplest case, proportional to the slab thickness and the number of incident photons and the mean target size presented by a slab atom to an x-ray photon.

Mathematically, We May Proceed as Follows:

1) Let dN be the change in the number of photons in the x-ray beam after the beam has passed through an infinitesimal distance dy. Because the number of photons decreases with every interaction, dN is a negative quantity.

2) At any depth within the phantom the number of interactions that will occur in the next incremental thickness dy is proportional to the remaining number of photons N at that depth and the distance of penetration dy. In mathematical terms, we have the following:

$$dN = -\mu N dy$$

where the symbol μ is the constant of proportionality and is known as the linear attenuation coefficient. It is defined by the above equation and has the following unit: 1/cm.

3) Rearranging the above equation, we perform the following integration:

$$\int_{N_0}^{N} dN/N = -\mu \int_{0}^{y} dy$$

which leads to the following relation:

$$\ln(N/N_0) = -\mu y$$

4) If we use the properties of logarithms and raise both sides of the last equation to the power "e," we obtain the x-ray attenuation equation:

$$N = N_0 e^{-\mu y}$$

5) For 50 KeV photons passing through 5 cm of soft tissue, we have the following:

$$\mu_{\text{soft tissue}} = 0.214 \text{ and } y = 5$$

Substituting these values into the last equation and rearranging the equation a bit, we obtain the following:

$$N/N_0 = e^{-(0.214 \times 5)} = 0.34$$

which shows that only 0.34, or 34%, of the initial number of photons in the 50 KeV beam remain (i.e. have not undergone an interaction) after traversing a 5-cm slab of tissue. In other words, *66% of the incident x-ray beam has interacted with a tissue atom.*

Appendix B

Relationship between photons, electromagnetic waves, wavelength and energy

Before 1900, all attempts to use current theories and concepts in physics to explain the measured energy distribution of radiation from a heated body had failed grievously. In that year a German physicist, Max Planck, introduced the concept of a "quantum," or discrete unit of energy, to resolve these discrepancies. According to Planck's theory, whenever radiation is emitted or absorbed by a hot object, the energy of that radiation is emitted or absorbed in discrete amounts, which he called *quanta.*

Mathematically a single such amount or energy quantum is given by the following equation:

$$(1) \quad E = hf$$

where f is the frequency of the radiation and h is a proportionality constant called, appropriately, Planck's constant. This quantum of energy has since received the name *photon.* Thus the energy of a photon varies directly as the frequency of the radiation. Because the frequency f and the wavelength w of any type of radiation are related by the simple expression

$$(2) \quad c = fw$$

where "c" is the speed of light (300,000,000 meters per second in a vacuum), then

$$(3) \quad E = hf = hc/w$$

This last result shows that the energy of a photon decreases as the wavelength of the radiation increases (e.g., photons of infrared light are less energetic than those of ultraviolet light because infrared wavelengths are longer than ultraviolet wavelengths). Einstein used these ideas to explain the emission of electrons from a metallic surface when visible light radiation was directed at it. This was called the *photoelectric effect.* The light-produced electrons, or photoelectrons, were found to have energies that depended on the wavelength of the focused light but were completely independent of the intensity or brightness of that light. This phenomenon could not be explained by traditional physics. However, it was fully explicable in terms of the new concept of radiation energy (quanta or photons) and the energy relation given in equation (3). That relation contains no reference to the brightness of the light. For his work in this area, Einstein received the Nobel Prize in Physics in 1921.

To summarize, photons are the particles associated with the electromagnetic (EM) radiation spectrum (within which visible light and x-rays are included). When energy is transferred from an EM wave through interaction with matter, the energy is transferred by photons in discrete, or integral, amounts. Each such discrete amount is directly proportional to the frequency of the EM radiation.

Appendix C
Compton interaction

The principle of conservation of mass-energy is that for an isolated system (i.e., a system on which no external energy source or energy drain is active), the total mass plus energy of all the particles composing the system remains constant. This restraint, however, does not prevent mass-energy transfers between individual particles.

The *linear momentum* of a particle is defined as the product of its mass and its velocity. A photon, which is the particle associated with electromagnetic radiation, moves at the speed of light; consequently, according to Einstein's theory of relativity, a photon must be a massless entity. Because of the equivalence between mass m and energy E given by the famous relation

$$E = mc^2$$

where c is the speed of light in a vacuum, we can associate a mass equivalent with the photon given by

$$E/c^2$$

Then the photon can be considered to have a linear momentum given by the product of the mass equivalent and the velocity of the photon.* The principle of conservation of linear momentum states that for an isolated system the sum of the linear momenta of all its particles is constant. Exchanges of linear momentum between particles within the system can, of course, occur.

---

*From Appendix C we have the following energy relation:
$$E = hc/w$$
Then the linear momentum expression for the photon becomes
$$p = (E/c^2)c = (hc/w)/c = h/w.$$

The Compton interaction is, most simply, a collision between an incident x-ray photon and the weakly bound outer electron of a target atom. Application of the conservation of mass-energy and the conservation of linear momentum principles to the x-ray photon and outer electron system leads to equations that can be used to predict the energies and angles of scattering of both particles following their collision. If the energy of the incident photon is E, we can write the following energy balance relation:

$$E = E' + K$$

where E is the photon's energy after the collision and K is the recoil energy of the "struck" electron.

We will now describe several important types of Compton interactions. These effects depend on the size of E and the angle at which the photon interacts with the electron.

Case 1: **The photon makes a head-on collision with the electron.**
    Result: The electron travels or scatters directly forward, and the photon backwards (180-degree scatter angle).
    Energy Situations
      a) $E \ll 511$ keV (low energy range):
        E' is approximately equal to E
        K is almost zero
      b) $E = 511$ keV:
        $E' = E/3$
        $K = (2/3)\,E$
      c) $E \gg 511$ keV (high energy range):
        E' is approximately zero
        $K = E$ to good approximation

Case 2: **The photon grazes the electron.**

> *Result:* The photon emerges from the colli-
> sion nearly undeflected from its ini-
> tial direction, and the electron scatters
> at right angles.
>
> *Energy Situation:*
>> E′ is approximately equal to E
>> K is approximately zero

Collisions of this nature, in which the incident photon loses little or no energy, are especially important in the planning of radiation shielding for therapeutic x-ray suites.

Appendix D

Periodic table of the elements

Outer Electrons located in	Period	Group I	Group II	Group III	Group IV	Group V	Group VI	Group VII	Group VIII		
K shell	1	1 **H** Hydrogen 1.09							2 **He** Helium 4.00		
L shell	2	3 **Li** Lithium 6.94	4 **Be** Beryllium 9.02	5 **B** Boron 10.82	6 **C** Carbon 12.01	7 **N** Nitrogen 14.09	8 **O** Oxygen 16.00	9 **F** Fluorine 19.00	10 **Ne** Neon 20.18		
M shell	3	11 **Na** Sodium 23.0	12 **Mg** Magnesium 24.32	13 **Al** Aluminum 26.97	14 **Si** Silicon 28.06	15 **P** Phosphorus 30.98	16 **S** Sulfur 32.06	17 **Cl** Chlorine 35.46	18 **A** Argon 39.99		
N shell	4	19 **K** Potassium 39.096	20 **Ca** Calcium 40.08	21 **Sc** Scandium 45.10	22 **Ti** Titanium 47.90	23 **V** Vanadium 50.95	24 **Cr** Chromium 52.01	25 **Mn** Manganese 54.93	26 **Fe** Iron 55.85	27 **Co** Cobalt 58.94	28 **Ni** Nickel 58.69
		29 **Cu** Copper 63.57	30 **Zn** Zinc 65.38	31 **Ga** Gallium 69.72	32 **Ge** Germanium 72.60	33 **As** Arsenic 74.91	34 **Se** Selenium 79.00	35 **Br** Bromine 79.92	36 **Kr** Krypton 83.7		
O shell	5	37 **Rb** Rubidium 85.48	38 **Sr** Strontium 87.63	39 **Y** Yttrium 88.92	40 **Zr** Zirconium 91.22	41 **Cb** Columbium 92.91	42 **Mo** Molybdenum 96.0	43 **Tc** Technetium 99	44 **Ru** Ruthenium 101.7	45 **Rh** Rhodium 102.9	46 **Pd** Palladium 106.7
		47 **Ag** Silver 107.88	48 **Cd** Cadmium 112.41	49 **In** Indium 118.70	50 **Sn** Tin 121.77	51 **Sb** Antimony 127.6	52 **Te** Tellurium 126.93	53 **I** Iodine 126.92	54 **Xe** Xenon 131.3		
P shell	6	55 **Cs** Cesium 132.9	56 **Ba** Barium 137.4	Rare Earths 57-71	72 **Hf** Hafnium 178.6	73 **Ta** Tantalum 180.9	74 **W** Tungsten 183.9	75 **Re** Rhenium 186.3	76 **Os** Osmium 190.2	77 **Ir** Iridium 193.1	78 **Pt** Platinum 195.2
		79 **Au** Gold 197.2	80 **Hg** Mercury 200.6	81 **Tl** Thallium 204.4	82 **Pb** Lead 207.2	83 **Bi** Bismuth 209.0	84 **Po** Polonium 210	85 **At** Astatine 211	86 **Rn** Radon 222		
Q shell	7	87 **Vi** Virginium 224	88 **Ra** Radium 226.05	Actinide Series 89-103							

Rare Earths Series

57 **La** Lanthanum 138.91	58 **Ce** Cerium 140.12	59 **Pr** Proseodymium 140.91	60 **Nd** Neodymium 144.24	61 **Pm** Promethium 147	62 **Sm** Samarium 150.35	63 **Eu** Europium 151.96	64 **Gd** Gadolinium 157.25	65 **Tb** Terbium 158.92	66 **Dy** Dysprosium 162.50	67 **Ho** Holmium 164.93	68 **Er** Erbium 167.26	69 **Tm** Thulium 168.93	70 **Yb** Ytterbium 173.04	71 **Lu** Lutetium 174.97
89 **Ac** Actinium 227	90 **Th** Thorium 232.04	91 **Pa** Protactinium 231	92 **U** Uranium 238.03	93 **Np** Neptunium 237	94 **Pu** Plutonium 242	95 **Am** Americium 243	96 **Cm** Curium 245	97 **Bk** Berkellum 249	98 **Cf** Californium 251	99 **Es** Einsteinium 254	100 **Fm** Fermium 255	101 **Md** Mendelevium 256	102 **No** Nobelium 254	103 **Lr** Lawrencium 257

Actinide Series

Appendix E

Metric System Equivalents for Length				
Length	Symbol	Power of ten fractional form	Power of ten decimal form	Scientific notation
terameter	T	1,000,000,000,000	1,000,000,000,000	10^{12} (m)
gigameter	G	1,000,000,000	1,000,000,000	10^{9} (m)
megameter	M	1,000,000	1,000,000	10^{6} (m)
kilometer	k	1000	1000	10^{3} (m)
hectometer	h	100	100	10^{2} (m)
dekameter	da	10	10	10^{1} (m)
meter	m	1	1	10^{0} (m)
decimeter	d	1/10	0.1	10^{-1} (m)
centimeter	cm	1/100	0.01	10^{-2} (m)
millimeter	mm	1/1000	0.001	10^{-3} (m)
micrometer	μm	1/1,000,000	0.00001	10^{-6} (m)
nanometer	nm	1/1,000,000,000	0.000000001	10^{-9} (m)
picometer	pm	1/1,000,000,000,000	0.000000000001	10^{-12} (m)

Appendix F

Consumer-Patient Radiation Health and Safety Act of 1981*

SUBTITLE-I—CONSUMER-PATIENT RADIATION HEALTH AND SAFETY ACT OF 1981

Short title
[42 USC 10001] note
Sec. 975. This subtitle may be cited as the "Consumer-Patient Radiation Health and Safety Act of 1981."

Statement of findings
[42 USC 10001]
Sec. 976. The Congress finds that . . .
(1) it is in the interest of public health and safety to minimize unnecessary exposure to potentially hazardous radiation due to medical and dental radiologic procedures;
(2) it is in the interest of public health and safety to have a continuing supply of adequately educated persons and appropriate accreditation and certification programs administered by state governments;
(3) the protection of the public health and safety from unnecessary exposure to potentially hazardous radiation due to medical and dental radiologic procedures and the assurance of efficacious procedures are the responsibility of state and federal governments;
(4) persons who administer radiologic procedures, including procedures at federal facilities, should be required to demonstrate competence by reason of education, training, and experience; and
(5) the administration of radiologic procedures and the effect on individuals of such procedures have a substantial and direct effect upon United States interstate commerce.

*Modified from Consumer-Patient Radiation Health and Safety Act of 1981, Chapter 107, Secs. 10001-8 (Aug. 13, 1981).

Statement of purpose
[42 USC 10002.]
Sec. 977. It is the purpose of this subtitle to-

(1) provide for the establishment of minimum standards by the federal government for the accreditation of education programs for persons who administer radiologic procedures and for the certification of such persons; and

(2) ensure that medical and dental radiologic procedures are consistent with rigorous safety precautions and standards.

Definitions
[42 USC 10003.]

Sec. 978. Unless otherwise expressly provided, for purposes of this subtitle, the term-

(1) "radiation" means ionizing and nonionizing radiation in amounts beyond normal background levels from sources such as medical and dental radiologic procedures;

(2) "radiologic procedure" means any procedure or article intended for use in-

(A) the diagnosis of disease or other medical or dental conditions in humans (including diagnostic x-rays or nuclear medicine procedures); or
(B) the cure, mitigation, treatment, or prevention of disease in humans that achieves its intended purpose through the emission of radiation;

(3) "radiologic equipment" means any radiation electronic product that emits or detects radiation and is used or intended for use to-

> (A) diagnose disease or other medical or dental conditions (including diagnostic x-ray equipment); or
>
> (B) cure, mitigate, treat, or prevent disease in humans that achieves its intended purpose through the emission or detection of radiation;

(4) "practitioner" means any licensed doctor of medicine, osteopathy, dentistry, podiatry, or chiropractic who prescribes radiologic procedures for other persons;

(5) "persons who administer radiologic procedures" means any person, other than a practitioner, who intentionally administers radiation to other persons for medical purposes and includes medical radiologic technologists (including dental hygienists and assistants), radiation therapy technologists, and nuclear medicine technologists;

(6) "Secretary" means the Secretary of Health and Human Services; and

(7) "State" means the several states, the District of Columbia, the Commonwealth of Puerto Rico, the Commonwealth of the Northern Mariana Islands, the Virgin Islands, Guam, American Samoa, and the Trust Territory of the Pacific Islands.

Promulgation of standards

[Regulation. 42 USC 10004.]

Sec. 979. (a) Within 12 months after the date of enactment of this act, the Secretary, in consultation with the Radiation Policy Council, the Administrator of Veterans' Affairs, the Administrator of the Environmental Protection Agency, appropriate agencies of the States, and appropriate professional organizations, shall by regulation promulgate minimum standards for the accreditation of educational programs to train individuals to perform radiologic procedures. Such standards shall distinguish between programs for the education of (1) medical radiologic technologists (including radiographers), (2) dental auxiliaries (including dental hygienists and assistants), (3) radiation therapy technologists, (4) nuclear medicine technologists, and (5) such other kinds of health auxiliaries who administer radiologic procedures as the Secretary determines appropriate. Such standards shall not be applicable to educational programs for practitioners.

[Regulation.]

(b) Within 12 months after the date of enactment of this act, the Secretary, in consultation with the Radiation Policy Council, the Administrator of Veterans' Affairs, the Administrator of the Environmental Protection Agency, interested agencies of the States, and appropriate professional organizations, shall by regulation promulgate minimum standards for the certification of persons who administer radiologic procedures. Such standards shall distinguish between certification of (1) medical radiologic technologists (including radiographers), (2) dental auxiliaries (including dental hygienists and assistants), (3) radiation therapy technologists, (4) nuclear medicine technologists, and (5) such other kinds of health auxiliaries who administer radiologic procedures as the Secretary determines appropriate. Such standards shall include minimum certification criteria for individuals with regard to accredited education, practical experience, successful passage of required examinations, and such other criteria as the Secretary shall deem necessary for the adequate qualification of individuals to administer radiologic procedures. Such standards shall not apply to practitioners.

Model Statute

[42 USC 10005.]

Sec. 980. In order to encourage the administration of accreditation and certification programs by the states, the Secretary shall prepare and transmit to the states a model statute for radiologic procedure safety. Such model statute shall provide that-

(1) it shall be unlawful in a state for individuals to perform radiologic procedures unless such individuals are certified by the state to perform such procedures; and

(2) any educational requirements for certification of individuals to perform radiologic procedures shall be limited to educational programs accredited by the state.

Compliance

[42 USC 10006.]

Sec. 981. (a) The Secretary shall take all actions consistent with law to effectuate the purposes of this subtitle.

(b) A state may utilize an accreditation or certification program administered by a private entity if-

> (1) such state delegates the administration of the state accreditation or certification program to such private entity;
>
> (2) such program is approved by the state; and
>
> (3) such program is consistent with the minimum federal standards promulgated under this subtitle for such program.

(c) Absent compliance by the states with the provisions of this subtitle within 3 years after the date of enactment of this act, the Secretary shall report to the Congress recommendations for legislative changes considered necessary to ensure the states' compliance with this subtitle.

[Report to Congress.]

(d) The Secretary shall be responsible for continued monitoring of compliance by the states with the applicable provisions of this subtitle and shall report to the Senate and the House of Representatives by January 1, 1982, and January 1 of each succeeding year the status of the states' compliance with the purposes of this subtitle.

(e) Notwithstanding any other provision of this section, in the case of a state that has, prior to the effective date of standards and guidelines promulgated pursuant to this subtitle, established standards for the accreditation of educational programs and certification of radiologic technologists, such state shall be deemed to be in compliance with the conditions of this section unless the Secretary determines, after notice and hearing, that such state standards do not meet the minimum standards prescribed by the Secretary or are inconsistent with the purposes of this subtitle.

Federal radiation guidelines

[42 USC 1000`7.)

Sec. 982. The Secretary shall, in conjunction with the Radiation Policy Council, the Administrator of Veterans' Affairs, the Administrator of the Environmental Protection Agency, appropriate agencies of the states, and appropriate professional organizations, promulgate Federal radiation guidelines with respect to radiologic procedures. Such guidelines shall-

(1) determine the level of radiation exposure due to radiologic procedures that is unnecessary and specify the techniques, procedures, and methods to minimize such unnecessary exposure;

(2) provide for the elimination of the need for retakes of diagnostic radiologic procedures;

(3) provide for the elimination of unproductive screening programs;

(4) provide for the optimum diagnostic information with minimum radiologic exposure; and

(5) include the therapeutic application of radiation to individuals in the treatment of disease, including nuclear medicine applications.

Applicability to federal agencies
[42 USC 10008.]

Sec. 983. (a) Except as provided in subsection (b), each department, agency, and instrumentality of the executive branch of the federal government shall comply with standards promulgated pursuant to this subtitle.

[Regulations.]

[38 USC 101 *et seq.*]

(b) (1) The Administrator of Veterans' Affairs, through the Chief Medical Director of the Veterans' Administration, shall, to the maximum extent feasible consistent with the responsibilities of such Administrator and Chief Medical Director under subtitle 38, United States Code, prescribe regulations making the standards promulgated pursuant to this subtitle applicable to the provision of radiologic procedures in facilities over which the Administrator has jurisdiction. In prescribing and implementing regulations pursuant to this subsection, the Administrator shall consult with the Secretary in order to achieve the maximum possible coordination of the regulations, standards, and guidelines, and the implementation thereof, which the Secretary and the Administrator prescribe under this subtitle.

[Report to congressional committees.]

(2) Not later than 180 days after standards are promulgated by the Secretary pursuant to this subtitle, the Administrator of Veterans' Affairs shall submit to the appropriate committees of Congress a full report with respect to the regulations (including guidelines, policies, and procedures thereunder) prescribed pursuant to paragraph (1) of this subsection. Such report shall include-

(A) an explanation of any inconsistency between standards made applicable by such regulations and the standards promulgated by the Secretary pursuant to this subtitle;

(B) an account of the extent, substance, and results of consultations with the Secretary respecting the prescription and implementation of regulations by the Administrator; and

(C) such recommendations for legislation and administrative action as the Administrator determines are necessary and desirable.

[Publication in Federal Register.]

(3) The Administrator of Veterans' Affairs shall publish the report required by paragraph (2) in the Federal Register.

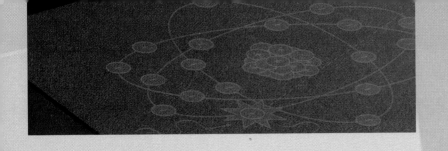

Index

Notes